Clinical Cases in Sleep Physical Therapy

Cristina Frange

Editor

Clinical Cases in Sleep Physical Therapy

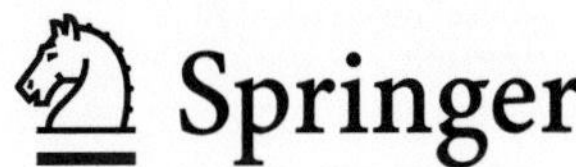 Springer

Editor
Cristina Frange
Neurology and Neurosurgery Department
Federal University of São Paulo (UNIFESP)
São Paulo, SP, Brazil

ISBN 978-3-031-38342-7   ISBN 978-3-031-38340-3   (eBook)
https://doi.org/10.1007/978-3-031-38340-3

This Springer imprint is published by the registered company Springer Nature Switzerland AG
The registered company address is: Gewerbestrasse 11, 6330 Cham, Switzerland

Paper in this product is recyclable.

Foreword 1

At the dawn of sleep medicine, the practitioners were most often psychiatrists. As more and more research explored the many facets of sleep and the impact of sleep disorders on disease and the impact of disease on sleep, more and more specialties entered the field. The goal was always to improve patient's lives.

Today practitioners of sleep medicine include specialists in psychiatry, neurology, respirology, cardiology, geriatrics, and pediatrics. With this beautifully illustrated book, Clinical Cases in Sleep Physical Therapy, Cristina Frange ushers an entire new profession into sleep medicine—Physiotherapy. She does this by showing that physiotherapists, all along, have been treating many disorders, which improved patients' sleep and overall health.

The clinical cases presented are a stunning array and can be used by physiotherapists and others to learn how physiotherapy can work in treating sleep disorders. The authors are not just from America and Europe, but span the entire globe, and highlight that some countries (e.g., Brazil) have become sleep powerhouses. The first two chapters are a broad overview of what modern physiotherapy is and what it has to offer to the sleep field. This is followed by a series of sections describing clinical cases that cover such important topics including insomnia, restless legs syndrome, circadian rhythm disorders, sleep bruxism, obstructive sleep apnea, central sleep apnea, and other sleep-breathing disorders including content on noninvasive ventilation. The book clearly shows and gives examples of how physiotherapists can help treating patients with these conditions.

Bravo to Cristina Frange, for ushering in physiotherapists into the sleep field!

Professor Emeritus Yale University   Meir Kryger, MD, FRCPC
New Haven, CT, USA

Foreword 2

It is with great pleasure that I write this foreword. Sleep is a universal reality in all alive creatures, and human sleep has been studied for hundreds of years. Since 1950, after a better understanding of neurophysiology, Sleep Medicine has been flourishing as a science. As better as we understand the clinical approach to sleep disturbances, better we realize that patients with sleep complaints must have multidisciplinary care. The involvement of physicians, physiotherapists, dentists, speech therapists, nutritionists, and psychologists is crucial for optimizing the well-being of these patients.

The role of physiotherapists has been concentrated for many years on respiratory approach in patients with obstructive sleep apnea with a focus on ventilation. The expertise in CPAP/Bilevel devices, complications, adherence, and follow-up was fundamental to building the actual knowledge and knowhow. However, many other contributions to the patients with sleep disturbances must be done by physiotherapists.

This book demonstrates how physiotherapists can contribute to the treatment, rehabilitation, and follow-up of patients suffering from sleep disturbances. The integration among physiotherapists, physicians, and other health professionals is highlighted with interesting case reports. These cases move the readers through good pieces of reality and the experiences of numerous authors.

As a professor of Neurology and Sleep Medicine, I have been defending the integration among all members of the team during the patient care process. Dr. Frange, who was my postdoctoral research fellow, is an over-standard researcher and practical physiotherapist. Her efforts to improve the scenario of care with a interdisciplinary approach have been seen in many papers and books, as well as in her clinical practice. I am proud of this book and endorse that all readers will learn as much as I have from these clinical histories.

Neurology and Neurosurgery Department, and Department of Psychobiology, Federal University of São Paulo (UNIFESP) São Paulo, SP, Brazil

Harvard Medical School Boston, MA, USA

Fernando Morgadinho Santos Coelho, MD, PhD

Preface

As physical therapy continues to evolve and advance as a health profession, new areas emerge. Sleep physiotherapy (PT) is one of these new areas that is in its embryonic stage. This book demonstrates the practice of sleep PT in several parts of the world, some that do not yet have the official recognition from their PT governing bodies.

Clinical Cases in Sleep Physical Therapy follows its companion book, *Sleep Medicine and Physical Therapy: a comprehensive guide for practitioners*, which was published in 2022. The first publication was an introduction to this new field, describing the most prevalent sleep disorders and the benefits of using an interdisciplinary approach that include PT. This second book is focused on the clinical practice of this new profession. Written by physiotherapists from several countries (Argentina, Australia, Brazil, Canada, Chile, India, Japan, Jordan, New Zealand, Switzerland, Turkey, and United States), this book explores in detail the clinical, evidence-based practice of sleep PT.

This book is divided into two main sections. The first section comprises two introductory chapters written by leading PT researchers and clinicians, promoting the role of PT in sleep health, and its use as a primary or adjunctive treatment for sleep disorders. The second section contains 28 case reports written by PTs, describing and illustrating different approaches of PT regarding sleep treatments. The case reports are divided into eight main clinical areas, some of them with less content than others, due to the short history of sleep PT, with more cases from areas that were first developed, such as sleep-breathing disorders. The history of sleep PT started back in the 1980s, with the development of positive airway pressure devices. Therefore, more than 40 years later, scientific evidence has been developed in this area, allowing more extensive chapters on sleep-breathing disorders (i.e., obstructive and central sleep apnea, other sleep-breathing disorders related to hypercapnic chronic obstructive pulmonary disease, as well as overlap syndrome and the congenital central alveolar hypoventilation syndrome), while there are only shorter and single chapters on circadian sleep-wake cycle disorder, restless legs syndrome, insomnia, and sleep bruxism. The chapters on insufficient sleep draw attention to the importance of healthy sleep for rehabilitation processes to occur. Taken together, these case studies clearly show the potential of the sleep PT along a biopsychosocial approach to deliver improved outcomes and more effective treatment to the patients.

São Paulo, Brazil   Cristina Frange
May 2023

Acknowledgments

Many people have been involved in the production of this book. All of the contributors and the Springer staff worked against the background of the COVID-19 pandemic. Many of us were working at hospitals and outpatient centers during these events. My special thanks to Dr. Elisa Çalisgan and Dr. Betül Akyol, who worked in the context of a major earthquake to deliver their chapter.

I am profoundly grateful to all of the contributors from around the world for believing in this project, sharing their expertise and clinical experience, and also the cultural aspects of their practice regarding sleep. Each of them is cited in the list of contributors, with the presence of each conferring authority to this book. My special thanks to Dr. Sandra Souza de Queiroz for critically reviewing my chapters.

I would also like to thank my incredible Springer Editor, Erica Ferraz and her team, Henry Rodgers, and all the staff at Springer, especially Anila Vijayan and ArulRonika Pathinathan for their work on the production of this book.

My gratitude to Dr. Lourdes DelRosso, and Mike Mutschelknaus, from whom I learned so much in the past year, through the extraordinary initiative I had the opportunity and the privilege to attend, the World Sleep Academy, from World Sleep Society.

Special thanks to Dr. Fernando Morgadinho Santos Coelho, Dr. Monica Levy Andersen, and Dr. Gilles Lavigne for their constant encouragement and belief in sleep physiotherapy.

Many thanks to the São Paulo Research Foundation (*Fundação de Amparo à Pesquisa do Estado de São Paulo* FAPESP), and to the Department of Neurology and Neurosurgery, Post-Graduate Program of Neurology and Neurosciences at the Federal University of São Paulo (*Universidade Federal de São Paulo*, UNIFESP).

To my son Matheus Frange, and my husband Mauricio Ribeiro da Silva, for their patience, support, and daily love. My gratefullness to Felicio Frange, Ilza Araújo e Lucimar Bello, examples of life and love.

To each one of the patients, who kindly permitted the sharing of their stories and personal experiences, making this book possible.

Contents

Editors and Contributors

About the Editor

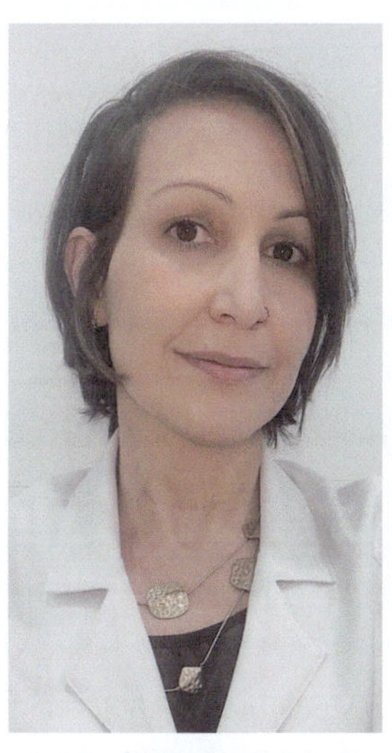 **Cristina Frange** is a Physiotherapist, specialized in Neurofunctional Physiotherapy, and certified in Sleep Physiotherapy (Brazilian Sleep Association/Brazilian Association of Cardiorespiratory Physiotherapy and Intensive Care Physiotherapy). She is a member of the Network for Health Promotion in Life and Work; of the Physiotherapy board of the Brazilian Sleep Association; and faculty of the World Sleep Academy (World Sleep Society). She holds a M.Sc. in Communication, Pontificia Universidade Católica de São Paulo (PUC/SP); a Ph.D. in Science, Department of Psychobiology, Division of Biology and Medicine of Sleep, Federal University of São Paulo (UNIFESP); and a Postdoctor de at Neurology and Neurosurgery Department, Post-Graduate Program in Neurology and Neurosciences, UNIFESP. Dr. Frange is a clinician (attends daily at her office, Frange Sleep Physiotherapy and Rehabilitation, in São Paulo, Brazil) and a researcher. She is passionate about learning, teaching and collaborating.

Contributors

Betül Akyol Department of Physical Education and Sport Malatya, Faculty of Sport Science, Inonu University, Malatya, Turkey

Mosab Aldabbas Centre for Physiotherapy and Rehabilitation Sciences, Jamia Millia Islamia, New Delhi, India

Al Azhar University, Gaza, Palestinian Authority

Mayis Aldughmi Department of Physiotherapy, School of Rehabilitation Sciences, University of Jordan, Amman, Jordan

Rafaela G. S. de Andrade Sleep Medicine, Pulmonary Division, Heart Institute, Faculdade de Medicina da Universidade Federal de São Paulo (InCor-FMUSP), São Paulo, SP, Brazil

Alberto Herrero Babiloni Division of Experimental Medicine, McGill University, Montreal, QC, Canada

Elisa Çalisgan Department of Physiotherapy and Rehabilitation, Faculty of Health Science, Kahramanmaras Sutcu Imam University, Kahramanmaras, Turkey

Luis Vasconcello-Castillo Department of Physical Therapy, University of Chile, Santiago, Chile

Carolina V. R. D'Aurea Department of Public Health, Universidade Católica de Santos, Santos, SP, Brazil

Elizabeth Dean Department of Physical Therapy, Faculty of Medicine, University of British Columbia, Vancouver, BC, Canada

Carlos Maria Franceschini Sleep and Mechanical Ventilation Unit, Cosme Argerich Hospital, Buenos Aires, Argentina

Cristina Frange Neurology and Neurosurgery Department, Federal University of São Paulo (UNIFESP), São Paulo, SP, Brazil

Sofia F. Furlan Sleep Laboratory, Faculty of Medicine, Heart Institute, University of São Paulo, São Paulo, SP, Brazil

Dany H. Gagnon School of Rehabilitation, Institut Universitaire sur la Réadaptation en Déficience Physique de Montréal of CIUSSS Centre-sud de Montréal, Université de Montréal, Montreal, QC, Canada

Mariana Gussoni Argentine Association of Respiratory Medicine (AAMR) and Argentine Society of Cardiorespiratory Kinesiology (SAKICARE), Buenos Aires, Argentina

Hiroya Honda Department of Physical Therapy, School of Rehabilitation Sciences, Seirei Christopher University, Hamamatsu, Shizuoka, Japan

Turhan Kahraman Department of Health Professions, Manchester Metropolitan University, Manchester,, UK

Department of Physiotherapy and Rehabilitation, Faculty of Health Sciences, Izmir Katip Celebi University, Izmir, Turkey

Jacqueline T. A. T. Lam School of Rehabilitation, Institut Universitaire sur la Réadaptation en Déficience Physique de Montréal of CIUSSS Centre-sud de Montréal, Université de Montréal, Montreal, QC, Canada

Gilles Lavigne Faculty of Dental Medicine, Research Center of CIUSSS Nord Ile de Montréal, Sleep and Trauma Unit and CHUM-Stomatology, Université de Montréal, Montreal, QC, Canada

Camila F. Leite Physical Therapy Department, Federal University of Ceara, Fortaleza, CE, Brazil

Mario A. Leocadio-Miguel Department of Psychology, Northumbria University, Newcastle upon Tyne, United Kingdom

Juliana A. Lino Federal University of Ceara, Fortaleza, CE, Brazil

Liliane P. S. Mendes Physiotherapy Department, Federal University of Minas Gerais, Belo Horizonte, MG, Brazil

Daiana M. Mortari Federal University of Rio Grande do Sul, Porto Alegre, RS, Brazil

Flávia B. Nerbass Sleep Laboratory, Pulmonary Division, University of Sao Paulo School of Medicine, Sao Paulo, SP, Brazil

Asiye T. Ozdogar Department of Physiotherapy and Rehabilitation, Faculty of Health Sciences, Van Yuzuncu Yil University, Van, Turkey

Maria José Perrelli Brazilian College of Systemic Studies (CBES), Curitiba, PR, Brazil

Vivien S. Piccin Sleep Medicine, Pulmonary Division, Heart Institute, Faculdade de Medicina da Universidade Federal de São Paulo (InCor-FMUSP), São Paulo, SP, Brazil

Amanda J. Piper Respiratory Support Service, Department of Respiratory and Sleep Medicine, Royal Prince Alfred Hospital, Camperdown, NSW, Australia

Sandra Souza de Queiroz Brazilian Sleep Association, São Paulo, SP, Brazil

Catherine F. Siengsukon Department of Physical Therapy, Rehabilitation Science, and Athletic Training, University of Kansas Medical Center, Kansas City, KS, USA

Margot Skinner Centre for Health and Rehabilitation Research, School of Physiotherapy, University of Otago, Dunedin, New Zealand

Cristina Staub Ausgeschlafen.ch and Pro Dormo, Zürich, Switzerland

Rodrigo Torres-Castro Department of Physical Therapy, University of Chile, Santiago, Chile

Melissa A. Ulhôa Faculty of Medicine, UNIVAÇO-AFYA, Ipatinga, MG, Brazil

Zubia Veqar Centre for Physiotherapy and Rehabilitation Sciences, Jamia Millia Islamia, New Delhi, India

Yoshinobu Yoshimoto Seirei Christopher University, Hamamatsu, Shizuoka, Japan

Abbreviations

AASM	American Academy of Sleep Medicine
ABC Scale	Activities-specific balance confidence scale
ADLs	Activities of daily life
AHA	American Heart Association
AHI	Apnea-hypopnea index
AROM	Active range of motion
ASV	Adaptive servo-ventilation
BBS	Berg balance scale
BDNF	Brain-derived neurotrophic factor
Bilevel	Bilevel ventilation
BMI	Body mass index
CBT-I	Cognitive-behavioral therapy for insomnia
CDC	Center for Disease Control and Prevention
CHF	Congestive heart failure
CNP	Chronic neck pain
CNS	Central nervous system
CO2	Carbon dioxide
COVID-19	Coronavirus disease 2019
CRSWD	Circadian rhythm sleep-wake disorders
CSB	Cheyne-Stokes breathing
CT	Computer assisted tomography
DISE	Drug-induced sleep endoscopy
DSM-V	Diagnostic and Statistical Manual for Mental Disorders, 5th Edition
EDS	Excessive daytime sleepiness
EEG	Electroencephalogram
EMG	Electromyogram
EOG	Electrooculogram
ESS	Epworth sleepiness scale
Ev/h	Events per hour of sleep
FSS	Fatigue severity scale
GERD	Gastroesophageal reflux disorder

HF	Heart failure
HR	Heart rate
Hz	Hertz
ICF	International Classification of Functioning, Disability and Health
ICSD	International Classification of Sleep Disorders
ICSD-3	International Classification of Sleep Disorders, 3rd Edition
IRLSSGS	International Restless Legs Syndrome Study Group scale
ISI	Insomnia severity index
LVEF	Left ventricular ejection fraction
mHIC	Modified Health Improvement Card
NCDs	Noncommunicable diseases
NDI	Neck disability index
NIV	Noninvasive ventilation
NPRS	Numerical pain rating scale
NREM	Non-REM sleep
O_2	Oxygen
OAI	Obstructive apnea index
ODI	Oxygen desaturation index
OSA	Obstructive sleep apnea
PAP	Positive airway pressure
PAR-Q	Physical Activity Readiness questionnaire
PCO_2	Pressure of arterial carbon dioxide
PD	Parkinson disease
PDQ-39	Parkinson's disease questionnaire
PDSS	Parkinson disease sleep scale
PhD	Philosopher doctor
PROM	Passive range of motion
PSG	Polysomnography
PSQI	Pittsburgh sleep quality index
PT	Physiotherapist
PTs	Physiotherapists
REM	Rapid eye movement
RERA	Respiratory effort related arousal
RLS	Restless legs syndrome
SB	Sleep bruxism
SBD	Sleep-breathing disorder
SE	Sleep efficiency
SHE	Sleep hygiene education
SL	Sleep latency
SOL	Sleep onset latency
Stage N1	NREM 1 sleep stage
Stage N2	NREM 2 sleep stage
Stage N3	NREM 3 sleep stage
Stage R	REM sleep stage
Stage W	Awake

SWS	Slow wave sleep
TECSA	Treatment-emergent central sleep apnea
TENS	Transcutaneous electrical nerve stimulation
TMD	Temporomandibular disorder
TMJ	Temporomandibular joint
TST	Total sleep time (sleep duration)
TUG	Timed up and go test
UA	Upper airway
WASO	Wake after sleep onset
WED	Willis-Ekbom disease
WHO	World Health Organization

Part I
Concepts

Chapter 1
A Twenty-First Century Physical Therapy Health and Lifestyle Framework to Maximize Sleep and Function

Elizabeth Dean ⓘ and Margot Skinner ⓘ

This book comprises a collection of case studies of patients with sleep complaints resulting from various pathologies and causes. It describes the physical therapy management to remediate disordered sleep in each case, with the ultimate goal of maximizing the patient's functional capacity and overall health and well-being.

Sleep is recognized as a complex process impacted not only by a primary disorder or pathology but also by confounding lifestyle practices and attributes [1]. The extent to which lifestyle practices and attributes contribute either primarily or secondarily to a patient's sleep disturbance is established through detailed assessment by the physical therapist. Findings are used to identify behavior change goals and strategies, which are discussed and agreed with the patient. Such an evidence-informed health and lifestyle framework [2, 3] is consistent with physical therapy practice in the twenty-first century [4–7], and the International Classification of Functioning, Disability and Health (ICF) (Fig. 1.1) [8], that has been long endorsed by World Physiotherapy [9].

Contemporary physical therapy is committed to the overall health of the patient [10]. Lifestyle-related non-communicable diseases (NCDs) are the leading causes of disability and premature death in high-income countries and increasingly in middle- and low-income countries [11]. Several NCDs, for example, cardiovascular disease, respiratory disease, stroke, obesity, and cancer, can disrupt sleep [12]. Thus, irrespective of a patient's presenting complaints, contemporary physical therapy practice includes assessment of smoking, alcohol use, nutritional status, body

E. Dean (✉)
Department of Physical Therapy, Faculty of Medicine, University of British Columbia, Vancouver, BC, Canada

M. Skinner
Centre for Health and Rehabilitation Research, School of Physiotherapy, University of Otago, Dunedin, New Zealand

C. Frange (ed.), *Clinical Cases in Sleep Physical Therapy*, https://doi.org/10.1007/978-3-031-38340-3_1

"

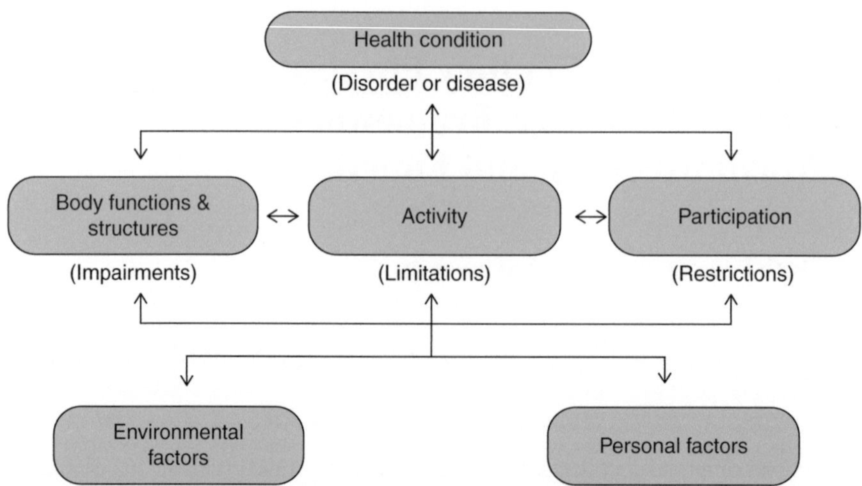

Fig. 1.1 International classification of functioning, disability, and health from the World Health Organization. ([8]; This figure has been modified and reprinted with permission of the World Health Organization (WHO), and all rights are reserved by the Organization)

mass, stress, and sleep, as well as sedentary behavior, inactivity, and structured exercise [4]. Healthy nutrition and exercise, in particular, go hand-in-hand [13].

Given that the relationship between sleep disorders and lifestyle practices and attributes is bidirectional, this chapter focuses on the literature related to the impact on sleep of lifestyle practices and attributes that also largely underlie NCDs. An established tool for assessing indexes and lifestyle behaviors, the modified Health Improvement Card (mHIC), is also described.

Chapter 2 outlines the literature specifically related to the contextual factors of the ICF, namely, environmental and personal factors that influence a night's sleep in an individual. Behavioral interventions that can be used by the physical therapist to modify one or more lifestyle practices or attributes to reverse adverse practices which compromise an individual's sleep and to promote healthy practices to maximize it are also described in that chapter and elsewhere [14–16].

Sleep Deprivation, Health, and Function

The health consequences of sleep deprivation have been well documented in the companion textbook [17] and other established evidence syntheses [18]. Comparable to other lifestyle factors, sleep deprivation is a metabolic oxidative stressor associated with chronic low-grade systemic inflammation (CLGSI), the common pathway for many chronic conditions [19]. Besides the traditional assessment of underlying pathophysiology associated with conditions and/or diseases contributing to sleep impairment, the physical therapist needs also to assess lifestyle practices and attributes. Lifestyle factors impact sleep independently, as well as in combination with underlying pathophysiology. Behavioral interventions can then be prescribed to maximize sleep quality and quantity. Adequate metabolic reserves and being well rested and restored are necessary conditions to maximize the benefits of exercise and minimize potential adverse effects in the sleep deprived individual.

Sleep is essential for health and for physiologic healing and repair [1, 20]. Sleep deprivation, on the other hand, is associated with various pathological, functional, and behavioral consequences [21] including high blood pressure, increased stress hormones, and lower immune function. Functional performance and capacity are reduced, along with impaired hand–eye coordination and reaction times. Sleep deprivation leads to daytime sleepiness, including the tendency to fall asleep during activities such as driving. All these contribute to making patients unsafe when navigating their environments. Sleep deprived individuals are more likely to be lethargic, mentally depressed, and disinterested in being active or exercising, which correspondingly compromises health and well-being. Even in the short term, sleep deprivation can increase susceptibility to viral infection and contribute to weight gain, heart disease, and diabetes [12]. Mortality risk increases with severity and duration of sleep deprivation [22].

Optimal Sleep Quantity and Quality

Generally, 7–9 h of uninterrupted sleep to enable a person to go through the sleep cycles is recommended for health and well-being in adults [23]. Young people and older adults require more or less sleep, respectively. Importantly, the clinician needs to appreciate that sleep is a behavior that is under stimulus control of the environment as well as a physiologic function. It needs to be regular and habitual to manifest its maximal benefits. The behavior of sleep is maximized by attention to sleeping hygiene practices and the environment where an individual sleeps [16]. These aspects and their assessments are detailed in the companion text [17].

Lifestyle Practices and Attributes That Impact Sleep

Targeted attention to patients' lifestyle practices and attributes within the health and lifestyle framework underpins physical therapy clinical practice guidelines, in general [2]. This section briefly reviews the impact of lifestyle practices and attributes on sleep specifically, and the need for the physical therapist to assess sleep and intervene by addressing not only the underlying pathology wherever possible but also those lifestyle practices and attributes factors that compromise sleep. By addressing these factors, sleep can be improved. Adverse lifestyle practices and attributes, along with sleep pathologies, are pro-inflammatory and have been well documented to contribute to CLGSI [24, 25]. CLGSI can be ameliorated with behavior change toward anti-inflammatory lifestyle practices. Topics include smoking, alcohol use, nutrition, body weight, and stress, as well as the level of conditioning including sedentariness, inactivity, and inadequate structured exercise.

Smoking

Because nicotine, a major constituent of tobacco, is a central nervous system stimulant, smoking contributes to insomnia [26]. Smokers often have problems falling and staying asleep and are more likely to develop breathing issues and experience restless leg syndrome, both of which interrupt sleep [27]. Smoking disturbs sleep cycles and leads to difficulty getting up in the morning and decreases alertness. Half of the people who smoke wake during the night with a nicotine craving [28]. Of some 1100 smokers surveyed in one study, 17% slept less than 6 h a night and 28% reported "disturbed" sleep quality [29]. Although exercise may offset the adverse effects of smoking on sleep, smoking cessation is the priority [30].

Alcohol Use

Alcohol depresses the central nervous system. It suppresses the all-important rapid eye movement sleep cycle, which is essential for physical and mental restoration and repair following sleep [31]. Alcohol reduces sleep latency onset, although alcohol may enable healthy people to fall asleep sooner and briefly sleep more deeply [32]. These findings have been supported in a questionnaire study in which men reported impaired sleep quality and duration, and general sleep disturbances, after consuming alcohol [33].

Nutritional Status

When it comes to health and the role of nutrition, an editorial published in the British Journal of Sports Medicine pitted exercise against diet; it summed it up—'You cannot outrun a bad diet' [34]. Nutritional quality impacts sleep, in turn, exercise capacity. For example, deficiency of key nutrients such as calcium, magnesium, and vitamins A, C, D, E, and K has each been associated with short sleep, differentially between men and women, likely mediated through the disruption of hormonal pathways [35]. Elements of the western-style diet have been reported to be deleterious to sleep. Low fiber and saturated fat are associated with lighter, less restorative sleep with more sleep arousals [36].

A healthy whole food plant-based Mediterranean diet (high in legumes, vegetables, fruit; and low in animal sourced foods, fat, sugar and salt, and processed foods) has been the most studied diet in the world, and has been reported to be among the healthiest [37, 38]. Its benefits have been attributed to the fact that a whole food plant-based diet is anti-inflammatory, whereas the standard western-style diet is pro-inflammatory contributing to NCDs [39]. Adherents to this diet have less disrupted nocturnal sleep compared with others [38–40]. They also have reported less anxiety and depression, conditions well known to disturb sleep [41]. Compared with the traditional western-style diet, the Mediterranean diet is higher in omega-3 fatty acids, which independently reduce symptoms of depression, and improve sleep and protect against cognitive deficits associated with sleep loss. This diet is also high in tryptophan, melatonin, magnesium, B vitamins and vitamin D; nutrients associated with several parameters linked with sound sleep [37].

Further, based on a sophisticated crossover design, the low-fat vegan diet was recently reported to surpass the Mediterranean diet in terms of general healthfulness and reduced disease risk [42]. The vegan diet was superior with respect to participants' body weight, lipid levels, and insulin sensitivity. Blood pressure decreased on both diets, but more so on the Mediterranean diet. These findings are consistent with the conclusions of the EAT Lancet Commission that the planet needs to shift to a whole food plant-based diet for individual, national, and planetary health [43]. Whether the consumption of a low-fat vegan diet specifically improves sleep beyond that reported with a Mediterranean diet when it is compared with other dietary regimes remains to be established.

That humans are vegan-by-design has been unequivocally supported by a detailed comparative analysis of the anatomy, physiology, and digestive/metabolism of carnivores, omnivores, and herbivores [44]. Not only have humans been shown to be dedicated herbivores, but there was no resemblance to omnivores—both plant and meat eaters—which is commonly believed by the public, health professionals, and dedicated so-called disease organizations. Substantial evidence has now been mounted that the cultural eating patterns of people in western countries, that include animal-sourced foods including meat, eggs, and dairy, are associated with many NCDs. These include chronic cardiovascular, respiratory, and metabolic diseases that are pandemic today [45] and frequently associated with breathing and sleep disorders [1].

In western countries, gastrointestinal dysfunction including gastroesophageal reflux disease (GERD) and 'heart burn' are also prevalent [46]. These often manifest when a person reclines, thus interfere with sleep. Such conditions are associated with a person's lifestyle practices and attributes including excess body weight, moderate/high alcohol consumption, smoking, and postprandial heavy exercise as well as lack of regular physical activity [47]. Eating habits such as consuming diets with heavy acid loads, irregular meal patterns, large volume of meals, and eating meals just before bedtime also contribute. Elements of the western-style diet have also been implicated, namely, fatty, fried food/products, acidic foods, coffee/tea, and carbonated beverages are triggers for GERD symptoms [47, 48]. The whole food plant-based diet because it is lean, green, and largely alkaline can offset gastroesophageal reflux, regurgitation, and heart burn [49].

Coffee, tea, and many soda drinks are caffeinated. Caffeine being a central nervous system stimulant can directly interfere with sleep induction [50]. Depending on the patient's sensitivity, caffeinated foods and beverages should be avoided several hours before bed. In addition, soda drinks typically have high content of sugar, an established energizer and stimulant, thus are best avoided before bed, or avoided altogether. Sugar is an oxidative stressor, pro-inflammatory, and increases C-reactive protein in an index of CLGSI [51].

Body Mass

Increased body mass is a major contributor to obstructive sleep apnea and related problems [52]. Fat deposits are commonly found in the tongue and around the neck and throat, as well as the waist and hips, and around internal organs. Reduced body mass can reduce these fat deposits, thus is recommended to reduce the severity of the apneic and hypopneic events [53, 54].

Insufficient sleep has been associated with obesity and increased waist circumference [55, 56]. In particular, increased waist circumference [56] is an indicator of numerous cardiovascular problems which, as they become more severe, compromise breathing and sleep.

Impaired sleep is associated with hypertension, potentially mediated through its association with increased body mass and associated hypoventilation during recumbency and rest [57, 58].

Stress

Western-style living is associated with high stress levels and sleep disturbance not only in adults but also in children [59]. The association of sleep and mental health can be bidirectional or a combination of both directions. Sleep can be disrupted by mental health issues most commonly anxiety and depression [60]; in turn, sleep deprivation can lead to anxiety and depression [60, 61]. A detailed assessment enables the physical therapist to establish the association between sleep and mental health in a given patient; which, in turn, informs targeted lifestyle behavior change interventions.

Sedentary Behavior, Inactivity, and Lack of Exercise

Traditionally, physical therapists have focused on sedentarism and inactivity as the basis for prescription of structured exercise in order to maximize the functional capacity of patients. With the adoption of the ICF however, physical therapists have recognized that functional capacity reflects other lifestyle practices and attributes including sleep, and underlying pathologies, and the reverse. Unless judiciously prescribed however, imposing exercise stress on a patient who is sleep deprived may not only exacerbate their symptoms but also further compromise their immune status by increasing a CLGSI response.

People with disrupted sleep are more likely to sit more and be less active, or not undertake regular structured exercise [1]. All three categories need to be assessed clinically in patients with sleep disorders. Imposing increased exercise load on sleep deprived individuals with the intent of improving exercise capacity is not likely to be effective and could be unsafe. First, the underlying causes of and contributors to disrupted sleep need to be identified and mitigated or largely reversed to prepare the patient physiologically for increased exercise stress.

Assessment of Lifestyle Practices and Attributes That Impact Sleep

This section highlights tools to assess sleep and describes the modified Health Improvement Card (mHIC) (Figs. 1.2a, b) [62]. The mHIC is a user-friendly tool for assessing basic lifestyle practices and attributes and serves as a basis for targeting and tailoring lifestyle behavior change programs.

Tools to Assess Sleep

There are several established tools for assessing and evaluating sleep quality and quantity objectively and subjectively which have been described in this text's companion volume [63, 64]. In addition, the Pittsburgh Sleep Quality Index [65, 66] is one of the most used tools for the subjective assessment of sleep quality, and is considered valid and reliable [67]. It is publicly accessible and can be completed online or on paper. The findings can then serve as a basis for behavioral change interventions which have been well described elsewhere [7–16].

The ICF check list provides a comprehensive framework for assessing functional health of individuals with sleep disorders in a clinical setting [68]. It enables the clinician to identify how various factors impact that individual's sleep and also provide an informed basis for targeted intervention.

The Modified Health Improvement Card

A useful easily administered assessment/evaluation tool for major lifestyle behaviors and attributes is the mHIC (Fig. 1.2). It provides a basis for targeting and tailoring education and interventions to effect positive lifestyle behavior change. The original HIC [69, 70] was developed by the World Health Professions Alliance

a

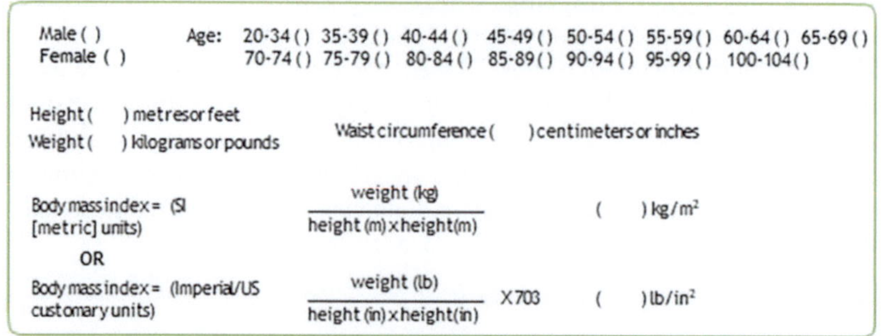

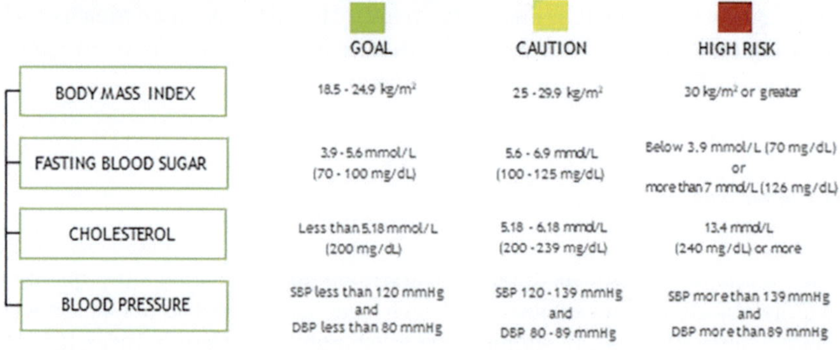

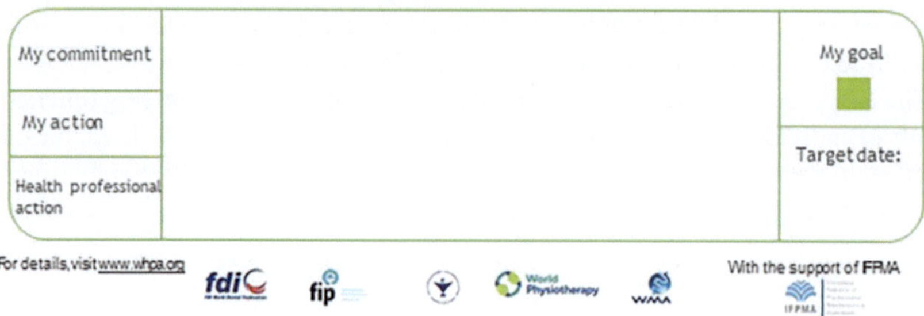

Fig. 1.2 (**a, b**) Modified health improvement card. ([62]; Modified and reprinted with permission World Health Professions Alliance

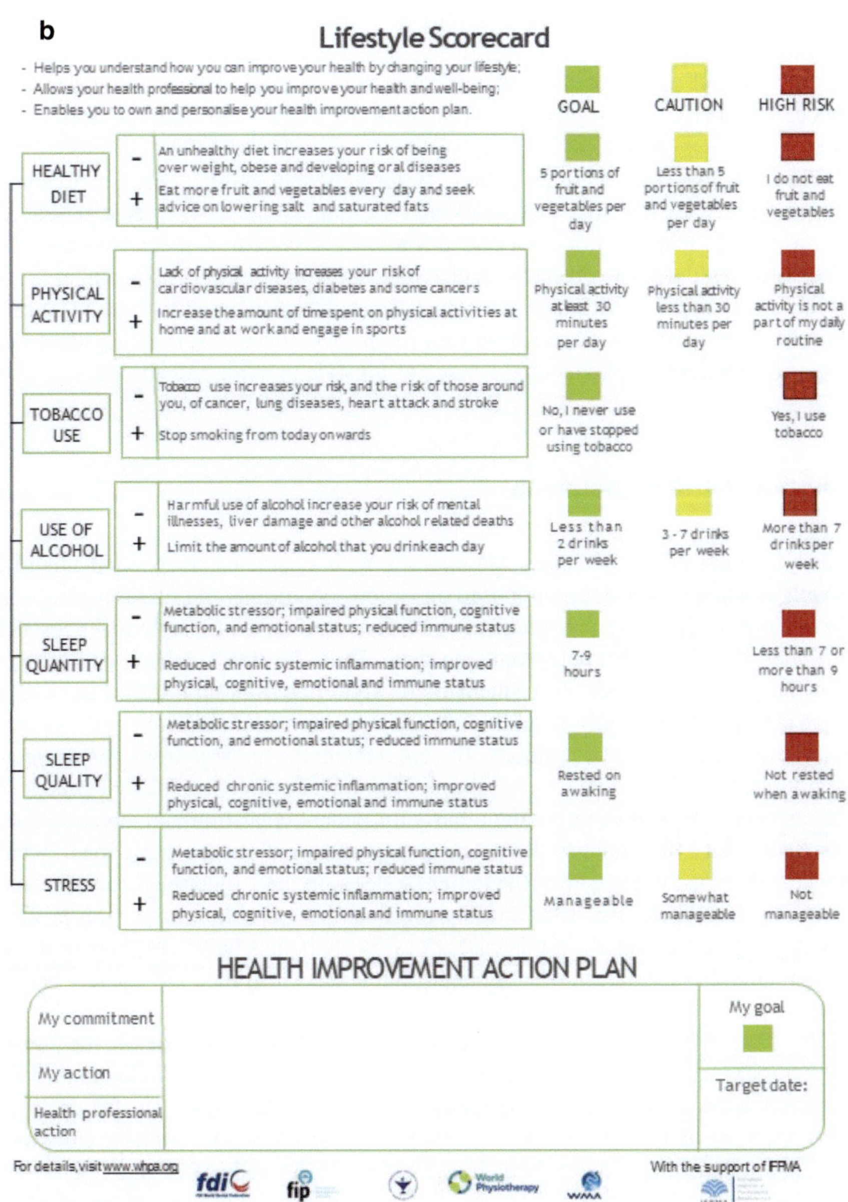

Fig. 1.2 (continued)

which consists of the world's five leading established health professions including nurses, physicians, and physical therapists. It has been modified to update its criteria for healthy and unhealthy lifestyle practices and attributes based on current evidence. The mHIC is designed to complement the assessment findings from dedicated sleep assessment tools.

The mHIC has three sections: patient's information, biometrics, and key lifestyle-related behaviors. Lifestyle behaviors and recommendations are rated based on degree of risk, that is, on a color-coded traffic light system of green (meeting the criteria for health for each behavior and associated with low NCD risk), amber (cautionary NCD disease risk), and red (unhealthy and associated with high NCD disease risk). The mHIC serves as a basis for patient education in that it clearly identifies targets for the patient's behavioral change of lifestyle practice and attributes.

Summary and Conclusion

Lifestyle practices and attributes can interfere with a patient's sleep independently, as well as when they are superimposed on various conditions and diseases affecting sleep. Conversely, pathophysiological conditions can impact lifestyle practices and attributes, thereby further compromising sleep. Thus, the physical therapist's assessment necessarily includes assessment of lifestyle practices and attributes, which impact sleep independently, in addition to the conventional assessment of the underlying pathophysiological conditions. To complement the findings from sleep assessment tools, the mHIC is an easy-to-use clinical tool for assessing lifestyle practices and attributes, as well as providing a basis for patient education and targeting specific health behavior changes. Behavior change interventions are prescribed by the physical therapist to maximize the patient's sleep, in turn, functional capacity and overall health. Alternatively, referral by physical therapists to other health professionals may be warranted. In this case, physical therapists have a responsibility to support those health behavior change initiatives instituted by other health professionals.

This chapter highlights the use of the health and lifestyle framework in the physical therapists' clinical practice guidelines, with special reference to individuals with sleep problems. It summarized the literature related to the impact on sleep of lifestyle practices and attributes, that also largely underlie NCDs, namely: smoking; alcohol use; nutritional status; body mass; and stress; as well as sedentary behavior, inactivity, and lack of structured exercise. Contemporary physical therapy practice warrants going beyond the traditional biomedical model and 'exercise as medicine' mantra, to maximizing functional capacity and performance through maximizing lifestyle attributes and practices including sleep. Physical therapy management of sleep disorders, based on the evidence-informed health and lifestyle framework that is consistent with twenty-first century physical therapy practice, can maximize several inter-related outcomes for patients with sleep disorders, that is, health-related, preventive, disease-specific, and functional.

References

1. Harvard Medical School Special Health. Improving sleep. Report. Boston, MA: Harvard Health Publishing; 2013.
2. Dean E, Lomi C. A health and lifestyle framework: an evidence-informed basis for contemporary physical therapist clinical practice guidelines with special reference to individuals with heart failure. Physiother Res Int. 2022;27:e1950. https://doi.org/10.1002/pri.1950.
3. Dean E, Fagevik Olsén M. A health and lifestyle framework for management of post covid-19 syndrome based on evidence-informed management of post-polio syndrome: a narrative review. Eur J Physiother. 2022;24:56–60. https://doi.org/10.1080/21679169.2021.2000150.
4. Dean E. Physical therapy practice in the 21st century: a new evidence-informed paradigm and implications. Invited Special Issue Editor. Physiother Theory Pract. 2009;25:327–462.
5. Dean E, Al-ObaidI S, Dornelas de Andrade A, Gosselink R, Umerah G, Al-Abdelwahab S, et al. The first physical therapy summit on global health: implications and recommendations for the 21st century. Physiother Theory Pract. 2011;27(8):531–47. https://doi.org/10.3109/09593985.2010.544052.
6. Dean E, Dornelas de Andrade A, O'Donoghue G, Skinner M, Umereh G, Beenen P, et al. The second physical therapy summit on global health: developing an action plan to promote health in daily practice and reduce the burden of non-communicable diseases. Physiother Theory Pract. 2014;30(4):261–75. https://doi.org/10.3109/09593985.2013.856977.
7. Dean E, Skinner M, Myezwa H, Mkumbuzi V, Mostert-Wentzel K, Perez DP, et al. Health competency standards in physical therapist practice. Phys Ther. 2019;99(9):1242–54.
8. World Health Organization. International classification of functioning, disability and health. Geneva: WHO; 2001. p. ea54r21.pdf. https://www.who.int/classifications/international-classification-of-functioning-disability-and-health. Accessed 2 Oct 2022.
9. World Physiotherapy. International classification of functioning, disability and health. n.d.. https://world.physio/resources/glossaryICF. Accessed 2 Oct 2022.
10. World Physiotherapy. Description of physical therapy. Policy statement. n.d.. https://world.physio/sites/default/files/2020-07/PS-2019-Description-of-physical-therapy.pdf. Accessed 2 Oct 2022.
11. World Health Organization. Non communicable diseases. n.d.. https://www.who.int/news-room/fact-sheets/detail/noncommunicable-diseases#:~:text=Key%20facts,%2D%20and%20middle%2Dincome%20countries. Accessed 2 Oct 2022.
12. Centers for Disease Control and Prevention. Sleep and chronic disease. n.d.. www.cdc.gov/sleep/about_sleep/chronic_disease.html. Accessed 3 Oct 2022.
13. Caprara G. Mediterranean-type dietary pattern and physical activity: the winning combination to counteract the rising burden of non-communicable diseases (NCDs). Nutrients. 2021;13(2):429. https://doi.org/10.3390/nu13020429.
14. Elvén M, Hochwälder J, Dean E, Söderlund A. A clinical reasoning model focused on clients' behaviour change with reference to physiotherapists: its multiphase development and validation. Physiother Theory Pract. 2015;31(4):231–43.
15. Dean E, Moffat M, Myezwa H, de Andrade D, Skinner M, Söderlund A. Toward core interprofessional health-based competencies to address the non-communicable diseases and their risk factors: curriculum content analysis. BMC Public Health. 2014;14:717. https://doi.org/10.1186/1471-2458-14-717.
16. Rodrigues D'Aurea CV, Soares Passos G, Frange C. Insomnia: physiotherapeutic approach. In: Frange C, Coelho FMS, editors. Sleep medicine and physical therapy: a comprehensive guide for practitioners. Basel: Springer Nature; 2022. p. 61–73. https://doi.org/10.1007/978-3-030-85074-6.
17. Frange C, Coelho FMS, editors. Sleep medicine and physical therapy: a comprehensive guide for practitioners. Basel: Springer Nature; 2022. https://doi.org/10.1007/978-3-030-85074-6.
18. Harvard Medical School. Guide. Understanding inflammation. Boston, MA: Harvard Health Publishing; 2018.

19. Harvard Medical School Special Health. Fighting inflammation. Report. Boston, MA: Harvard Health Publishing; 2020.
20. Frange C, Santos Coelho FM. Sleep: definition, concept, new area for physical therapy. In: Frange C, Coelho FMS, editors. Sleep medicine and physical therapy: a comprehensive guide for practitioners. Basel: Springer Nature; 2022. p. 3–11. https://doi.org/10.1007/978-3-030-85074-6.
21. Levy Andersen ML, Tufik S. Brief history of sleep medicine and its importance for overall health. In: Frange C, Coelho FMS, editors. Sleep medicine and physical therapy: a comprehensive guide for practitioners. Basel: Springer Nature; 2022. p. 21–7. https://doi.org/10.1007/978-3-030-85074-6.
22. Ikehara S, Iso H, Date C, Kikuchi S, Watanabe Y, Wada Y, et al. Association of sleep duration with mortality from cardiovascular disease and other causes for Japanese men and women: the JACC Study. Sleep. 2009;32(3):295–301.
23. Consensus Conference Panel, Watson NF, Badr MS, Belenky G, Bliwise DL, Buxton OM, Buysse D, et al. Recommended amount of sleep for a healthy adult: A Joint Consensus Statement of the American Academy of Sleep Medicine and Sleep Research Society. J Clin Sleep Med. 2015;11(6):591–2. https://doi.org/10.5664/jcsm.4758.
24. Harvard University. How sleep deprivation can cause inflammation. n.d.. https://www.health.harvard.edu/sleep/how-sleep-deprivation-can-cause-inflammation. Accessed 2 Oct 2022.
25. Meier-Ewert HK, Ridker PM, Rifai N, Regan MM, Price NJ, Dinges DF, et al. Effect of sleep loss on C-reactive protein, an inflammatory marker of cardiovascular risk. J Am Coll Cardiol. 2004;43(4):678–83.
26. Jaehne A, Loessl B, Bárkai Z, Riemann D, Hornyak M. Effects of nicotine on sleep during consumption, withdrawal and replacement therapy. Sleep Med Rev. 2009;13(5):363–77. https://doi.org/10.1016/j.smrv.2008.12.003.
27. Dias Gomes AC, Santos Coelho FM. Restless legs syndrome (Willis-Ekbom Disease) and periodic leg movements of sleep: an overview. In: Frange C, Coelho FMS, editors. Sleep medicine and physical therapy: a comprehensive guide for practitioners. Basel: Springer Nature; 2022. p. 3–11. https://doi.org/10.1007/978-3-030-85074-6.
28. Branstetter SA, Krebs NM, Muscat JE. Nighttime waking to smoke, stress, and nicotine addiction. Behav Sleep Med. 2022;20(6):706–15. https://doi.org/10.1080/15402002.2021.1992408.
29. Cohrs S, Rodenbeck A, Riemann D, Szagun B, Jaehne A, Brinkman J, et al. Impaired sleep quality and sleep duration in smokers—results from the German Multicenter Study on Nicotine Dependence. Addict Biol. 2014;19(3):486–96. https://doi.org/10.1111/j.1369-1600.2012.00487.x.
30. Purani H, Friedrichsen AA. Sleep quality in cigarette smokers: associations with smoking-related outcomes and exercise. Addict Behav. 2019;90:71–6. https://doi.org/10.1016/j.addbeh.2018.10.023.
31. Sleep Foundation. Alcohol and sleep. n.d.. www.sleepfoundation.org/nutrition/alcohol-and-sleep. Accessed 2 Oct 2022.
32. Ebrahim IO, Shapiro CM, Williams AJ, Fenwick PB. Alcohol and sleep I: effects on normal sleep. Alcohol Clin Exp Res. 2013;37(4):539–49. https://doi.org/10.1111/acer.12006.
33. Park S, Oh M, Lee B, Kim H, Lee W, Lee J, et al. The effects of alcohol on quality of sleep. Kor J Fam Med. 2015;36(6):294–9.
34. Malhotra A, Noakes T, Phinney S. It is time to bust the myth of physical inactivity and obesity: you cannot outrun a bad diet. Br J Sports Med. 2015;49(15):967–8. https://doi.org/10.1136/bjsports-2015-094911.
35. Ikonte CJ, Mun JG, Reider CA, Grant RW, Mitmesser SH. Micronutrient inadequacy in short sleep: analysis of the NHANES 2005-2016. Nutrients. 2019;11(10):2335. https://doi.org/10.3390/nu11102335.
36. St-Onge M-P, Roberts A, Shechter A, Choudhury AR. Fiber and saturated fat are associated with sleep arousals and slow wave sleep. J Clin Sleep Med. 2016;12(1):19–24. https://doi.org/10.5664/jcsm.5384.

37. Harvard Medical School. Special health report. The diet review. Boston, MA: Harvard Health Publishing; 2020.
38. Scoditti E, Tumolo MR, Garbarino S. Mediterranean diet on sleep: a health alliance. Nutrients. 2022;14(14):2998. https://doi.org/10.3390/nu14142998.
39. Harvard Medical School. Foods that fight inflammation. Designing your diet to lower disease risk. Boston, MA: Harvard Health Publishing; 2021.
40. St-Onge M-P, Mikic A, Pietrolungo CE. Effects of diet on sleep quality. Adv Nutr. 2016;7(5):938–49. https://doi.org/10.3945/an.116.012336.
41. Psaltopoulou T, Sergentanis TN, Panagiotakos DB, Sergentanis IN, Kosti R, Scarmeas N. Mediterranean diet: relationship with anxiety and depression. Ann Neurol. 2014;75(4):614. https://doi.org/10.1002/ana.23990.
42. Barnard ND, Alwarith J, Rembert E, Brandon L, Nguyen M, Goergen A, et al. A Mediterranean diet and low-fat vegan diet to improve body weight and cardiometabolic risk factors: a randomized cross-over trial. Am J Clin Nutr. 2021;5:1–13. https://doi.org/10.1080/07315724.2020.1869625.
43. Report of the EAT Lancet Commission. Healthy diets from sustainable food systems. 2019. https://eatforum.org/content/uploads/2019/07/EAT-Lancet_Commission_Summary_Report.pdf. Accessed 30 Sep 2022.
44. Mills M. The comparative anatomy of eating. n.d.. https://www.adaptt.org/documents/Mills%20The%20Comparative%20Anatomy%20of%20Eating1.pdf.
45. GBD 2019 Risk Factors Collaborators. Global burden of 87 risk factors in 204 countries and territories, 1990–2019: a systematic analysis for the Global Burden of Disease Study 2019. Lancet. 2020;396:1223–49.
46. Harvard Medical School. The sensitive gut. Boston, MA: Harvard Health Publishing; 2022.
47. Zhang M, Hou Z-H, Huang Z-B, Chen X-L, Liu F-B. Dietary and lifestyle factors related to gastroesophageal reflux disease: a systematic review. Ther Clin Risk Manag. 2021;17:305–23. https://doi.org/10.2147/TCRM.S296680.
48. Müller A, Zimmermann-Klemd AM, Lederer A-K, Hannibal L, Kowarschik S, Huber R, et al. A vegan diet Is associated with a significant reduction in dietary acid load: post hoc analysis of a randomized controlled trial in healthy individuals. Int J Environ Res Public Health. 2021;18(19):9998. https://doi.org/10.3390/ijerph18199998.
49. Bhatia SJ, Reddy DN, Ghoshal UC, Jayanthi V, Abraham P, Choudhuri G, et al. Epidemiology and symptom profile of gastroesophageal reflux in the Indian population: report of the Indian Society of Gastroenterology Task Force. Indian J Gastroenterol. 2011;30(3):118–27. https://doi.org/10.1007/s12664-011-0112-x.
50. O'Callaghan F, Muurlink O, Reid N. Effects of caffeine on sleep quality and daytime functioning. Risk Manag Healthc Pol. 2018;11:263–71. https://doi.org/10.2147/RMHP.S156404.
51. Vgontzas AN, Zoumakis E, Bixler EO, Lin H-M, Follett H, Kales A, et al. Adverse effects of modest sleep restriction on sleepiness, performance, and inflammatory cytokines. J Clin Endocrinol Metab. 2004;89(5):2119–26.
52. Mortimore IL, Marshall I, Wraith PK, Sellar RJ, Douglas NJ. Neck and total body fat deposition in nonobese and obese patients with sleep apnea compared with that in control subjects. Am J Respir Crit Care Med. 1998;157(1):280–3. https://doi.org/10.1164/ajrccm.157.1.9703018.
53. Fattal D, Hester S, Wendt L. Body weight and obstructive sleep apnea: a mathematical relationship between body mass index and apnea-hypopnea index in veterans. J Clin Sleep Med. 2022;18:2723. https://doi.org/10.5664/jcsm.10190.
54. Arora T. Sleep doesn't waste time, It's good for the waist line. Sleep. 2015;38(8):1159–60. https://doi.org/10.5665/sleep.4884.
55. Wu Y, Zhai L, Zhang D. Sleep duration and obesity among adults: a meta-analysis of prospective studies. Sleep Med. 2014;15(12):1456–62. https://doi.org/10.1016/j.sleep.2014.07.018.
56. Sperry SD, Scully ID, Gramzow RH, Jorgensen RS. Sleep duration and waist circumference in adults: a meta-analysis. Sleep. 2015;38(8):1269–76. https://doi.org/10.5665/sleep.4906.

57. Palagini L, Bruno RM, Gemignani A, Baglioni C, Ghiadoni L, Riemann D. Sleep loss and hypertension: a systematic review. Curr Pharm Des. 2013;19(13):2409–19. https://doi.org/10.2174/1381612811319130009.

58. Chunnan L, Shang S. Relationship between sleep and hypertension: findings from the NHANES (2007-2014). Int J Environ Res Public Health. 2021;18(15):7867. https://doi.org/10.3390/ijerph18157867.

59. Pires GN, Bezerra AG, Tufik S, Andersen ML. Effects of acute sleep deprivation on state anxiety levels: a systematic review and meta-analysis. Sleep Med. 2016;24:109–18. https://doi.org/10.1016/j.sleep.2016.07.019.

60. Nutt D, Wilson S, Paterson L. Sleep disorders as core symptoms of depression. Dialogues Clin Neurosci. 2008;10(3):329–36. https://doi.org/10.31887/DCNS.2008.10.3/dnutt.

61. Harvard Medical School Special Health. Anxiety and stress. Report. Boston, MA: Harvard Health Publishing; 2018.

62. Dean E, Söderlund A. Lifestyle medicine to address orthopaedic conditions: rationale and practice. In: Tatta J, Garner G, editors. Lifestyle medicine and orthopaedic physical therapy practice. Minneapolis, MN: Orthopedic Physical Therapy Products; 2022.

63. Frange C, Figueiro Reis MJ, Lottenberg Vago E, Santos Coelho FM. Subjective assessment of sleep. In: Frange C, Coelho FMS, editors. Sleep medicine and physical therapy: a comprehensive guide for practitioners. Basel: Springer Nature; 2022. p. 381–400. https://doi.org/10.1007/978-3-030-85074-6.

64. Figueiro Reis MJ, Lottenberg Vago E, Frange C, Santos Coelho FM. Objective assessment of sleep. In: Frange C, Coelho FMS, editors. Sleep medicine and physical therapy: a comprehensive guide for practitioners. Basel: Springer Nature; 2022. p. 401–10. https://doi.org/10.1007/978-3-030-85074-6.

65. SnoozeUniversity. Pittsburgh sleep quality index online calculator. n.d.. https://www.snoozeuniversity.com/psqi/. Accessed 3 Oct 2022.

66. Perelman School of Medicine at the University of Pennsylvania. Pittsburgh Sleep Quality Index (PSQI). n.d.. https://www.med.upenn.edu/cbti/assets/user-content/documents/Pittsburgh%20Sleep%20Quality%20Index%20(PSQI).pdf.

67. Backhaus J, Junghanns K, Broocks A, Riemann D, Hohagen F. Test-retest reliability and validity of the Pittsburgh Sleep Quality Index in primary insomnia. J Psychosom Res. 2002;53(3):737–40. https://doi.org/10.1016/s0022-3999(02)00330-6.

68. Gradinger F, Glassel A, Gugger M, Cieza A, Braun N, Khatami R, et al. Identification of problems in functioning of people with sleep disorders in a clinical setting using the International Classification of Functioning Disability and Health (ICF) Checklist. J Sleep Res. 2011;20(3):445–53. https://doi.org/10.1111/j.1365-2869.2010.00888.x.

69. World Health Professions Alliance. Health improvement card. 2014. http://www.ifpma.org/fileadmin/content/Publication/2011/ncd_Health-Improvement-Card_web-1.pdf. Accessed 5 Oct 2022.

70. World Health Professions Alliance. WHPA health improvement card. User guide for health professionals. 2017. http://www.whpa.org/ncd_health_improvement_card_professionals.pdf. Accessed 5 Oct 2022.

Chapter 2
Physiotherapists: Sleep Health Promoters

Mayis Aldughmi ⓘ, Cristina Frange, and Catherine F. Siengsukon ⓘ

Role of Physiotherapists in Promoting Sleep Health

Physical therapists (PTs) are health care professionals who are well positioned and experienced to promote health across different populations and age groups [1]. Their role is vital in encouraging their patients to adjust various lifestyle behaviors as seen in Chap. 1 [1]. PTs help in preventing, reducing the risk factors, and treating various conditions including non-communicable diseases (NCDs) [1]. They use various strategies, modalities, and non-invasive hands-on interventions when they treat their patients, such as physical activity and exercise therapy [1], kinesiotherapy, manual therapies, electrotherapeutic and needling modalities, education and self-management. Educating patients about the role of PTs as health promoters is key for the success of improving the patient's overall health and wellness.

Promoting sleep health is no different from the lifestyle behaviors in which PTs can play a vital role in [2–4]. In June 2020, the American Physical Therapy Association (APTA) house of delegates officially adopted the position "The Role of the Physical Therapist and the American Physical Therapy Association in Sleep Health" [5]. In part, it states:

M. Aldughmi (✉)
Department of Physiotherapy, School of Rehabilitation Sciences, University of Jordan, Amman, Jordan

C. Frange
Neurology and Neurosurgery Department, Federal University of São Paulo (UNIFESP), São Paulo, SP, Brazil

C. F. Siengsukon
Department of Physical Therapy, Rehabilitation Science, and Athletic Training, University of Kansas Medical Center, Kansas City, KS, USA

C. Frange (ed.), *Clinical Cases in Sleep Physical Therapy*,
https://doi.org/10.1007/978-3-031-38340-3_2

Physical therapists are part of an interdisciplinary team of licensed health services providers in prevention and management of sleep impairments and promotion of healthy sleep behaviors.

This position was an important step that recognized the professional role of the physical therapist in promoting sleep health. Recently, a presidential advisory from the American Heart Association (AHA) added *"sleep health"* as an essential life factor for cardiovascular health [6].

Despite acknowledging the importance of sleep for health, the prevalence of sleep disturbances is rising across the globe. Up to 70 million adults in the United States alone experience sleep disturbances [7]. The most reported health complaint among adults is sleep insufficiency [1]. The Center for Disease Control and Prevention (CDC) considered insufficient sleep as a public health epidemic due to its negative impact on health [8]. Furthermore, numerous studies have been conducted to estimate the prevalence of sleep disturbances since the outbreak of the COVID-19 virus [9]. A recent systematic review and metanalysis of data from 49 countries worldwide concluded that the prevalence of sleep disturbances increased by 43% during the lockdown and decreased to 38% after lockdown [9]. Also, the study found that four out of ten individuals who were mostly children, adolescents, and patients infected with the disease reported a sleep problem during the pandemic.

PTs who are professional health promoters and movement specialists need to recognize the consequences of poor sleep on rehabilitation outcomes and the overall well-being of their patients. They need to be well equipped with knowledge regarding the common assessment and screening tools of sleep quality, and what are the management strategies they can utilize to help their patients improve their sleep quality. Their role as sleep health promoters is of high importance and should become a standard of clinical care in PT.

Relevance of Sleep to PT Practice

Sleep Issues in Various Populations Commonly Treated by PTs

The prevalence of sleep disturbances is frequent in different populations that are commonly treated by PTs. Sleep disturbances such as sleep onset delay, sleep apnea, and frequent nocturnal wakings are common in children with neurodevelopmental conditions (NDC), including children with cerebral palsy (CP), down syndrome (DS), autism spectrum disorders (ASD), and pediatric cancer patients [10, 11]. Poor sleep is also highly prevalent among individuals with neurologic conditions such as stroke [12, 13], Parkinson's disease [14, 15], Alzheimer's disease [16, 17], and multiple sclerosis [18, 19]. Sleep disturbance in these populations is often primary from brain lesions in areas that control sleep, or secondary from common factors and symptoms such as side effects from medications administered to control their neurologic symptoms, pain, spasticity, bowel and bladder dysfunctions, anxiety, or breathing difficulties [1]. Furthermore, individuals who undergo orthopedic surgeries and those with low back pain can also suffer from various sleep disturbances [20, 21].

In addition to that, it is well documented in the literature that older adults commonly have sleep disturbances [22]. It is important to note that sleep architecture changes with the normal aging process; it is the consequences of aging such as medication use and psychosocial factors that make older adults vulnerable to sleep problems [22]. Considering the variety of patients often receive PT services, providing sleep education and promoting sleep health and wellness should be prioritized by PTs, to reduce the risk of developing sleep disturbances that can negatively impact the quality of life of these individuals.

Sleep Issues Among Individuals Treated in Various PT Practice Settings

Sleep disruption is a common complaint for many individuals receiving PT but is particularly a prevalent issue for people receiving care in hospital settings. Hospitalized patients are at high risk for developing sleep–wake dysfunction [23], which refers to disruption of the normal sleep–wake relationship that can result from factors such as a reduced number of hours of sleep or inappropriate timing between wake and sleep. For instance, neurologic adult patients in the hospital suffer from frequent night-time awakenings and sleep an average of 5 h per night [24]. Patients who are in a critical state in intensive care units often have more sleep disruptions, such as decreased total sleep time and abnormal sleep architecture manifested by increased NREM N1 and N2 sleep stages, and reduced NREM N3 sleep stage [23]. Around 55% reduction in sleep hours has been previously reported among pediatric patients in intensive care units [25]. Also, reduced total sleep time, sleep fragmentation, and later bedtimes are factors that have been previously linked with sleep disruption among young, hospitalized children [26].

Evidence suggests that sleep–wake dysfunction can become exacerbated by hospitalization if there is a preexisting sleep disorder such as sleep-disordered breathing (SDB) or hypersomnia disorders [27]. Unfortunately, when present, sleep–wake dysfunction can have detrimental health consequences on hospitalized patients [23, 28, 29]. Sleep–wake dysfunction among hospitalized patients is believed to be caused by both intrinsic and extrinsic factors [30]. Intrinsic factors which can vary among patients include pain, discomfort, pre-existing sleep disorder, psychiatric conditions such as depression and anxiety, bowel and bladder issues, and delirium [23, 31]. On the other hand, extrinsic factors are related to the environment surrounding the patient, such as room bright lights, noise (from medical staff, equipment alarms, visitors, hospital roommates), repetitive clinical examinations day and night, losing normal bedtime routine, rooms without windows and medication use [23, 26].

Sleep alterations are also common in individuals in long-term care facilities and nursing homes [32, 33]. Sleep patterns shift follows admission of elderly individuals into long-term care facilities [32, 34]. These individuals reported interrupted sleep approximately twice as frequently as pre-admission as well as a 60% reduction in the number of hours slept, increase in nap frequency during the day following admission compared to pre-admission, and around one-third of the residents have symptoms of insomnia [32]. In addition, nursing home residents who suffer from sleep disturbances often exhibit lower levels of physical activity or a sedentary state, decreased social interaction and communication, and an increase in interpersonal conflicts compared to those with no sleep problems which could lead to a spiraling decline in function and health [34]. Physical, psychosocial, and environmental factors have been previously reported that increase the incidence of sleep disturbances among residents of long-term care facilities and nursing homes [32]. Ideally the hospital and long-term care settings should be modified to encourage a healthy sleeping environment, in addition to routine sleep quality assessment and management to improve their sleep quality.

Impact of Sleep Disturbances on Rehabilitation Outcomes

Sleep disturbances among the variety of patients who receive PT services may worsen their condition, prolong recovery periods, and affect functional rehabilitation outcomes. Evidence suggests that the presence of sleep disorders among various neurological conditions reduces the participation of these patients in physical therapy activities, hence affecting recovery process [35–37]. For instance, individuals with stroke who commonly suffer from sleep apnea, insomnia, and excessive daytime sleepiness report poor quality of life and impaired performance of activities of daily life (ADLs) and functional activities [38]. Excessive daytime sleepiness among individuals with multiple sclerosis is highly associated with fatigue which in turn impact their daily functional activities [39]. Furthermore, evidence suggests that sleep disturbances impact motor skill learning and cognitive function [40, 41]. PTs incorporate in their treatments learning new skills and tasks that require the patient's attention, working memory, problem-solving, and mental flexibility. Therefore, participation in therapy and functional outcomes will be negatively affected in patients with poor sleep quality or quantity.

Among hospitalized patients, sleep–wake disorders were linked with prolonged recovery and length of stay, and poor perceptions of wellness and hospital care [23, 24]. Sleep deprivation and sleep–wake disorders may lead to serious detrimental effects on immune function, pain modulation, the hypothalamic-pituitary-adrenal axis, and autonomic function [27]. In fact, evidence suggests that among hospitalized patients, reduced sleep duration and deprivation were independently associated with hyperglycemia and impaired fasting glucose [42]. Furthermore, sleep deprivation may increase the likelihood of the development of delirium, which affects up to

50% of hospitalized older adults, specifically men who are older than 80 years old [43]. Compared to those without delirium, hospitalized older adults with delirium have a higher risk of prolonged hospital stay, institutionalization post discharge, and higher mortality rates 6 months post-discharge [44].

Obstructive sleep apnea (OSA) is the most studied sleep disorder among hospitalized patients that can significantly impact clinical outcomes [45]. Evidence suggests that patients post-surgeries who suffer from OSA are more likely to be transferred to the intensive care unit with prolonged hospital stay, mainly due to hypoxemia that resulted from OSA [46]. Similarly, pregnant women who suffer from OSA have an increased risk for cardiovascular and maternal morbidity, and consequently in-hospital death [47].

PTs can have an active role in preventing the risk for developing sleep disturbances among various conditions. They need to be aware of the critical need for quality and quantity sleep for patients to heal, modulate pain, learn, develop new skills and abilities, and function at their greatest potential.

Considering management strategies to improve sleep quality may offer a new venue of targeted treatment for PTs that could lead to improvement in patients' function and overall quality of life.

Physiotherapeutic Interventions to Improve Sleep

Considering sleep's critical role for proper body function, healing, and recovery, what should be the PT's role regarding sleep? Several international associations publicly released their views on the role of PT regarding sleep health as well as clinical practice guidelines to guide PTs in respect to the assessment and management of common sleep issues. The APTA 2020 house position [5] clearly stated that the PT should use the best available evidence to:

> Screen for sleep dysfunction; Identify impairments related to sleep dysfunction; Implement and progress therapeutic interventions to address impairments that interfere with sleep; Educate society, patients and clients, caregivers and providers on healthy sleep behaviors and the relationship between sleep, pain, physical activity, function, health, and wellbeing; Monitor and, if indicated, manage sleep quality and quantity in patients and clients to enhance physical therapy outcomes; and Refer to sleep medicine professionals as indicated.

Also, the Brazilian Sleep Association published in 2022 clinical practice guidelines as recommendations for PTs to manage sleep disorders, reviewing the literature so far and suggesting further investigations in the field [48].

In addition to that, practical sleep health and wellness information for PTs was previously published in an attempt to spread the knowledge among PTs about the critical role of sleep and its impact on rehabilitation outcomes, and what they can do in terms of assessment and management of sleep [2, 4]. This section will provide an overview and summary of evidence about the management strategies PTs can utilize to improve sleep quality among their patients.

Sleep Hygiene Education

Sleep Hygiene Education (SHE) is a set of behavioral and environmental recommendations provided to an individual for the purpose of promoting healthy sleep. It was first used in the late 1970s for the treatment of insomnia and is considered the most commonly used non-pharmacological treatment for individuals with sleep problems [49, 50]. The most common covered areas in SHE include lifestyle behavior modifications (caffeine, tobacco, and alcohol consumption), noise, stress, and sleep regularity [51].

Improved sleep quality following SHE was shown among adolescents and university students, individuals with chronic low back pain and hemodialysis [52–54]. Although SHE alone can be effective in improving sleep, evidence suggests that if SHE was combined with other treatments, this may provide more favorable outcomes. For example, patients with cancer receiving chemotherapy had improved sleep following SHE combined with reflexology [55].

In addition to that, the mode of delivery of SHE might impact its effectiveness. A 2021 study that explored SHE on hospitalized patients did not offer SHE in the form of a leaflet or booklet instructions. Instead, SHE was delivered in a form of a bundle containing scripts with SHE prompts, and a sleep package that includes earplugs, eye masks, and non-caffeinated tea [56]. Sleep quality improved significantly in their sample.

Although SHE seems to improve sleep quality, other treatments might be more superior in improving sleep. A 2018 systematic review and meta-analysis on the efficacy of SHE for treating insomnia [57] showed that compared to SHE, Cognitive Behavioral Therapy for Insomnia (CBT-I) treated insomnia more significantly. Similar findings were found among postmenopausal women [58] and patients with traumatic brain injury [59].

More studies are needed to explore effect of SHE on various populations and its impact on rehabilitation outcomes.

Exercise Therapy

The benefits of exercise on various body functions and systems are well known, and physical activity is considered one of the most areas of focus for health promotion and wellness among PTs [4]. The impact of exercise therapy on sleep quality is well documented among healthy adults [60–65].

Evidence suggests that a single bout of exercise can increase sleep efficiency and slow wave sleep (SWS or NREM N3 sleep stage), and at the same time decrease sleep latency and wake after sleep onset among healthy young adults [63, 66]. The mechanisms by which exercise improve sleep are still under investigation; a combination of factors such as improved mood, melatonin-mediated factors, heart rate variability changes, increases in growth hormone, changes in autonomic dysfunction, changes in body core temperature, boosting of immunologic system, change of important neurotransmitters related to sleep, increase sleep pressure, and increased brain-derived neurotrophic factor (BDNF) levels might explain these positive effects [67–69].

The intensity and timing of exercise need to be taken into consideration when prescribed to improve sleep quality. A 2019 systematic review on the effect of physical activity on sleep showed that a moderate intensity physical exercise seems the optimal intensity to improve sleep quality among healthy individuals of all age groups [65]. On the contrary, vigorous late night exercise showed negative impacts on sleep, probably due to increased body temperature induced by exercise that interferes with the normal sleep mechanisms [70]. A 2018 systematic review and meta-analysis on the effect of evening exercise (within 4 h before bedtime) on sleep among healthy individuals [62] showed that evening exercise improved sleep quality except for vigorous intensity exercise, which seem to impair sleep efficiency, total sleep time, and sleep latency. Therefore, one can conclude that it is the intensity of exercise in the evening that may improve or impair sleep.

Among older adults, a 2022 systematic review and network meta-analysis that aimed to compare the efficacy of exercise types on sleep quality showed a combined exercise program specifically muscle endurance training and walking was the optimal form of exercise to improve sleep quality. In addition to that, multi-component exercise therapy to improve sleep quality gained attention in recent years, as there is no optimal type of exercise to recommend for improving sleep. Low impact multi-component mind-body exercises such as Tai-chi and Yoga showed positive impact on sleep among middle aged and older adults compared to conventional exercise [64, 71–74].

The effect of exercise on sleep disorders such as insomnia and OSA is being studied in the literature [60, 61, 75–77]. Findings from a 2021 systematic review showed that regular exercises such as walking and cycling as well as mind-body exercise such as Yoga improved self-reported insomnia severity and daytime sleepiness among adults with insomnia [60]. Another 2020 systematic review and meta-analysis that aimed to explore the effect of exercise on adults with OSA showed that exercise training improved sleep quality and quality of life and simultaneously decreased daytime sleepiness among adults with OSA [77]. Several attempts were made to explore the impact of exercise on sleep among adults with various conditions who commonly suffer from sleep disturbances. A 2020 review [78] on the impact of exercise on sleep among individuals with neurodegenerative disease showed that exercise has promising results in improving self-reported sleep among those with Alzheimer's disease and Parkinson's disease, but additional research is needed to understand which type of exercise is most effective. Another 2022 review on the effect of exercise on sleep and fatigue among individuals with chronic stroke concluded that there is preliminary evidence that exercise improves sleep and reduces fatigue in this population, but there were concerns on the quality of these studies in terms of bias [79]. A 6-week aerobic moderate intensity exercise program improved sleep quality and increased serotonin levels among individuals with multiple sclerosis [80]. Another study in multiple sclerosis also showed that both a 12-week moderate intensity aerobic exercise program and a low intensity stretching and walking program improved self-reported sleep quality [81]. More research is needed in this area, but findings so far show promising results that exercise training can improve sleep quality among individuals with various neurological conditions.

Other populations that had their sleep quality improved after exercise training include children with autism [82], individuals with breast cancer [83], and individuals with low back pain [84, 85].

Based on the evidence reviewed in this section, it is of no surprise that sleep associations recommend exercise therapy as a low cost, low risk, non-pharmacological, and easily administered treatment for poor sleep [86]. Exercise training seems to improve sleep quality among various populations from all age groups; PTs therefore can utilize exercise therapy in their routine plan of care as a target to improve sleep quality.

Cognitive Behavioral Therapy

The most recommended first line of treatment for individuals with insomnia disorder is Cognitive Behavioral Therapy for Insomnia (CBT-I) [87]. CBT-I is a psychological and behavioral evidence-based intervention that targets thoughts and behaviors about sleep [1]. It consists of multiple components including sleep restriction, sleep hygiene education, stimulus control, relaxation techniques, and cognitive therapy [88]. Evidence suggests that CBT-I can have an immediate and long-lasting effects on sleep quality and quantity [89].

Traditionally CBT-I is delivered face to face as an individual session or within a group by a certified professional (psychologist) [1]. However, researchers have recently utilized digital CBT-I which can be delivered via telephone, mobile apps, and websites [90]. A systematic review and network meta-analysis study in 2022 explored the efficacy of digital CBT-I; it found that the number one mode of delivery was web-based CBT-I with a therapist which improved sleep efficiency and duration and decreased sleep latency and wake after sleep onset [90].

A 6-week CBT-I intervention was shown to be feasible with positive effects on self-reported sleep quality among individuals with multiple sclerosis [91]. Findings from another study on individuals with multiple sclerosis found that CBT-I increased sleep efficiency and decreased total sleep time measured using actigraphy [92]. A systematic review and meta-analysis on the efficacy of CBT-I on several non-motor symptoms including sleep in Parkinson's disease found that a CBT-I intervention of more than 8 weeks showed moderate positive effects on sleep among this population [93]. Other populations that had improved sleep quality following CBT-I include older adults with osteoarthritis [94], pregnant women [95], individuals with chronic pain [96], fibromyalgia [97], type 2 diabetes [98], stable heart failure [99], breast cancer [100], and hemodialysis [101].

Recognizing the benefits of the biopsychosocial model in PT practice is gaining recognition [102]. CBT-I components (sleep hygiene education, sleep restriction, stimulus control, relaxation, etc.) offer a venue in which PTs can incorporate the biopsychosocial model into their practice to promote sleep health [103].

Future Directions

The field of sleep PT is growing and is yet in its embryonic state worldwide. Many sleep-related disorders may have positive outcomes with non-pharmacological treatment provided by PTs, as standalone therapies or in adjunction with physician and other health professionals care. Willis-Ekbom disease (Restless Legs Syndrome), circadian rhythm sleep–wake disorders and sleep-breathing disorders, such as upper airway resistance syndrome, are still a challenge for PTs to treat, due to the lack of evidence-based treatments guidelines and recommendations. We need to invest on research for this field to grow.

Summary and Conclusion

This chapter highlighted the role of PTs in sleep health promotion and wellness. It summarized the evidence regarding the conditions with sleep disturbances that PTs commonly treat, and in different practice settings. Also, the impact of sleep disturbances on rehabilitation outcomes among various conditions was highlighted. There are different feasible treatment strategies that can be utilized by PTs to improve sleep quality among their patients. Education, physical and behavioral strategies are the main pillars of intervention that can be used by PTs to promote sleep health. PTs need to continuously update their knowledge on sleep treatment interventions as research in this area is growing in a fast pace.

References

1. Magnusson DM, et al. Population health, prevention, health promotion, and wellness competencies in physical therapist professional education: results of a modified Delphi study. Phys Ther. 2020;100(9):1645–58.
2. Siengsukon CF, Al-Dughmi M, Stevens S. Sleep health promotion: practical information for physical therapists. Phys Ther. 2017;97(8):826–36.
3. Albakri U, Drotos E, Meertens R. Sleep health promotion interventions and their effectiveness: an umbrella review. Int J Environ Res Public Health. 2021;18(11):5533.
4. Bezner JR. Promoting health and wellness: implications for physical therapist practice. Phys Ther. 2015;95(10):1433–44.
5. Association, APT. The Role of the Physical Therapist and the American Physical Therapy Association in Sleep Health HOD P06-20-39-09. 2020.
6. Lloyd-Jones DM, et al. Life's essential 8: updating and enhancing the American Heart Association's construct of cardiovascular health: a presidential advisory from the American Heart Association. Circulation. 2022;146(5):e18–43.
7. Altevogt BM, Colten HR. Sleep disorders and sleep deprivation: an unmet public health problem. Washington, DC: National Academies Press (US); 2006.
8. Control, C.f.D. and Prevention. Insufficient sleep is a public health epidemic. 2015. http://www.cdc.gov/features/dssleep/index.html#References.

9. Jahrami HA, et al. Sleep disturbances during the COVID-19 pandemic: a systematic review, meta-analysis, and meta-regression. Sleep Med Rev. 2022;62:101591.

10. Sheikh IN, Roth M, Stavinoha PL. Prevalence of sleep disturbances in pediatric cancer patients and their diagnosis and management. Children. 2021;8(12):1100.

11. Halstead EJ, et al. Sleep disturbances and patterns in children with neurodevelopmental conditions. Front Pediatr. 2021;9:637770.

12. Cai H, Wang X-P, Yang G-Y. Sleep disorders in stroke: an update on management. Aging Dis. 2021;12(2):570.

13. Khot SP, Morgenstern LB. Sleep and stroke. Stroke. 2019;50(6):1612–7.

14. Minakawa EN. Bidirectional relationship between sleep disturbances and Parkinson's disease. Front Neurol. 2022;13:927994.

15. Xu Z, et al. Progression of sleep disturbances in Parkinson's disease: a 5-year longitudinal study. J Neurol. 2021;268:312–20.

16. Borges CR, et al. Alzheimer's disease and sleep disturbances: a review. Arq Neuropsiquiatr. 2019;77:815–24.

17. Sunkaria A, Bhardwaj S. Sleep disturbance and Alzheimer's disease: the glial connection. Neurochem Res. 2022;47(7):1799–815.

18. Foschi M, et al. Sleep-related disorders and their relationship with MRI findings in multiple sclerosis. Sleep Med. 2019;56:90–7.

19. Kołtuniuk A, et al. Sleep disturbances, degree of disability and the quality of life in multiple sclerosis patients. Int J Environ Res Public Health. 2022;19(6):3271.

20. Uchmanowicz I, et al. The influence of sleep disorders on the quality of life in patients with chronic low back pain. Scand J Caring Sci. 2019;33(1):119–27.

21. Beetz G, et al. Relevance of sleep disturbances to orthopaedic surgery: a current concepts narrative and practical review. JBJS. 2021;103(21):2045–56.

22. Miner B, Kryger MH. Sleep in the aging population. Sleep Med Clin. 2020;15(2):311–8.

23. Morse AM, Bender E. Sleep in hospitalized patients. Clocks Sleep. 2019;1(1):151–65.

24. Thomas KP, et al. Sleep rounds: a multidisciplinary approach to optimize sleep quality and satisfaction in hospitalized patients. J Hosp Med. 2012;7(6):508–12.

25. Hardin KA. Sleep in the ICU: potential mechanisms and clinical implications. Chest. 2009;136(1):284–94.

26. Meltzer LJ, Davis KF, Mindell JA. Patient and parent sleep in a children's hospital. Pediatr Nurs. 2012;38(2):64.

27. Young JS, et al. Sleep in hospitalized medical patients, part 1: factors affecting sleep. J Hosp Med. 2008;3(6):473–82.

28. Truong KK, et al. Timing matters: circadian rhythm in sepsis, obstructive lung disease, obstructive sleep apnea, and cancer. Annal Am Thorac Soc. 2016;13(7):1144–54.

29. Rampes S, et al. Postoperative sleep disorders and their potential impacts on surgical outcomes. J Biomed Res. 2020;34(4):271.

30. Dobing S, et al. Sleep quality and factors influencing self-reported sleep duration and quality in the general internal medicine inpatient population. PLoS One. 2016;11(6):e0156735.

31. Ünsal A, Demir G. Evaluation of sleep quality and fatigue in hospitalized patients. Int J Caring Sci. 2012;5(3):311–9.

32. Kim DE, Yoon JY. Factors that influence sleep among residents in long-term care facilities. Int J Environ Res Public Health. 2020;17(6):1889.

33. Valenza MC, et al. Nursing homes: impact of sleep disturbances on functionality. Arch Gerontol Geriatr. 2013;56(3):432–6.

34. Garms-Homolovà V, Flick U, Röhnsch G. Sleep disorders and activities in long term care facilities—a vicious cycle? J Health Psychol. 2010;15(5):744–54.

35. Kalmbach DA, et al. Poor sleep is linked to impeded recovery from traumatic brain injury. Sleep. 2018;41(10):zsy147.

36. Fleming MK, et al. Sleep disruption after brain injury is associated with worse motor outcomes and slower functional recovery. Neurorehabil Neural Repair. 2020;34(7):661–71.

37. Drerup M, et al. Therapeutic approaches to insomnia and fatigue in patients with multiple sclerosis. Nat Sci Sleep. 2021;13:201–7.
38. Iddagoda MT, et al. Post-stroke sleep disturbances and rehabilitation outcomes: a prospective cohort study. Intern Med J. 2020;50(2):208–13.
39. Devos H, et al. Real-time assessment of daytime sleepiness in drivers with multiple sclerosis. Mult Scler Relat Disord. 2021;47:102607.
40. Aricò D, et al. Effects of NREM sleep instability on cognitive processing. Sleep Med. 2010;11(8):791–8.
41. Kempler L, Richmond JL. Effect of sleep on gross motor memory. Memory. 2012;20(8):907–14.
42. DePietro RH, et al. Association between inpatient sleep loss and hyperglycemia of hospitalization. Diabetes Care. 2017;40(2):188–93.
43. Watson PL, Ceriana P, Fanfulla F. Delirium: is sleep important? Best Pract Res Clin Anaesthesiol. 2012;26(3):355–66.
44. Leukoff S, Evans D, Liptzin B. Delirium: the occurrence and persistence of symptoms among elderly hospitalised patients. Arch Intern Med. 1992;152(2):334–40.
45. Bolona E, Hahn PY, Afessa B. Intensive care unit and hospital mortality in patients with obstructive sleep apnea. J Crit Care. 2015;30(1):178–80.
46. Kaw R, et al. Postoperative complications in patients with obstructive sleep apnea. Chest. 2012;141(2):436–41.
47. Louis JM, et al. Obstructive sleep apnea and severe maternal-infant morbidity/mortality in the United States, 1998-2009. Sleep. 2014;37(5):843–9.
48. Frange C, et al. Practice recommendations for the role of physiotherapy in the management of sleep disorders: the 2022 Brazilian Sleep Association Guidelines. Sleep Sci. 2022;15(4):515.
49. Hauri PJ. Sleep hygiene, relaxation therapy, and cognitive interventions. In: Case studies in insomnia. Boston, MA: Springer; 1991. p. 65–84.
50. Sivertsen B, et al. Sleep problems in general practice: a national survey of assessment and treatment routines of general practitioners in Norway. J Sleep Res. 2010;19(1 Pt I):36–41.
51. Irish LA, et al. The role of sleep hygiene in promoting public health: a review of empirical evidence. Sleep Med Rev. 2015;22:23–36.
52. Cho S, Kim G-S, Lee J-H. Psychometric evaluation of the sleep hygiene index: a sample of patients with chronic pain. Health Qual Life Outcomes. 2013;11:1–7.
53. Lin C-Y, et al. A cluster randomized controlled trial of a theory-based sleep hygiene intervention for adolescents. Sleep. 2018;41(11):zsy170.
54. Dietrich SK, et al. Effectiveness of sleep education programs to improve sleep hygiene and/or sleep quality in college students: a systematic review. JBI Evid Synth. 2016;14(9):108–34.
55. Zengin L, Aylaz R. The effects of sleep hygiene education and reflexology on sleep quality and fatigue in patients receiving chemotherapy. Eur J Cancer Care. 2019;28(3):e13020.
56. Herscher M, et al. A sleep hygiene intervention to improve sleep quality for hospitalized patients. Jt Comm J Qual Patient Saf. 2021;47(6):343–6.
57. Chung K-F, et al. Sleep hygiene education as a treatment of insomnia: a systematic review and meta-analysis. Fam Pract. 2018;35(4):365–75.
58. Drake CL, et al. Treating chronic insomnia in postmenopausal women: a randomized clinical trial comparing cognitive-behavioral therapy for insomnia, sleep restriction therapy, and sleep hygiene education. Sleep. 2019;42(2):zsy217.
59. Bogdanov S, Naismith S, Lah S. Sleep outcomes following sleep-hygiene-related interventions for individuals with traumatic brain injury: a systematic review. Brain Inj. 2017;31(4):422–33.
60. Xie Y, et al. Effects of exercise on sleep quality and insomnia in adults: a systematic review and meta-analysis of randomized controlled trials. Front Psychiatry. 2021;12:664499.
61. Lowe H, et al. Does exercise improve sleep for adults with insomnia? A systematic review with quality appraisal. Clin Psychol Rev. 2019;68:1–12.
62. Stutz J, Eiholzer R, Spengler CM. Effects of evening exercise on sleep in healthy participants: a systematic review and meta-analysis. Sports Med. 2019;49(2):269–87.

63. Park I, et al. Exercise improves the quality of slow-wave sleep by increasing slow-wave stability. Sci Rep. 2021;11(1):4410.
64. Hasan F, et al. Comparative efficacy of exercise regimens on sleep quality in older adults: a systematic review and network meta-analysis. Sleep Med Rev. 2022;65:101673.
65. Wang F, Boros S. The effect of physical activity on sleep quality: a systematic review. Eur J Physiother. 2021;23(1):11–8.
66. Youngstedt SD, O'connor PJ, Dishman RK. The effects of acute exercise on sleep: a quantitative synthesis. Sleep. 1997;20(3):203–14.
67. Szuhany KL, Bugatti M, Otto MW. A meta-analytic review of the effects of exercise on brain-derived neurotrophic factor. J Psychiatr Res. 2015;60:56–64.
68. Hartescu I, Morgan K, Stevinson CD. Increased physical activity improves sleep and mood outcomes in inactive people with insomnia: a randomized controlled trial. J Sleep Res. 2015;24(5):526–34.
69. Sellami M, et al. The effect of exercise on glucoregulatory hormones: a countermeasure to human aging: insights from a comprehensive review of the literature. Int J Environ Res Public Health. 2019;16(10):1709.
70. Kubitz KA, et al. The effects of acute and chronic exercise on sleep: a meta-analytic review. Sports Med. 1996;21:277–91.
71. Riemann D, et al. European guideline for the diagnosis and treatment of insomnia. J Sleep Res. 2017;26(6):675–700.
72. Buric I, et al. What is the molecular signature of mind–body interventions? A systematic review of gene expression changes induced by meditation and related practices. Front Immunol. 2017;8:670.
73. Wang W-L, et al. The effect of yoga on sleep quality and insomnia in women with sleep problems: a systematic review and meta-analysis. BMC Psychiatry. 2020;20:1–19.
74. Ai J-Y, et al. Effects of multi-component exercise on sleep quality in middle-aged adults. Int J Environ Res Public Health. 2022;19(23):15472.
75. Aiello KD, et al. Effect of exercise training on sleep apnea: a systematic review and meta-analysis. Respir Med. 2016;116:85–92.
76. Stavrou VT, et al. Obstructive sleep apnea syndrome: the effect of acute and chronic responses of exercise. Front Med. 2021;8:806924.
77. Lins-Filho OL, et al. Effect of exercise training on subjective parameters in patients with obstructive sleep apnea: a systematic review and meta-analysis. Sleep Med. 2020;69:1–7.
78. Memon AA, Coleman JJ, Amara AW. Effects of exercise on sleep in neurodegenerative disease. Neurobiol Dis. 2020;140:104859.
79. Tai D, et al. Can exercise training promote better sleep and reduced fatigue in people with chronic stroke? A systematic review. J Sleep Res. 2022;31(6):e13675.
80. Al-Sharman A, et al. The effects of aerobic exercise on sleep quality measures and sleep-related biomarkers in individuals with Multiple Sclerosis: a pilot randomised controlled trial. NeuroRehabilitation. 2019;45(1):107–15.
81. Siengsukon CF, et al. Randomized controlled trial of exercise interventions to improve sleep quality and daytime sleepiness in individuals with multiple sclerosis: a pilot study. Mult Scler J Exp Transl Clin. 2016;2:2055217316680639.
82. Tse AC, et al. Effects of exercise on sleep, melatonin level, and behavioral functioning in children with autism. Autism. 2022;26(7):1712–22.
83. Kreutz C, Schmidt ME, Steindorf K. Effects of physical and mind–body exercise on sleep problems during and after breast cancer treatment: a systematic review and meta-analysis. Breast Cancer Res Treat. 2019;176:1–15.
84. Eadie J, et al. Physiotherapy for sleep disturbance in people with chronic low back pain: results of a feasibility randomized controlled trial. Arch Phys Med Rehabil. 2013;94(11):2083–92.
85. Akodu AK, Akindutire OM. The effect of stabilization exercise on pain-related disability, sleep disturbance, and psychological status of patients with non-specific chronic low back pain. Kor J Pain. 2018;31(3):199–205.

86. Spiegel K, et al. Effects of poor and short sleep on glucose metabolism and obesity risk. Nat Rev Endocrinol. 2009;5(5):253–61.
87. Qaseem A, et al. Management of chronic insomnia disorder in adults: a clinical practice guideline from the American College of Physicians. Ann Intern Med. 2016;165(2):125–33.
88. Edinger JD, et al. Behavioral and psychological treatments for chronic insomnia disorder in adults: an American Academy of Sleep Medicine clinical practice guideline. J Clin Sleep Med. 2021;17(2):255–62.
89. Van Straten A, et al. Cognitive and behavioral therapies in the treatment of insomnia: a meta-analysis. Sleep Med Rev. 2018;38:3–16.
90. Hasan F, et al. Comparative efficacy of digital cognitive behavioral therapy for insomnia: a systematic review and network meta-analysis. Sleep Med Rev. 2022;61:101567.
91. Siengsukon CF, et al. Feasibility and treatment effect of cognitive behavioral therapy for insomnia in individuals with multiple sclerosis: a pilot randomized controlled trial. Mult Scler Relat Disord. 2020;40:101958.
92. Williams-Cooke C, et al. The impact of cognitive behavioral therapy for insomnia on sleep log and actigraphy outcomes in people with multiple sclerosis: a secondary analysis. Nat Sci Sleep. 2021;13:1865–74.
93. Luo F, et al. Efficacy of cognitive behavioral therapy on mood disorders, sleep, fatigue, and quality of life in Parkinson's disease: a systematic review and meta-analysis. Front Psychiatry. 2021;12:793804.
94. Vitiello MV, et al. Cognitive behavioral therapy for insomnia improves sleep and decreases pain in older adults with co-morbid insomnia and osteoarthritis. J Clin Sleep Med. 2009;5(4):355–62.
95. Kalmbach DA, et al. A randomized controlled trial of digital cognitive behavioral therapy for insomnia in pregnant women. Sleep Med. 2020;72:82–92.
96. Selvanathan J, et al. Cognitive behavioral therapy for insomnia in patients with chronic pain–a systematic review and meta-analysis of randomized controlled trials. Sleep Med Rev. 2021;60:101460.
97. Martínez MP, et al. Cognitive-behavioral therapy for insomnia and sleep hygiene in fibromyalgia: a randomized controlled trial. J Behav Med. 2014;37:683–97.
98. Alshehri MM, et al. The effects of cognitive behavioral therapy for insomnia in people with type 2 diabetes mellitus, pilot RCT part II: diabetes health outcomes. BMC Endocr Disord. 2020;20(1):1–9.
99. Redeker NS, et al. Effects of cognitive behavioral therapy for insomnia on sleep-related cognitions among patients with stable heart failure. Behav Sleep Med. 2019;17(3):342–54.
100. Ma Y, et al. Efficacy of cognitive behavioral therapy for insomnia in breast cancer: a meta-analysis. Sleep Med Rev. 2021;55:101376.
101. Chen H-Y, et al. Cognitive-behavioral therapy for sleep disturbance decreases inflammatory cytokines and oxidative stress in hemodialysis patients. Kidney Int. 2011;80(4):415–22.
102. Dantas DS, et al. Biopsychosocial model in health care: reflections in the production of functioning and disability data. Fisioterapia em Movimento. 2020;33:1.
103. Nielsen M, et al. Physical therapist–delivered cognitive-behavioral therapy: a qualitative study of physical therapists' perceptions and experiences. Phys Ther. 2014;94(2):197–209.

Part II
Clinical Cases: Insufficient Sleep

Chapter 3
Treating Pain to Secondarily Treat Sleep-Related Issues

Zubia Veqar (iD) **and Mosab Aldabbas** (iD)

Introduction

Chronic neck pain (CNP) is one of the most common types of chronic musculoskeletal pain [1]. It was defined as pain in the cervical arca with or without referred pain to upper limbs that lasts for at least 3 months [2]. The precise etiology of CNP is not yet well documented; however, it is linked with and complicated by different physiological and psychological factors. Sleep disturbance is one of the factors that are believed to be associated with CNP [3, 4]. Sleep is an essential element for health, and obtaining sufficient sleep is important for various physiological functions [5]. During sleep, the brain cycles through four stages that include Non-Rapid Eye Movement (NREM) which encompasses N1, N2, and N3 sleep stages, and Rapid-Eye-Movement (REM) sleep stage. These sleep stages cycle around 4–6 times, lasting around 90 min each [6].

Sleep disturbance is a broad term that encompasses problems of initiating and maintaining sleep. Sleep disturbance has become an increasingly prominent symptom in CNP patients and is significantly associated with the intensity of pain [4]. In our previous work, PSG findings have found that CNP patients had shorter total sleep time (TST), decreased time spent in deep sleep (REM sleep stage), and increased amount of time spent in light sleep (N1 sleep stage) compared to healthy participants, and these disruptions were associated with pain intensity [7].

Conservative treatment is the mainstay for the treatment of CNP. Training of neck muscles was shown to be an essential approach to improve the clinical outcomes in short- and long-term benefits for CNP patients [8]. Manual therapy is another approach that has proven its effectiveness in alleviating neck pain [9].

Z. Veqar (✉)
Centre for Physiotherapy and Rehabilitation Sciences, Jamia Millia Islamia, New Delhi, India

M. Aldabbas
Centre for Physiotherapy and Rehabilitation Sciences, Jamia Millia Islamia, New Delhi, India

Al Azhar University, Gaza, Palestinian Authority

C. Frange (ed.), *Clinical Cases in Sleep Physical Therapy*,
https://doi.org/10.1007/978-3-031-38340-3_3

Specifically, there has been growing interest in evaluating the effect of myofascial release therapy in the treatment of neck pain [10]. Myofascial release therapy was shown to be more efficient than manual therapy in improving the range of motion and quality of life in CNP patients [10]. Furthermore, incorporating interferential current therapy into rehabilitation programs was found to increase the efficacy of exercises in alleviating the intensity of pain and disability compared to exercise alone in CNP patients [11]. Although myofascial release therapy and neck exercises were effective in the treatment and management of CNP as well as in improving quality of life, sleep quality as a primary outcome has rarely been examined in clinical trials in CNP patients. These treatment strategies have been shown to be effective in improving sleep quality in CNP patients; however, this improvement was established only via subjective measures [12–15]. It could be reasonable that, when sleep disturbances are present, they can be essential contributing variables to the clinical presentation of CNP patients. Therefore, the aims of this case report are to describe the results from an evaluation of a patient with CNP that includes a comprehensive evaluation of objective sleep measurement by PSG and sleep quality assessment by the Pittsburgh Sleep Quality Index (PSQI), and to describe a physiotherapy intervention that includes active exercises and myofascial release to minimize the impact of sleep disturbances. The focus of the physiotherapy intervention was on (1) sleep architecture, (2) self-reported sleep quality, and (3) pain intensity.

Patient Information

M.C.G., a 38-year-old man, came to the physiotherapy clinic with CNP.

Chief Complaint

The patient reported a 2.5-year history of slowly progressive neck pain with short periods of relief which sometimes went till the trapezius of both the sides. This pain hampered his ability to sleep. His average pain score on a visual analogue scale was found to be 7/10 and his worst imaginable pain was experienced to be 9.5/10. The patient reported difficulties in maintaining sleep and frequent awakening during the night (2–4) times. He also complaint of waking up unrefreshed with grogginess along with neck pain.

Aggravating and Relieving Factors

The patient reported that his neck pain increased with most neck activities (specifically neck extension and rotation). He reported difficulty in sitting and working on a chair for greater than 40–45 min. Maintaining straight back and doing physical activities for more than 30 min were reported to be aggravating factors. Lying supine and prone, gentle massage, and taking a hot bath were reported to be relieving factors.

Previous Intervention

One year prior to his physiotherapy visit, the patient received three different treatments options that included (pain medications, anti-inflammatory medicine, and steroid injections). The patient reported significant relief after treatment, but the improvement did not last for more than 2–3 months after each treatment.

Diagnostic Assessment

Physical Examination

Visual examination found (1) a forward head posture, (2) a protracted scapula, (3) a kyphotic thoracic spine, (4) increased extension in the upper cervical spine, and (5) protracted shoulders.

Cervical active range of motion: The patient had 41-degree flexion, 52 extensions, 28/30 side bending to the left and right, respectively, and 75°/80° of rotation to the right and left, respectively. Passive range of motion was not assessed as it led to an increase in pain.

Shoulder active range of motion: Shoulder motions were assessed and were painless and had full range. The patient reported an increase in pain intensity in the upper trapezius muscle with shoulder flexion.

Manual muscle testing was not performed because resisted movement aggravated the pain.

Sleep and Pain Assessment

Polysomnography

At baseline, a 2-night protocol was performed to avoid "first-night" effects. On the second night, the PSG recordings included electroencephalogram (EEG), electro-oculogram (EOG), and submental electromyography (EMG) electrodes. Data from the second night were used for assessing sleep architecture at baseline. After completing 7 weeks of intervention, the patient was assessed for his sleep through the same procedure of PSG recording used at baseline. Detailed PSG protocol, electrode placement, and scoring can be found in our previous work [7]. Table 3.1 explains the parameters derived from PSG.

Subjective Sleep Quality

Self-reported sleep quality was evaluated by the Pittsburgh Sleep Quality Index (PSQI) [16] which is a 19-item questionnaire assessing sleep across seven dimensions over the last month with 21 being highest and 0 being the lowest score.

Table 3.1 Sleep architecture parameters

Variable	Definition
Total sleep time (TST, minutes)	The total amount of time from the sleep onset until the awakening or amount of time in NREM and REM
Sleep efficiency (S. %)	The ratio of TST/total time in bed/100
Sleep onset latency (SOL, minutes)	The total time between lights out and the onset of sleep or the first epoch of the N1 stage, following those six epochs of N1 or a deep stage of NREM
Non-rapid eye movement (approximately 75% of TST)	Percentage of time spent in Stage 1 (N1), Stage 2 (N2), and Stage 3 (N3, slow wave slep, SWS)
Rapid eye movement (approximately 25% of TST)	Percentage of time spent in Stage R (REM sleep)
Wakefulness (W, %)	Percentage of time spent in wakefulness

Subjects scoring from 0 to 4 are considered to be good sleepers, whereas five or more are considered as poor sleepers.

Pain Intensity and Disability

Pain intensity and disability were assessed by the Numerical Pain Rating Scale (NPRS) and the Neck Disability Index (NDI). They were measured at the time of recruitment and after 7 weeks of intervention [17].

Physiotherapeutic Intervention

The goal of the physiotherapy intervention was to address the identified physical and sleep impairments in an attempt to improve the sleep quality and to reduce the severity of pain.

The patient received a total of 30 sessions distributed over 7 weeks of progressive resistance-endurance exercises for the neck and shoulder muscles. The patient started the session with 10–15 min of warm up on the treadmill followed by 5 min of general body stretching. The treatment began with a hot pack for 15 min followed by gentle neck isometric exercises. The patient engaged in a variety of neck-shoulder exercises, including chin tucks, cranio-cervical flexion, cervical flexion, and upper back extensions in supine and prone positions, respectively. Exercises for the shoulders were done standing up (shoulder shrugging and abduction). To prevent excessive loading of the cervical spine during the first few sessions, no external resistance was added to the exercises. TheraBand was utilized to do exercises for the neck and shoulders, while dumbbells were used for the shoulders. On the basis of patient feedback and tolerance, the exercise's intensity and repetitions were gradually increased. Training for neck endurance and resistance was done while seated, supine, and prone (Fig. 3.1). The session's length was gradually extended from 30 to 35 min to 50–60 min.

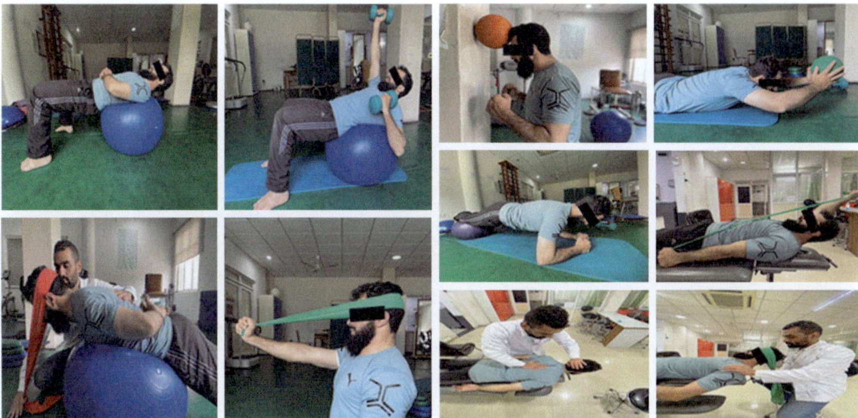

Fig. 3.1 Groups of selected neck strength-endurance exercises. (Original Figure. Reprinted with permission from M.C.G.)

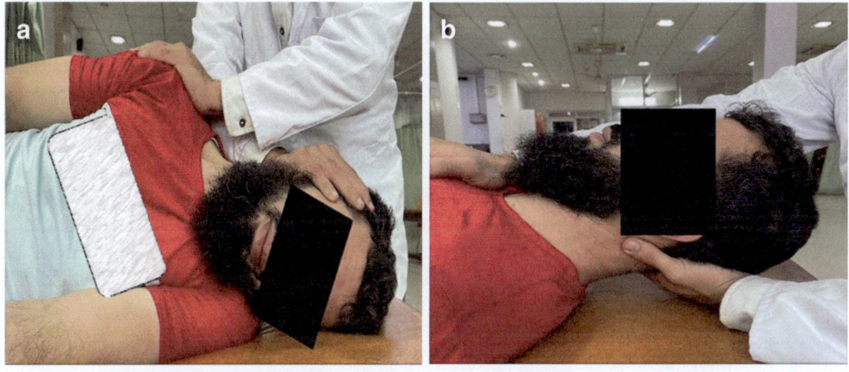

Fig. 3.2 (**a**) Cross-hand release of lateral neck muscles: the patient is placed in a side-lying position and the therapist stands at the corner of the table. The therapist places one hand on the anterolateral aspect of the shoulder and the other hand on the lateral side of the neck. Lean toward the patient to reach the tissue depth barrier, wait and apply sustained pressure; (**b**) Cross-hand release of the anterior cervical spine muscles: The patient is placed in a supine position and the therapist is sitting on a chair on the head side, with one hand on the posterior aspect of the head to support it and the other hand on the patient sternal area. The patient is instructed to relax and leave the head weight on the therapist hand, while the other hand sinks into the sternal area or to the barrier of tissue resistance, wait and follow the subtle yielding of the tissue. As the patient's neck softens, gently draw the patient's head toward you and at the same time apply a gentle pressure toward the feet with another hand [18]. Technique applied for at least 5 min. (Original Figure. Reprinted with permission from M.C.G.)

Additionally, the patient received myofascial release therapy focused on the neck muscles (Figs. 3.2 and 3.3), especially (the upper trapezius muscle and the suboccipital muscles) [18, 19]. Each session of the release lasted for about 50–60 min. A combined therapeutic device, which included interferential therapy, was applied for

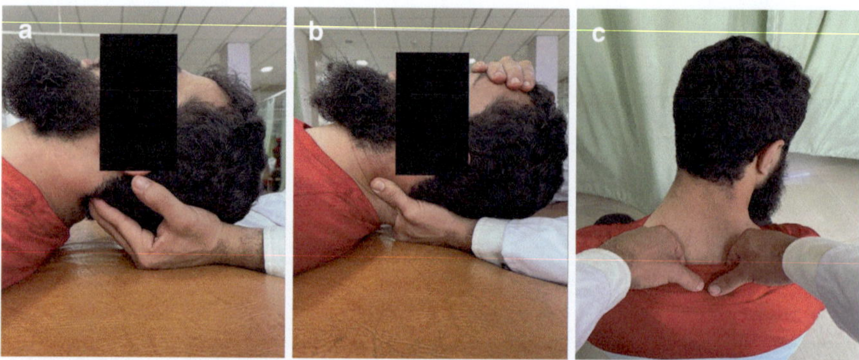

Fig. 3.3 (**a**) Cervical wedge technique: the patient is placed in a supine lying position with the therapist standing at the head of the treatment table. The therapist uses the fingertips of both hands to identify the space and texture of tissues between and beside the spinous processes of two vertebrae and at the suboccipital area. The therapist fingertips reach into areas of restriction while maintaining the hands in a relaxed position. Wait for joints to open in response to the pressure of the fingertips, rather than trying to push your fingertips inside; (**b**) Mother cat technique: this technique aims to relax and surrender the posterior neck fascia. The therapist wraps his hand around the back of the cervical spine, while the patient is supine lying. The full hand of the therapist gathers and grasps the outer layers of the neck tissues. The therapist applies gentle posterior traction to the outer layers of the muscles within these, particularly trapezius muscle, and deep and superficial fasciae. Permit the tissues to slowly slide out from under the therapist hands. Repeat the technique several times; (**c**) Upper Trapezius Release: The patient is in the sitting on a low stool with hips being higher than the knees. The therapist stands behind the patient. The therapist works bilaterally with soft fists, sinking, and taking up a line of tension into the middle part of the trapezius muscle. Then, the therapist carries the tension toward the trapezius muscle attachments at the acromial processes. Repeat the technique 2–3 times Repeat this technique while the patient slowly drops his head forward and rotates his head and neck from side to side ([19]; Original Figure. Reprinted with permission from M.C.G.)

Fig. 3.4 Interferential current application. (Original Figure. Reprinted with permission from M.C.G.)

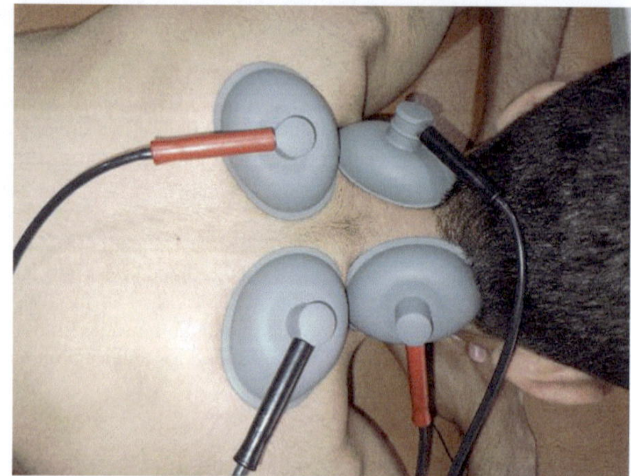

15 min; the electrodes were positioned in opposition to the cervical spine (C5-C6-C7). The intensity of the interferential therapy was adjusted for each patient's sensitivity (Fig. 3.4).

Findings

In the clinical results that have been evaluated, the patient has significantly improved. After receiving treatments for 7 weeks, he reported a tremendous improvement in the severity of his neck pain. On a NPRS scale, the level of pain dropped from 7 before therapy to 2 after. He showed improvement in his sleep quality, as seen by his PSQI dropping from 8 to 3 which indicated that the pain alleviation was followed by an improvement in sleep architecture. The disability was likewise reduced from 31% to 14%. After therapy, nighttime awakenings were reported to be (1–2) times which is less than before (2–4) times.

The results of the PSG performed before and after 7 weeks of physiotherapy intervention also showed improvements in sleep architecture parameters. The total sleep time increased from 402 to 415 min, sleep efficiency increased from 92.3% to 96%, and sleep onset latency decreased from 26 to 18 min. The percentage of N1 sleep decreased from 18% to 9%, while the percentage of N2 sleep increased from 40% to 45%. The percentage of N3 sleep decreased from 21% to 18%, while the percentage of REM sleep increased from 13% to 20%. Wakefulness did not show any significant changes and remained at 8%.

Discussion

The current case report provides new evidence that physiotherapy treatments enhanced sleep quality and sleep architecture in patients with CNP with sleep disturbance. In this case report, the patient recorded both subjective and objective sleep problems prior to treatment. After 7 weeks of therapy, the patient sleep quality was improved according to his own self-reported sleep patterns.

Sleep architecture has also improved as he spent less time in light sleep (N1) and more time in deep sleep (REM). Additionally, TST and sleep efficiency have increased, while SOL has decreased.

Following neck stabilization and progressive resistance-endurance exercises, CNP patients reported a significant increase in their self-reported sleep quality. This could be linked to a decrease in pain intensity, which in turn may enhance sleep quality [12]. There isn't yet information on how people with CNP are affected by changes in sleep architecture. Roehrs et al. [20] observed that hyperalgesia was connected with REM deprivation and cumulative sleep loss. This may be linked to the high score on pain reported by the patient, who also had insufficient amount of sleep in REM. Our PSG findings have revealed that the patient spent more time in the superficial sleep. This also was evident in musculoskeletal pain patients [21]. We could assume that an improvement in sleep architecture is accompanied by a decrease in the intensity of CNP based on the findings of this case study. This was also noted in a prior study that found better and more consistent sleep was related to pain relief [22].

Sleep continuity measures, which describe the distribution and amount of sleep compared to wakefulness, including sleep initiation and maintenance [23], showed significant changes. These changes encompass the proportions of wakefulness, TST, SE, and SOL, and they were altered before the treatment. However, following 7 weeks of physiotherapy intervention, there was a decrease in SOL from 26 minutes before the treatment to 18 minutes after the treatment. TST showed an increase from 402 minutes before the treatments to 415 minutes after the treatments. The proportions of TST and SOL after the physiotherapy treatment, as determined by reference data for Polysomnography (PSG), are considered to be normal [24].

Patients with CNP frequently have impaired physical and mental performance. Exercises for the neck and MFR possess mental and physical effects that could improve sleep by improving blood flow, strengthening the body's core, and promoting muscle relaxation while easing musculoskeletal pain [25, 26]. These results suggest that clinical conditions like CNP and other musculoskeletal problems can have a deleterious impact on sleep architecture, which may either cause or intensify pain. The results of this case report further suggest that a decrease in the intensity of CNP may have a favorable effect on the PSG-measured sleep architecture.

In conclusion, this chapter provides a detailed case study of a patient with chronic neck pain with sleep disturbances and demonstrates an evidence-based approach to managing this condition using physiotherapy. The discussion of the assessment and treatment strategies used in this case provides valuable insights for clinicians and researchers working in this field.

References

1. Ylinen J. Physical exercises and functional rehabilitation for the management of chronic neck pain. Eur Medicophys. 2007;43(1):119.
2. Hoy D, March L, Woolf A, Blyth F, Brooks P, Smith E, Vos T, Barendregt J, Blore J, Murray C, Burstein R. The global burden of neck pain: estimates from the global burden of disease 2010 study. Ann Rheum Dis. 2014;73(7):1309–15.
3. Van Looveren E, Bilterys T, Munneke W, Cagnie B, Ickmans K, Mairesse O, Malfliet A, De Baets L, Nijs J, Goubert D, Danneels L. The association between sleep and chronic spinal pain: a systematic review from the last decade. J Clin Med. 2021;10(17):3836.
4. Artner J, Cakir B, Spiekermann JA, Kurz S, Leucht F, Reichel H, Lattig F. Prevalence of sleep deprivation in patients with chronic neck and back pain: a retrospective evaluation of 1016 patients. J Pain Res. 2012;28:1–6.
5. Mashaqi S, Gozal D. Normal sleep in humans. In: Pediatric sleep medicine: mechanisms and comprehensive guide to clinical evaluation and management. Cham: Springer; 2021. p. 3–15.
6. Rundo JV, Downey R III. Polysomnography. Handb Clin Neurol. 2019;160:381–92.
7. Aldabbas MM, Tanwar T, Ghrouz A, Iram I, Warren Spence D, Pandi-Perumal SR, Veqar Z. A polysomnographic study of sleep disruptions in individuals with chronic neck pain. J Sleep Res. 2022;31(5):e13549.
8. Cheng CH, Su HT, Yen LW, Liu WY, Cheng HY. Long-term effects of therapeutic exercise on nonspecific chronic neck pain: a literature review. J Phys Ther Sci. 2015;27(4):1271–6.
9. Miller J, Gross A, D'Sylva J, Burnie SJ, Goldsmith CH, Graham N, Haines T, Brønfort G, Hoving JL. Manual therapy and exercise for neck pain: a systematic review. Man Ther. 2010;15(4):334–54.

10. Rodríguez-Fuentes I, De Toro FJ, Rodríguez-Fuentes G, de Oliveira IM, Meijide-Faílde R, Fuentes-Boquete IM. Myofascial release therapy in the treatment of occupational mechanical neck pain: a randomized parallel group study. Am J Phys Med Rehabil. 2016;95(7):507–15.
11. Albornoz-Cabello M, Pérez-Mármol JM, Barrios Quinta CJ, Matarán-Peñarrocha GA, Castro-Sánchez AM, de la Cruz Olivares B. Effect of adding interferential current stimulation to exercise on outcomes in primary care patients with chronic neck pain: a randomized controlled trial. Clin Rehabil. 2019;33(9):1458–67.
12. Akodu AK, Nwanne CA, Fapojuwo OA. Efficacy of neck stabilization and Pilates exercises on pain, sleep disturbance and kinesiophobia in patients with non-specific chronic neck pain: a randomized controlled trial. J Bodyw Mov Ther. 2021;26:411–9.
13. Akodu AK, Akindutire OM. The effect of stabilization exercise on pain-related disability, sleep disturbance, and psychological status of patients with non-specific chronic low back pain. Kor J Pain. 2018;31(3):199–205.
14. Cabrera-Martos I, Rodríguez-Torres J, López-López L, Prados-Román E, Granados-Santiago M, Valenza MC. Effects of an active intervention based on myofascial release and neurodynamics in patients with chronic neck pain: a randomized controlled trial. Physiother Theory Pract. 2022;38(9):1145–52.
15. Zibiri RA, Akodu AK, Okafor UA. Effects of muscle energy technique and neck stabilization exercises on pain, psychological status, and sleep disturbance in patients with non-specific chronic neck pain. Mid E J Rehabil Health. 2019;6(2):e87192.
16. Buysse DJ, Reynolds CF III, Monk TH, Berman SR, Kupfer DJ. The Pittsburgh Sleep Quality Index: a new instrument for psychiatric practice and research. Psychiatry Res. 1989;28(2):193–213.
17. Cleland JA, Childs JD, Whitman JM. Psychometric properties of the Neck Disability Index and Numeric Pain Rating Scale in patients with mechanical neck pain. Arch Phys Med Rehabil. 2008;89(1):69–74.
18. Clarke S. Myofascial release. A step-by-step guide to more than sixty techniques. J Austr Trad Med Soc. 2014;20(3):220–1.
19. Luchau T. Advanced myofascial techniques: volume 2: neck, head, spine and ribs. London: Jessica Kingsley Publishers; 2016.
20. Roehrs T, Hyde M, Blaisdell B, Greenwald M, Roth T. Sleep loss and REM sleep loss are hyperalgesic. Sleep. 2006;29(2):145–51.
21. Diaz-Piedra C, Catena A, Sanchez AI, Miró E, Martínez MP, Buela-Casal G. Sleep disturbances in fibromyalgia syndrome: the role of clinical and polysomnographic variables explaining poor sleep quality in patients. Sleep Med. 2015;16(8):917–25.
22. Roehrs T, Roth T. Sleep and pain: interaction of two vital functions. Semin Neurol. 2005;25(1):106–16.
23. Hall M, Greeson J, Pantesco E. Sleep as a biobehavioral risk factor for cardiovascular disease. New York, NY: Springer; 2018.
24. Hertenstein E, Gabryelska A, Spiegelhalder K, Nissen C, Johann AF, Umarova R, Riemann D, Baglioni C, Feige B. Reference data for polysomnography-measured and subjective sleep in healthy adults. J Clin Sleep Med. 2018;14(4):523–32.
25. Kaka B, Ogwumike OO. Effect of neck stabilization and dynamic exercises on pain, disability and fear avoidance beliefs in patients with non-specific neck pain. Physiotherapy. 2015;101:e704.
26. Castro-Sánchez AM, Matarán-Peñarrocha GA, Granero-Molina J, Aguilera-Manrique G, Quesada-Rubio JM, Moreno-Lorenzo C. Benefits of massage-myofascial release therapy on pain, anxiety, quality of sleep, depression, and quality of life in patients with fibromyalgia. Evid Based Complement Alternat Med. 2010;2011:561753.

Chapter 4
Good Sleep Prevents Falls?

Yoshinobu Yoshimoto and Hiroya Honda

Introduction

Sleep disorders are associated with falls among community-dwelling older adults with disabilities [1, 2]. Cognitive Behavioral Therapy for Insomnia (CBT-I) has been reported to be the standard treatment of choice for insomnia [3]. It has also been shown to be effective in improving sleep disorders in older adults [4]. We suggested that since CBT-I could improve sleep disorders, it might have reduced the risk of falls. The efficacy of CBT-I in preventing falls in older adults with disabilities remains unclear. In this case report, we performed physical therapy in an adult with disabilities requiring care, who showed a reduction in complaints of sleep, pain, and number of falls after CBT-I, exercise, and pacing combined.

Patient Information

The patient was an 87-year-old woman, S.B.S. In February 2018, she fell while walking at her home and was immediately transferred to a hospital, diagnosed with the first lumbar vertebral fracture. The patient underwent conservative therapy for treatment. Although the patient was treated at home, she had post-injury severe back

Y. Yoshimoto (✉)
Seirei Christopher University, Hamamatsu, Shizuoka, Japan

H. Honda
Department of Physical Therapy, School of Rehabilitation Sciences, Seirei Christopher University, Hamamatsu, Shizuoka, Japan

C. Frange (ed.), *Clinical Cases in Sleep Physical Therapy*,
https://doi.org/10.1007/978-3-031-38340-3_4

pain and showed decreased mobility and physical activity. In March 2018, her post-injury back pain did not abate. In addition, the patient experienced loss of appetite and complaint of poor sleep. She was admitted to hospital and diagnosed with hyponatremia and anxiety neurosis. From the time of admission in March 2018, she received physical therapy with the goal of returning home. She was discharged from the hospital in October 2018 and underwent physical therapy at our facility to prevent falls. The patient had a medical history of lumbar spinal canal stenosis and cataracts.

Clinical Findings

The patient reported: *"I am afraid I am going to fall when I walk inside my home."* Walking at home required supervision by family members while using handrails, furniture, and other supportive objects to prevent falls. The results of gait observation showed that the gait manifested trunk sway to the left and right-side stance in the stance phase, with a short stride length and slow walking speed. The results of the initial assessment are presented in Table 4.1.

Diagnostic Assessment

Sleep

She reported: *"I can't sleep at night because of the pain and the feeling of something rushing over me."* The total score of the Pittsburgh Sleep Quality Index (PSQI) was 10 points (Table 4.1). The patient had a sleep disorder with a cutoff value of 5.5 points. In the Japanese version of the PSQI, it has been reported that a cutoff value of 5.5 points increases the sensitivity and specificity of primary insomnia and other symptoms [15]. The analysis of the sleep quality (PSQI) showed poor sleep efficiency and use of sleeping medication. Specifically, "sleep efficiency" in the past month was 63.3%, with a sleep latency of approximately 30 min and supine sleep time from awakening to waking up for more than 1 h. Although the patient left the bed several times in the middle of the night to urinate, she went to bed immediately after lying down and had no difficulty falling asleep. The patient used a benzodiazepine anti-anxiety drug (diazepam 2 mg, once a day before bedtime). She further described her condition, *"I cannot sleep without my medicine."*

Table 4.1 Results of the initial and final assessments

Assessment item	Initial assessment	Final assessment
Age, years	87	88
Sex	Female	
Number of Drugs	8	8
Body Mass Index, kg/m^2	22.2	22.4
Care Support Level[a]	Care level 1	Care level 1
History of Falls (1 year)	1	0
Timed Up and Go test, s[b]	20.2	18.3
5 m Maximal Walking Speed, m/min[c]	0.68	0.81
Five Times Sit to Stand Test, s[d]	16.8	12.2
One-Leg Standing Time with Eyes, s[e]	5.1	2
Mini-Mental State Examination, score[f]	23	24
Mini Nutritional Assessment-SF, score[g]	12	11
Geriatric Depression Scale 15, score[h]	2	3
Numerical Rating Scale, score[i]	5	3
Pain Catastrophizing Scale, score[j]	43	40
Pittsburgh Sleep Quality Index, score[k]	10	6
C1; Sleep Quality, score	1	1
C2; Sleep Latency, score	1	0
C3; Sleep Duration, score	1	0
C4; Sleep Efficiency, score	3	1
C5; Sleep Disturbance, score	1	0
C6; Use of Sleeping Medication, score	3	3
C7; Daytime Dysfunction, score	0	1
Sleep Efficiency, %[l]	63.3	76.2

[a] Levels of support and care required under Japan's long-term care insurance system (7 levels: Support 1–2, Care 1–5) [5]

[b] The time required to "turn around," "walk to a chair," and "sit down" at the maximum speed (cut-off point; $\geq$12.6 s) [6]

[c] Walking speed when walking 5 m (cut-off point; 1.0 m/s) [7]

[d] The time required to stand up 5 times from a sitting position in a chair (cut-off point; $\geq$12 s) [8]

[e] Both hands were placed on the hips, and the time from the point when one leg is raised to the point when the leg reaches the floor is measured (cut-off point; $\leq$12.7 s) [9]

[f] Overall score: from 0 to 30 points, with a score >24 indicate preserved cognitive function and <24 impaired cognitive function [10]

[g] Overall score: from 0 to 14 points, with a score >12 indicate good nutritional status, and <12 malnutrition or fear of malnutrition [11]

[h] Overall score: from 0 to 15 points, with a score <6 indicate non-depression symptoms, and >6 depression symptoms [12]

[i] Overall score: from 0 to 10 points, with a score <5 indicate non-pain or mild pain, and >5 moderate-to-severe pain [13]

[j] Overall score: from 0 to 52 points, with a score <30 indicate low severity of catastrophic thinking, and >30 high severity of catastrophic thinking [14]

[k] Overall score: from 0 to 21 points. Scores $\geq$5 indicate poor sleep, and <5 good sleep quality [15]

[l] The ratio between the amount of time spent asleep (in minutes) by the total amount of time in bed (in minutes), a normal sleep efficiency is considered to be $\geq$85%

Chronic Pain

The patient had a history of chronic pain associated with back pain that persisted for more than 6 months since the first lumbar vertebral fracture. The Numerical Rating Scale (NRS, 0–10), an assessment of chronic pain (Table 4.1), showed that the mean intensity of lumbar pain within 24 h was 5 points, revealing moderate chronic pain. The Pain Catastrophizing Scale (PCS) score was 43 points, with a cutoff value of 30 points, indicating catastrophic cognition related to pain.

Problems Related to the Risk of Fall

The problems associated with this case were summarized in Fig. 4.1. The factors associated with an increased risk of falling were sleep disorder [1, 2] and decreased physical function, including decreased standing balance [9], decreased gait ability [16], and chronic pain [17].

Physiotherapeutic Intervention

Cognitive Behavioral Therapy for Insomnia

Sleep hygiene education (SHE) was provided. A booklet of SHE, originally developed based on the principles of stimulus-control [18] and sleep restriction [19] therapies, was distributed to the patient and her family (Table 4.2). After introducing the booklet, the physical therapist counseled the patient on a regular basis. Considering counseling, the patient was asked to verbally describe her sleep situation and the physical therapist listened to the patient's story. The physical therapist encouraged reflections on the sleep situation and offered sleep advice, as needed. The counseling sessions were conducted once every 2 weeks for 5–10 min each, for a period of 1 year (approximately 24 sessions).

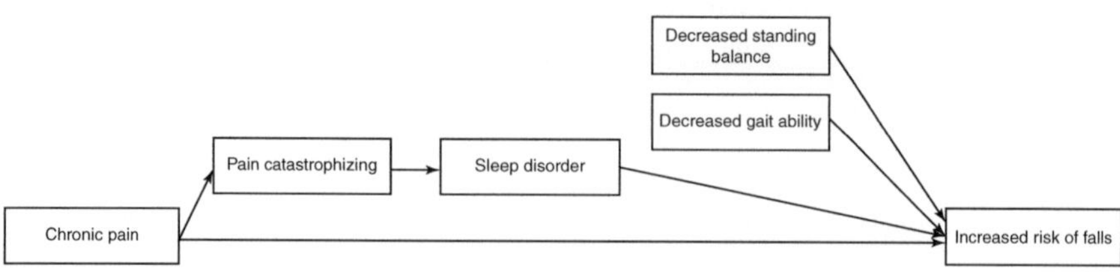

Fig. 4.1 Physical therapy content for preventing falls. (Original figure)

Table 4.2 Sleep hygiene education booklet content (excerpts)

Sleep hygiene education recommendations	Precautions
1. Reduce your time in bed	The goal is not to reduce the actual hours of sleep, but to reduce the amount of time spent awake in bed
2. Get up at the same time of day every day of the week, no matter how poorly you slept the night before	The later the wake-up time is, the lower the need for sleep the next night is. Therefore, always get up on time, even if you sleep well
3. Do not go to bed unless you are sleepy	Decide in advance on activities to do when you are not sleepy (e.g., reading, doing crosswords, organizing photo albums, folding laundry, etc.)
4. Do not stay in bed unless you are asleep	If the patient is awake during the night and more than 30 min have elapsed, he/she should perform the activity or other activity determined in 3. However, it is not recommended to look at the clock to check if 30 min have elapsed

SHE was provided to maintain and strengthen the patient's circadian rhythm, including constant wake-up time and outdoor walking training for gradual exposure to sunlight [20, 21]. Although not limited to this case, the facility's hours of operation are 9:30–16:30, and the facility's staff provides transportation from the patient's home to the facility on a regular schedule. While using the facility, the patient's waking up time was 7:30–8:00 daily, and by using the facility 3 times a week, the patient was able to keep her waking up time as consistent as possible. We also encouraged the patient to wake up at the same time as much as possible, even on days off the facility. During hours of facility use, in addition to rehabilitation, the patient was encouraged to engage in activities such as craft work, recreation, and interaction with other facility users. In addition, an environment was created in collaboration with nurses and care workers to promote daytime wakefulness. Outdoor walking program included walking exercises for approximately 20–30 min under supervision of a physical therapist, together with other users who were able to walk outdoors on their own.

Exercise and Pacing

Exercise was performed to improve standing balance and walking ability. The exercise consisted of circuit training and group work out, including balance and walking exercises, with exercise intensity within the pain tolerance range. Exercise frequency was 3 times a week using our facility for approximately 60 min each time for 1 year (approximately 72 sessions). In addition, pacing was used for chronic pain management, and daily physical activity was adjusted to be constant.

Follow-Up and Outcomes

Changes, before and after interventions, are presented in Table 4.1. The patient did not fall during the 1-year intervention period. The patient was able to walk independently at home, and the trunk sway to the left or right-side stance that occurred during hands-free walking decreased. After the intervention, the PSQI improved from 10 to 6 points, indicating improved sleep quality. Sleep efficiency sub-item improved from 3 to 1 point, changing from 63.3% to 76.2% sleep efficiency. The patient's sleep-inducing medication was unchanged, and after the intervention, she expressed that *"I did not intend to stop taking the sleeping medication because I sleep well thanks to it."*

Discussion

This case-report describes the treatment course of a case in which CBT-I was performed as one of the measures to prevent falls in an older adult with disability and pain, and sleep efficiency improved during the year of intervention.

A previous prospective study examining the association between sleep efficiency and falls in community-dwelling older adults with disabilities reported that decreased sleep efficiency was associated with falls [1]. It has also been suggested that older people with decreased sleep efficiency could experience increased wakefulness at night. This insomnia might induce falls associated with decreased daytime arousal, falls due to increased physical activity at night, and falls associated with side effects of sleep-inducing drugs. These mechanisms also suggest that decreased sleep efficiency in older adults with disabilities would be associated with an increased risk of falls, which is consistent with the present results, indicating that an association between decreased sleep efficiency and the number of falls.

If decreased sleep efficiency is associated with falls, it might be natural to suggest that CBT-I could reduce the risk of falls by improving sleep efficiency. Although we could not find any previous studies examining the effect of CBT-I on preventing falls in older adults, there are several previous studies examining whether CBT-I was effective in improving sleep efficiency. The effect of CBT-I in older patients with insomnia who received CBT-I, including SHE, sleep restriction, stimulus control, and cognitive therapy, 6 times a week for 50 min per session for 6 weeks improved sleep efficiency [22]. Another study of older adults reported that the intervention group, which used a modified, simplified approach to traditional CBT-I, 4 times a week for 45 min each time for 4 weeks, improved sleep efficiency compared with the control group [23]. The CBT-I used in this case study comprised simplified intervention contents compared with that in previous studies, with less frequent implementation and time per session. However, our intervention might be unique in that it was implemented over an extended period of 1 year. In older adults with disabilities with reduced mental and physical function, this approach might be simpler than that of the general CBT-I. Long-term implementation may lead to improved sleep efficiency and reduced risks of falls.

The possibility that approaches other than CBT-I reduced the number of falls cannot be ruled out. In our case, balance and walking exercises may have improved physical function and reduced the number of falls. In addition, a previous study that evaluated fall-related factors in older adults with disabilities [2] reported that chronic pain was associated with falls, either directly or indirectly, through the mediating effect of sleep disorders. Furthermore, reduction in chronic pain through exercise and pacing may have affected sleep efficiency and decreased the number of falls in our patient. Recent reports have indicated that a combined approach of exercise and CBT-I might improve sleep disorders [24].

First, it might be difficult for older adults with disabilities with reduced physical and mental functions to self-manage their sleep. One of the goals of a typical CBT-I was to improve patients' ability to self-manage their sleep disorders to acquire and maintain proper sleep habits. Accordingly, multiple approaches could be used, including reflecting on one's own sleep status using sleep diaries, learning and modifying proper sleep, and controlling stimuli that inhibit or promote sleep. However, as in the present case, older adults with disabilities might have difficulties in continuously performing self-monitoring (visual and cognitive abnormalities), reflecting on their own sleep habits and solving problems, and being encouraged to get out of bed when waking up in the middle of the night (increased risk of falling). The fact that patients themselves would not realize that sleep disorders might be linked to an increased risk of falls was another factor that makes self-management difficult. When CBT-I is administered to older adults with disabilities, it is necessary to devise content that could be practiced by patients themselves versus content that could be supervised continuously by the staff involved in support. Second, reducing sleeping medication use (by physicians) might be difficult in older adults with disabilities. However, this patient recognized that sleeping medications were essential for comfortable sleep.

Patient Perspective

S.B.S. commented positively on using our facility and exercising: *"I feel better physically now that I am allowed to come to this facility and they do rehabilitation for me."* However, there were no comments on sleep guidance. Additionally, the patient did not seem aware that sleep guidance was being provided.

References

1. Yoshimoto Y, Honda H, Take K, Tanaka M, Sakamoto A. Sleep efficiency affecting the occurrence of falls among the frail older adults. Geriatr Nurs. 2021;42:1461–6. https://doi.org/10.1016/j.gerinurse.2021.10.001.
2. Honda H, Ashizawa R, Kiriyama K, Take K, Hirase T, Arizono S, et al. Chronic pain in the frail elderly mediates sleep disorders and influences falls. Arch Gerontol Geriatr. 2022;99:104582. https://doi.org/10.1016/j.archger.2021.104582.

3. Riemann D, Baglioni C, Bassetti C, Bjorvatn B, Dolenc Groselj L, Ellis JG, et al. European guideline for the diagnosis and treatment of insomnia. J Sleep Res. 2017;26:675–700. https://doi.org/10.1111/jsr.12594.

4. Huang K, Li S, He R, Zhong T, Yang H, Chen L, et al. Efficacy of cognitive behavioral therapy for insomnia (CBT-I) in older adults with insomnia: a systematic review and meta-analysis. Austral Psychiatry. 2022;30:592–7. https://doi.org/10.1177/10398562221118516.

5. Yamada M, Arai H. Long-term care system in Japan. Annal Geriatr Med Res. 2020;24:174. https://doi.org/10.4235/agmr.20.0037.

6. Kojima G, Masud T, Kendrick D, Morris R, Gawler S, Treml J, et al. Does the timed up and go test predict future falls among British community-dwelling older people? Prospective cohort study nested within a randomised controlled trial. BMC Geriatr. 2015;15:1–7. https://doi.org/10.1186/s12877-015-0039-7.

7. Kyrdalen IL, Thingstad P, Sandvik L, Ormstad H. Associations between gait speed and well-known fall risk factors among community-dwelling older adults. Physiother Res Int. 2019;24:e1743. https://doi.org/10.1002/pri.1743.

8. Lusardi MM, Fritz S, Middleton A, Allison L, Wingood M, Phillips E. Determining risk of falls in community dwelling older adults: a systematic review and meta-analysis using posttest probability. J Geriatr Phys Ther. 2017;40:1. https://doi.org/10.1519/jpt.0000000000000099.

9. Jalali MM, Gerami H, Heidarzadeh A, Soleimani R. Balance performance in older adults and its relationship with falling. Aging Clin Exp Res. 2015;27:287–96. https://doi.org/10.1007/s40520-014-0273-4.

10. Escobar JI, Burnam A, Karno M, Forsythe A, Landsverk J, Golding JM. Use of the Mini-Mental State Examination (MMSE) in a community population of mixed ethnicity: cultural and linguistic artifacts. J Nerv Ment Dis. 1986;174:607–14. https://doi.org/10.1097/00005053-198610000-00005.

11. Rubenstein LZ, Harker JO, Salvà A, Guigoz Y, Vellas B. Screening for undernutrition in geriatric practice: developing the short-form mini-nutritional assessment (MNA-SF). J Gerontol Ser A Biol Med Sci. 2001;56:M366–72. https://doi.org/10.1093/gerona/56.6.m366.

12. Sheikh JI, Yesavage JA. Geriatric Depression Scale (GDS): recent evidence and development of a shorter version. Clin Gerontol J Aging Ment Health. 1986;5:165. https://psycnet.apa.org/doi/10.1300/J018v05n01_09.

13. Williamson A, Hoggart B. Pain: a review of three commonly used pain rating scales. J Clin Nurs. 2005;14(7):798–804.

14. Sullivan MJ. The pain catastrophizing scale. User Manual. 2009. https://sullivan-pain-research.mcgill.ca/pdf/pcs/PCSManual_English.pdf.

15. Doi Y, Minowa M, Uchiyama M, Okawa M, Kim K, Shibui K, et al. Psychometric assessment of subjective sleep quality using the Japanese version of the Pittsburgh Sleep Quality Index (PSQI-J) in psychiatric disordered and control subjects. Psychiatry Res. 2000;97:165-172. https://doi.org/10.1016/S0165-1781(00)00232-8.

16. Kojima G, Masud T, Kendrick D, Morris R, Gawler S, Treml J, et al. Does the timed up and go test predict future falls among British community-dwelling older people? Prospective cohort study nested within a randomised controlled trial. BMC Geriatr. 2015;15:38. https://doi.org/10.1186/s12877-015-0039-7.

17. Honda H, Ashizawa R, Take K, Hirase T, Arizono S, Yoshimoto Y. Effect of chronic pain on the occurrence of falls in older adults with disabilities: a prospective cohort study. Physiother Theory Pract. 2022;6:1–9. https://doi.org/10.1080/09593985.2022.2141597.

18. Bootzin RR, Epstein D, Wood JM, Hauri P. Case studies in insomnia. Stimulus control instructions. New York, NY: Plenum; 1991. p. 19–28.

19. Spielman AJ, Saskin P, Thorpy MJ. Treatment of chronic insomnia by restriction of time in bed. Sleep. 1987;10:45–56.

20. Chung KF, Lee CT, Yeung WF, Chan MS, Chung EWY, Lin WL. Sleep hygiene education as a treatment of insomnia: a systematic review and meta-analysis. Fam Pract. 2018;35:365–75. https://doi.org/10.1093/fampra/cmx122.

21. Capezuti E, Sagha Zadeh R, Pain K, Basara A, Jiang NZ, Krieger AC. A systematic review of non-pharmacological interventions to improve nighttime sleep among residents of long-term care settings. BMC Geriatr. 2018;18:1–8. https://doi.org/10.1186/s12877-018-0794-3.
22. Sivertsen B, Omvik S, Pallesen S, Bjorvatn B, Havik OE, Kvale G, et al. Cognitive behavioral therapy vs zopiclone for treatment of chronic primary insomnia in older adults: a randomized controlled trial. JAMA. 2006;295:2851–8. https://doi.org/10.1001/jama.295.24.2851.
23. Martin JL, Song Y, Hughes J, Jouldjian S, Dzierzewski JM, Fung CH, et al. A four-session sleep intervention program improves sleep for older adult day health care participants: results of a randomized controlled trial. Sleep. 2017;40:zsx079. https://doi.org/10.1093/sleep/zsx079.
24. Gencarelli A, Sorrell A, Everhart CM, Zurlinden T, Everhart DE. Behavioral and exercise interventions for sleep dysfunction in the elderly: a brief review and future directions. Sleep Breath. 2021;25:2111–8. https://doi.org/10.1007/s11325-021-02329-9.

Chapter 5
Sleep and Psyche: Life is a Versatile Game

Cristina Staub

Introduction

Sleep problems and mental disorders are strongly related [1, 2]. It is not always obvious which problem was present first. Often there are several factors that lead to a loss of inner balance regarding sleep and psyche [3]. During the corona lockdown, many people were unexpectedly exposed to such factors, so their resilience was not optimal: Suddenly, many people had to remain isolated in their homes. They only moved within a few square meters and were irritated by media reports [4–6]. Some were unable to work at all during the lockdown and became lost in time and space. Others worked on computers in home offices, but also no longer adhered to the circadian rhythms of our chronobiology. The consequences were a decline in physical fitness, in social and cognitive skills, and often also in mental health. With holistic treatments, good results can be achieved within a short time against the Corona Lockdown Syndrome.

Patient Information

At the beginning of the lockdown, older people, in particular, turned up, suffering from isolation and lack of exercise. Over time, however, more and more younger people appeared who showed somatic, neuropsychological, and psychological symptoms. Representative of these, the story of a 30-year-old woman is documented here.

C. Staub (✉)
Ausgeschlafen.ch and Pro Dormo, Zürich, Switzerland

© The Author(s), under exclusive license to Springer Nature Switzerland AG 2023
C. Frange (ed.), *Clinical Cases in Sleep Physical Therapy*,
https://doi.org/10.1007/978-3-031-38340-3_5

Before lockdown, the patient performed service tasks, exercised three times a week, and met regularly with friends. She lived with colleagues in a comfortable shared apartment. She led a normal life.

Because of the lockdown, everyone was at home most of the time: They had to perform certain professional tasks at home, so they could not gain distance from work. Also, because more free time was spent at home, they had less control over contact with roommates. There was also a lack of specific activities to achieve inner balance.

After a few weeks, the woman visited her family doctor because of inner restlessness and increasing discomfort in her neck and head. The doctor prescribed physical therapy for her.

Clinical Findings

During the first consultation, it was immediately obvious that the patient frequently ground her teeth and that the masseter muscle was very pronounced. Palpation revealed trigger points in the masseter muscle but also in the temporalis muscle and the pterygoid muscles bilaterally. Dental damage was not present: It is possible that the bruxism symptoms had developed after lockdown onset. In addition, trigger points also existed in the levator scapulae, scalene, and sternocleidomastoid muscles bilaterally with overall increased muscle tone and superficial respiration.

Timeline

Initially, two treatments were carried out weekly, followed by one weekly, and then further treatments at longer intervals. A total of 17 appointments took place, which, if possible, lasted longer than the usual 30 min. On the days without treatment, the patient consciously performed activation and relaxation exercises.

Diagnostic Assessment

The affected patient suffered from significant pain (numerical rating scale, NRS: 7 out of 10 points) and intense grinding (NRS: 7 out of 10 points), fatigue (fatigue severity scale, FSS: 4.7 out of 7 points; [7]), from impaired sleep quality (NRS: 5 out of 10 points). She rated her psychological well-being as 6–7 out of 10 points (NRS). She could hardly relax (NRS: 4 out of 10 points).

Physiotherapeutic Intervention

Already during the first treatment, the most important tips of cognitive behavioral therapy against sleep disorders were taught: During psychoeducation, the patient received the usual tips of sleep hygiene education. The patient already followed most of the rules. At most, dimmed lights burned in the evening and at night, the bedroom was cool and quiet, and the patient did not look at the clock at night. However, she used the bedroom not only for sleeping: it was the only room she had to herself, so she spent many hours working in it. Newly, she covered the work surface with a cloth in the evening to shut down the working day.

However, although she also performed other sleep rituals and tried to maintain a regular sleep-wake rhythm, she was unable to increase her ability to relax before treatment began. She could not let go and kept biting her teeth hard.

This is where accessing the person through the body is helpful. The patient was placed on the treatment couch in the most relaxing way possible. Breathing remained superficial for the time being, however, and muscle tension was hardly reduced.

Manual stimulation often reduces sympathetic activity in such cases. The patient was asked if she could tolerate a neck massage, but also a facial massage. During the massage, the various trigger points were also treated.

For a massage to have a lasting effect, the patient must be mentally intentional about it: The feeling of relaxation must be felt and stored so that it can be recalled over and over again afterward and in the following days, as this leads to being stored in the brain for the long term. The patient also consciously breathed out pent-up tension.

Scents have a supporting effect. Olfactory stimuli can also influence emotions during sleep. For example, anise, jasmine, vanilla, or cinnamon have a relaxing effect on most people; patients must choose the scent individually.

However, if patients do start to brood at night, they can listen to an audio file that will help them fall back asleep. Again, it is crucial that patients choose the file individually: Would they rather listen to quiet music, a technical reading, a funny story, or even jokes?

An exhausted body usually sleeps more deeply than one without enough challenges. Therefore, the patient was shown intensive strengthening exercises during several treatments, which she repeated independently at home several times a week. In addition, she should get some fresh air every day if possible.

To counteract the grinding, the patient let the air out slowly several times a day with the pursed lips breathing, slightly inflating her cheeks. In the coachman's seat, this breathing is particularly relaxing.

In order to feel the body pleasantly again and again, the patient newly performed stretches several times a day. Of course, with bruxism, the muscles of the neck and shoulder girdle must also be stretched. Afterward, the upper body should be straightened up again, preferably combined with stretches of the pectoralis muscle.

Supplementary nutritional tips were given to the patient: In particular, plants and herbs with relaxing effects (i.e., valerian, lemon balm, St. John's wort, or chamomile) should be consumed in the evening and rather some activating substances (xanthines, ginkgo) in the morning.

Follow-Up and Outcomes

Muscle tone and breathing normalized. The pain score decreased to 3, the grinding score to 4, and the FSS score to 2.3 points. The NRS regarding sleep quality increased to 9 points and regarding psychological well-being to 8–9 points. She was able to relax more deeply (9 points) and was satisfied with the treatment (NRS: 10 out of 10 points).

Discussion

Especially in the case of complex complaints, it is worthwhile to make the examination as holistically as possible and to comprehensively include daytime and nighttime behavior.

Unfortunately, sleep is often not taken into account in patients with pain and/or psychological complaints. However, the simple screening questionnaire (Fig. 5.1) could sometimes already provide clues to possible causes and for the further procedure [3]: The questions on the left explore the problem, the questionnaires, which are listed on the right in each case, provide information about the subjective severity of the disease. In addition, the possible objective examinations regarding sleep disorders are listed on the right.

To assess psychological problems, questionnaires such as the Beck Depression Inventory (BDI-II) [8] or the Perceived Stress Questionnaire 20 (PSQ-20) [9] can be used. However, like the sleep log or a pain or tinnitus diary, overly detailed questionnaires have the disadvantage that the patients deal with the problem too intensively and too often, which can intensify the complaints.

According to Riemann et al. [10], cognitive behavioral therapy for insomnia (CVT-I) is recommended for patients with insomnia. Sleep medications should be taken for a maximum of 4 weeks.

To achieve more restful sleep and pain reduction as efficiently as possible, many comprehensive treatments are given simultaneously.

Cognitive behavioral therapy information can and should be taught for sleep problems. Additionally, the body should be involved. After all, the body and psyche form a unit: Body and psyche are influenced by sleep regulation processes (a) and depend on synaptic connections (b).

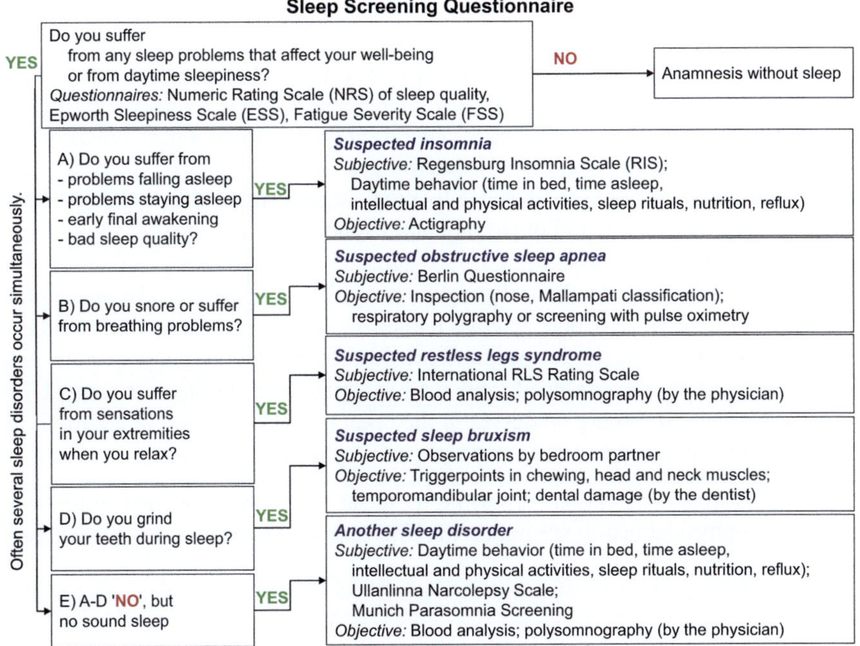

Fig. 5.1 Sleep screening questionnaire [3]. Original figure (All rights reserved Staub, 2020)

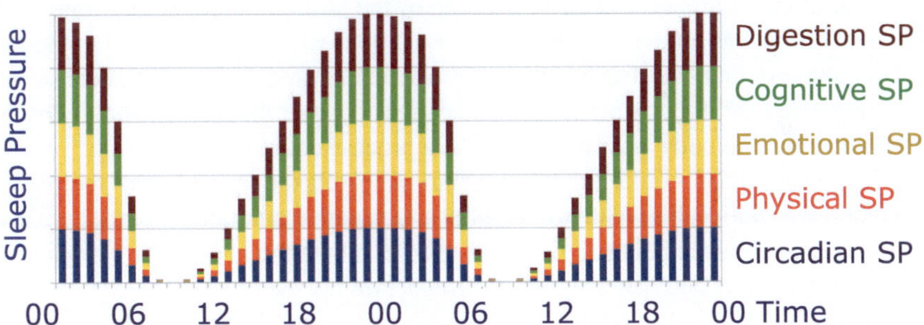

Fig. 5.2 A multifactorial model for sleep regulation [3]. *SP* sleep pressure. Original figure (copyright Staub, 2020)

(a) Sleep regulation processes: The most accepted scientific model of sleep regulation [11] includes only a homeostatic and a circadian process, with the two curves shifted in time and subtracted to obtain sleep pressure. However, there is no physiological reason for the temporal shift and subtraction of the curves, and homeostatic pressure is more complex. In the multifactorial model (Fig. 5.2), many parameters are taken into account (e.g., the hormone leptin for digestion, amyloid β for cognition, adenosine and stress hormones for emotions, and growth hormone for physical questions), all curves are left in the correct place in the time axis, and all are added to a sleep pressure [3]. This model can be used to explain the effects of an irregular and sedentary lifestyle on health: Sleep pressure decreases, sleep regeneration processes no longer function efficiently, and health progressively deteriorates.

By means of correctly dosed activation, targeted relaxation, balanced nutrition, and optimization of environmental factors, sleep and health can be maximally promoted.

(b) Synaptic connections: By involving the body, thought cycles can be interrupted: The strength of synaptic activity related to worry and sleep disturbance is reduced; in return, more receptors are formed at other synapses, more neurotransmitters are produced, and new synaptic connections are formed [3]. Thus, sleep-promoting processes in the brain can be activated. In addition, the patient's mood can be influenced by specific physical exercises.

Versatile treatment options are to be tried out in a playful manner until sleep, mental and physical health are improved. The case study conveys that hope should not be given up.

Patient Perspective

I was emotional, sad, and indignant because of the circumstances at that time. The deep relaxation was totally missing, which I did not realize, because I did not know that feeling. At first, the treatments were exhausting and unfamiliar because we went into a new field. I was often tired and exhausted after the massage on my back, neck, and jaw. The body was revitalized, so a process could start.

After some time I could quickly get into deep relaxation. Only the feeling of relaxation was noticeable, with no thoughts and negative emotions more. There is a big difference between being actively involved in relaxation and not. In this case, it was something new and had a significant impact on my everyday life.

In many areas of life, physical and cognitive relaxation is crucial. This is something I had actually tried but not learned the years before. Deep relaxation has helped me to a great advantage. I am totally grateful for that. It is not just about performance, but actually much more about relaxation, and regeneration. My performance is only as good as my recovery.

I believe that deep relaxation is the antidote to stress. I think the body can develop a certain immunity to stress so that the highs and lows do not have to be so high and low.

References

1. Palagini L, Domschke K, Benedetti F, Foster RG, Wulff K, Riemann D. Developmental pathways towards mood disorders in adult life: is there a role for sleep disturbances? Review article. J Affect Disord. 2019;243:121–32.
2. Vodovotz Y, Barnard N, Hu FB, et al. Prioritized research for the prevention, treatment, and reversal of chronic disease: recommendations from the lifestyle medicine research summit. Review Front Med (Lausanne). 2020;7:585744.
3. Staub C. In collaboration with Droth B and Vanderlinden J. Daytime Behavior & Sleep. Healthy lifestyle book. Ausgeschlafen.ch; 2021.
4. Peters E, Hübner J, Katalinic A. Stress, Copingstrategien und gesundheitsbezogene Lebensqualitätwährend der Corona-Pandemie im April 2020 in Deutschland [stress, coping strategies and health-related quality of life duringthe corona pandemic in April 2020 in Germany]. Dtsch Med Wochenschr. 2021;146(2):e11–20.
5. Schwinger M, Trautner M, Kärchner H, Otterpohl N. Psychological impact of Corona lockdown in Germany: changes in need satisfaction, well-being, anxiety, and depression. Int J Environ Res Public Health. 2020;17(23):9083.
6. Veer IM, Riepenhausen A, Zerban M. Psycho-social factors associated with mental resilience in the Corona lockdown. Transl Psychiatry. 2021;11:67.
7. Krupp LB, LaRocca NG, Muir-Nash J, Steinberg AD. The fatigue severity scale. Application to patients with multiple sclerosis and systemic lupus erythematosus. Arch Neurol. 1989;46(10):1121–3.
8. Beck AT, Steer RA, Ball R, Ranieri W. Comparison of Beck depression inventories -IA and-II in psychiatric outpatients. J Pers Assess. 1996;67(3):588–97.
9. Fliege H, Rose M, Arck P, Levenstein S, Klapp BF. Validierung des "Perceived Stress Questionnaire" (PSQ) an einer deutschen Stichprobe. Diagnostica. 2001;47(3):142–52.
10. Riemann D, Baum E, Cohrs S, Crönlein T, Hajak G, Hertenstein E, Klose P, Langhorst J, Mayer G, Nissen C, Pollmächer T, Rabstein S, Schlarb A, Sitter H, Weeß H-G, Wetter T, Spiegelhalder K. S3-Leitlinie Nicht erholsamer Schlaf/Schlafstörungen. Kapitel "Insomnie bei Erwachsenen". Update 2016. Somnologie. 2017;211:2–44.
11. Borbély AA. A two process model of sleep regulation. Hum Neurobiol. 1982;1:195–204.

Part III
Clinical Cases: Insomnia

Chapter 6
Insomnia Complaints, Positional Pain, and Unfavorable Sleep Habits

Carolina V. R. D'Aurea ⓘ

Introduction

There is a close bidirectional relationship between insomnia and chronic pain, with pain being able to impair the quantity and quality of sleep, while an altered sleep pattern can initiate or worsen pain [1–3]. Therefore, it is imperative that the physiotherapist understands the different approaches that can be used to evaluate and improve the patient's sleep so that together they can create the best treatment plan [4, 5].

Patient Information

Patient C.L.L was a sedentary, 38-year-old, upper-middle class single male living in São Paulo, with grade I obesity, and complaints of neck and lumbar pain, that interfered with sleep, resulting in nonrestorative sleep and daytime sleepiness.

The patient reported having neck, lumbar, and gluteal pain during the day and throughout the night for approximately 5 years, and that in the previous 3 years, the pain was getting worse, causing him to frequently wake up during the night and being unable to easily go back to sleep (sleep maintenance insomnia). He complained of not being able to find a comfortable sleeping position. He worked from home for approximately 12 h a day, sitting and rarely taking breaks, spending most

C. V. R. D'Aurea (✉)
Department of Public Health, Universidade Católica de Santos, Santos, SP, Brazil

C. Frange (ed.), *Clinical Cases in Sleep Physical Therapy*,
https://doi.org/10.1007/978-3-031-38340-3_6

of his time on the computer or cell phone. He reported that the pain increased in intensity the longer he remained seated or when lying on his stomach and decreased when he moved or lay on his side. The pain occurred daily, starting in the lumbar region and gradually intensifying as the musculature stiffened, spreading to the cervical and gluteal region.

The patient did not practice any regular physical exercise. Although he stated that he liked to swim, he did not do this with any regularity. He reported having some physical complaints since childhood. He was not using any medication regularly, only sporadically for pain control. He is a moderate drinker and tried to maintain healthy eating habits. His aim was to sleep at least 8 h a day, but ideally would like to be able to sleep for at least 10 h. He had no regular sleep and wake-up times and said that he used his cell phone until bedtime, and even used it if he woke up in the middle of the night.

From family history, both parents presented with long-term pain complaints, with the father having severe pain in the neck region, and the mother having wrists, shoulders, and ankles joints pain.

The patient reported having previously had acupuncture, massage, Rolfing, and physiotherapy to treat pain, including lower back pain, but that it was unsuccessful.

Clinical Findings

A physical examination of the standing patient revealed that he presented an anterior head position, increased tension and trigger points in the trapezius region, the elevation of the shoulders, decreased lumbar lordosis, pelvic retroversion, significant shortening of the hamstrings, slightly valgus knees, and slightly flat feet.

When sitting down, he did not support the pressure on ischial tubercles and kept the spine flexed, maintaining himself in hyperkyphosis not to exacerbate pain. He most used his cell phone close to the umbilical region, which constantly overloaded the cervical region.

Timeline

The physiotherapeutic treatment timeline can be seen in Fig. 6.1.

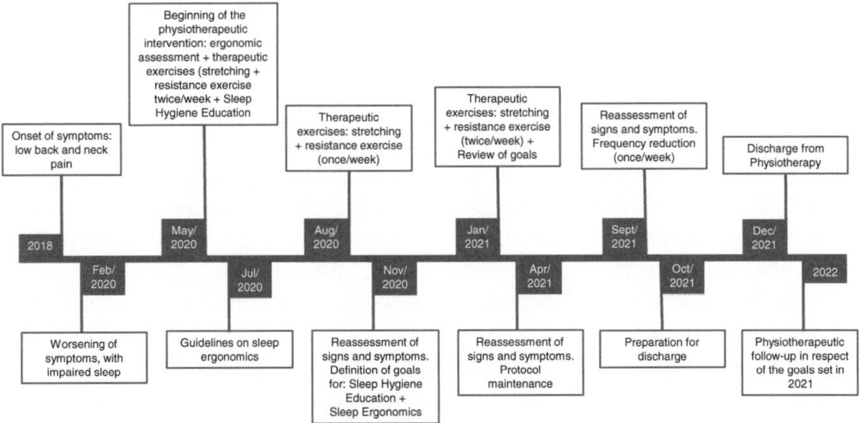

Fig. 6.1 Timeline depicting the episode of care

Diagnostic Assessment

In the first evaluation, in May 2020, the Epworth Sleepiness Scale (ESS [6], Pittsburgh Sleep Quality Index (PSQI) [7], Insomnia Severity Index (ISI) [8], and Morningness-Eveningness Questionnaire (MEQ) [9] questionnaires were applied. Overall, the patient presented with excessive daytime sleepiness (ESS = 17), poor sleep quality (PSQI = 11), clinically moderate insomnia (ISI = 17), and being an extreme evening type (MEQ = 21).

Physiotherapeutic Intervention

Beginning of the physiotherapeutic intervention—May 2020: In the first session, after a very detailed anamnesis, an ergonomic analysis of the patient's work environment was performed. We then talked about posture and automatic daily movements, the importance of body awareness for postural control and physical exercise to maintain an elongated, strong musculature capable of absorbing the stresses throughout the day, and how those changes would affect his pain-sleep/insomnia issue. The height of the computer monitor was adjusted, and support was improved for the forearms to avoid overloading the shoulders and trapezius region. Finally, a small pillow was added to improve the chair's lumbar support.

Mobility work was then started, mainly aimed at the lumbar region and hips. This involved passive stretching of the posterior chain and isometric strengthening of the paravertebral, lumbar, gluteal, pelvic, and abdominal muscles. The main focus was on teaching the patient to activate the musculature rather than strengthening it. This work was carried out every 15 days, lasting 90 min.

In the first session, the patient also received guidance on sleep in respect of its functions, the consequences of sleep deprivation and insufficient sleep, chronotype, and advice on sleep hygiene education (SHE) [1] that could help him to improve the quality of his sleep. The main SHE guidelines were:

1. Maintain regular schedules of sleep and waking times, even during weekends;
2. Use the bed only for sleeping. Go to bed only when sleepy. Do not use it for other activities such as working and eating;
3. Get some exposure to sunlight in the morning, as it promotes awakening;
4. Practice regular physical activity and avoid sedentary behavior;
5. Avoid drinking alcoholic beverages at least 4 h before bedtime. The consumption of alcoholic beverages, in general, helps to induce sleep, but impairs sleep quality;
6. Control caffeine intake throughout the day. Try to drink the last cup of any beverage containing caffeine by 14 h;
7. Avoid napping during the day. If necessary, naps should be taken after lunch and should not exceed 30 min;
8. Avoid using electronic devices close to bedtime. Melatonin, one of the hormones that helps to induce sleep, is secreted in the absence of light. Try to avoid such devices from 1 to 2 h before sleep;
9. Avoid eating large amounts of food very close to bedtime. The digestive system has reduced function at night and fastening is important;
10. Build a pre-sleep routine to tell your brain you're getting ready for sleep. Reduce activities, especially the most stressful ones, and do low-intensity activities such as reading, having a hot bath, relaxation, stretching, meditation, or any other activity that signals your body that you intend to sleep.

Sleep Ergonomics—July 2020: The patient reported a slight improvement in symptoms throughout the day, but still complained about them during the nighttime period, as he woke up in the prone position with low back and neck pain. During this period, the patient's room and postures adopted while sleeping were evaluated. He reported that he always slept in the prone position and had great difficulty sleeping in the lateral decubitus.

It was decided to change the mattress to a semi-orthopedic one. The pillow was also changed, as the old one was too high, making cervical alignment difficult. He was recommended to use a pillow between the knees to allow better hip-knee alignment and to prevent lumbar rotation.

Increased frequency—August 2020: At this stage, sessions happened weekly. The focus was on muscle strengthening exercises, and stretching became active or assisted. The patient was given a set of exercises to be performed 2–3 times a week.

First Reassessment—November 2020: Pain had decreased, but daytime sleepiness still interfered with the patient's daily routine—(ESS = 13). One of the main problems was difficulty in maintaining lateral decubitus throughout the night. Some other possible positions were tried but without success. It was decided to try placing a tennis ball in the sternal region of the patient's pajamas to see if this could help, and this produced a positive result with the patient finally being able to remain longer on his side as when he turned onto his sternum, the ball exerted some pressure on the region causing him to return to his initial position.

At this time, follow-up goals were also set and the ergonomic and SHE recommendations were reinforced, e.g.: stop using cell phone 15 to 30 min before going to sleep, and not use it during the night; bedtime by 01:00 and wake-up time by 10:00; exposition to natural light when waking-up; use the tennis ball placed on the sternum and a pillow between the knees.

Review of the protocol and increase in the frequency of sessions—January 2021: The patient was feeling much better in all aspects, but he decided to increase the frequency of sessions to twice a week, as he felt much better on the days when he performed the session. The patient presented better in all questionnaires: no more excessive daytime sleepiness (ESS = 8), still poor sleep quality, but much better than January (PSQI = 8), and clinically nonsignificant insomnia (ISI = 7).

In this phase, the patient performed the exercises 5 times a week—2 sessions lasting 90 min being guided by the physiotherapist, and 3 sessions lasting approximately 20 to 30 min without assistance. We also adjusted SHE recommendations: stop using cell phone 30 min before bed and do not use it during the night; bedtime at 00:30, turning off the lights, perform stretching and breathing techniques in bed, and wake-up time at 9:30 AM; exposition to natural light when waking up; maintain the sleep ergonomics recommendations.

Second Reassessment—April 2021: There was a significant improvement in respect of all of the patient's initial complaints—sometimes with a whole week going to bed without any complaints. He was sleeping better, without waking up during the night, the daytime drowsiness had reduced a lot and he felt that he had more energy throughout the day. The decision was to maintain the aforementioned recommendations: exercises + follow-up in respect of SHE and ergonomic goals.

Third Reassessment—September 2021: The patient had no physical complaints and reported good quantity of sleep (between 8.5 and 9 h per night) and quality.

By this stage, he had excellent body awareness and maintained good exercise discipline throughout the week. We, therefore, decided to reduce the frequency of assisted sessions to once a week, continue the follow-up, and prepare for discharge. I suggested that he start practicing some other form of exercise and he opted for swimming once a week.

Preparation for Discharge—October 2021: The reduction in physical therapy sessions and the start of swimming were going very well. It was decided to follow up every 15 days and try to increase the frequency of physical exercise to twice a week: either 2 days of swimming or 1 day of swimming and 1 day of resistance training and stretching.

Discharge—December 2021: By the discharge day, the patient felt confident about performing the exercises and understood that the ergonomic recommendations related to work and activities throughout the day, including sleep, would be forever and that the habits acquired through the SHE recommendations would need to be maintained to ensure good quality sleep. The questionnaires showed that the patient was better with good sleep quality (PSQI = 4), without insomnia (ISI = 0), and without sleepiness (ESS = 5). We then decided to an online monitoring session, with a reduction in frequency over the months.

Follow-up for 1 year—2022: Weekly in the first month, every 15 days in the second and third months, and monthly until the end of the year. The purpose of this follow-up was to understand how the patient was and to make him comfortable and confident that he was being assisted whenever he needed it. In the online consultations, we revisited some points and adjusted when necessary.

Discussion

Recently, a guideline with recommendations was created [5], with the aim of highlighting the various methods and techniques that physiotherapists can use to assess and treat their patients' sleep. What is clearly known is that an altered sleep pattern can influence health and, in cases of pain, can aggravate symptoms and delay the rehabilitation process [2, 3].

In this case, we obtained positive results with the adoption of therapeutic exercises, associated with improved ergonomics and SHE. Physical exercise has been shown to have many benefits, including improving sleep quality [10–12]. Although there is no protocol on type, intensity and frequency of exercise, it is clear that regular practice can improve sleep patterns [12]. In relation to ergonomics, there is no ideal pillow or mattress, but the adoption of simple measures and a focus on improving posture and sleep positions can generate both physical and sleep-related benefits [13, 14]. Regarding the tennis ball, this has been commonly used in cases of obstructive sleep apnea to prevent patients from sleeping on their backs [15]. The benefits of improved SHE through following sleep hygiene guidelines have been widely recognized, especially when used with other therapies [16].

Personalized treatment using a range of techniques and the careful follow-up of the patients, which made them feel safe and cared for, were the two main pillars of this treatment and were largely responsible for the positive outcomes. The methodology used in this case helped the patient to better understand sleep and pain problems, and the relation between them, as well as the various nonpharmacological techniques and methods that can be used in the treatment. The information and advice that they received during the treatment period gave the patient the independence to stipulate their own goals and reach a successful conclusion.

Patient Perspective

"I realized I needed help as I always had some kind of pain, and it got to the point where I was in pain every day. My sleep started to be affected and sleep is something I've always enjoyed. This made me decide to seek help, although I started the physiotherapy without a lot of confidence that it would improve my condition as I had already tried other treatments and they had not helped me.

The most interesting thing was when the physiotherapist started talking about sleep, at first, I thought there might be too much information about sleep but the physiotherapist explained to me that sleep was important as it has a very important relationship with pain, with one affecting the other. I had nothing to lose, so I decided to give physiotherapy a try. To my surprise, I gained a lot - a life without pain, without medication and a good quality of sleep. Before the treatment, I thought that I slept well up until the pain episodes got really bad, but I can see that I was wrong, as I can say now that I really know what it's like to sleep well! I appreciate the treatment and follow up that I received and being taught so many things - things I think I can take on for life."

References

1. Nitter AK, Pripp AH, Forseth KO. Are sleep problems and non-specific health complaints risk factors for chronic pain? A prospective population-based study with 17 year follow-up. Scand J Pain. 2012;3(4):210–7.
2. Frange C, Babiloni AH, Lam JTAT, Lavigne GJ. Sleep and chronic pain interlaced influences: guidance to physiotherapy practice. In: Frange C, Coelho FMS, editors. Sleep medicine and physical therapy. Cham: Springer; 2022. https://doi.org/10.1007/978-3-030-85074-628.
3. Ostovar-Kermani T, Arnaud D, Almaguer A, Garcia I, Gonzalez S, Mendez Martinez YH, Surani S. Painful sleep: insomnia in patients with chronic pain syndrome and its consequences. Folia Med (Plovdiv). 2020;62(4):645–54. https://doi.org/10.3897/folmed.62.e50705.
4. Siengsukon CF, Al-Dughmi M, Stevens S. Sleep health promotion: practical information for physical therapists. Phys Ther. 2017;97(8):826–36.
5. Frange C, Franco AM, Brasil E, Hirata RP, Lino JA, Mortari DM, et al. Practice recommendations for the role of physiotherapy in the management of sleep disorders: the 2022 Brazilian sleep association guidelines. Sleep Sci. 2022;15(4):515–73.
6. Bertolazi AN, Fagondes SC, Hoff LS, Pedro VD, Menna Barreto SS, Johns MW. Portuguese-language version of the Epworth sleepiness scale: validation for use in Brazil. J Bras Pneumol. 2009;35(9):877–83.
7. Bertolazi AN, Fagondes SC, Hoff LS, Dartora EG, Miozzo IC, de Barba ME, et al. Validation of the Brazilian Portuguese version of the Pittsburgh sleep quality index. Sleep Med. 2011;12(1):70–5.
8. Bastien CH, Vallieres A, Morin CM. Validation of the insomnia severity index as an outcome measure for insomnia research. Sleep Med. 2001;2(4):297–307.
9. Horne JA, Ostberg O. A self-assessment questionnaire to determine morningness-eveningness in human circadian rhythms. Int J Chronobiol. 1976;4(2):97–110.
10. Lowe H, Haddock G, Mulligan LD, Gregg L, Fuzellier-Hart A, Carter LA, et al. Does exercise improve sleep for adults with insomnia? A systematic review with quality appraisal. Clin Psychol Rev. 2019;68:1–12.

11. Xie Y, Liu S, Chen XJ, Yu HH, Yang Y, Wang W. Effects of exercise on sleep quality and insomnia in adults: a systematic review and meta-analysis of randomized controlled trials. Front Psych. 2021;12:664499. https://doi.org/10.3389/fpsyt.2021.664499; PMID: 34163383; PMCID: PMC8215288.
12. D'Aurea CVR, Frange C, Poyares D, Souza AAL, Lenza M. Physical exercise as a therapeutic approach for adults with insomnia: systematic review and meta-analysis. Einstein (Sao Paulo). 2022;20:eAO8058.
13. Jeon MY, Jeong H, Lee S, Choi W, Park JH, Tak SJ, et al. Improving the quality of sleep with an optimal pillow: a randomized, comparative study. Tohoku J Exp Med. 2014;233(3):183–8.
14. Yim JE. Optimal pillow conditions for high-quality sleep: a theoretical review. Indian J Sci Technol. 2015;8(5):135–9.
15. Eijsvogel MM, Ubbink R, Dekker J, Oppersma E, de Jongh FH, van der Palen J, et al. Sleep position trainer versus tennis ball technique in positional obstructive sleep apnea syndrome. J Clin Sleep Med. 2015;11(2):139–47.
16. Chung KF, Lee CT, Yeung WF, Chan MS, Chung EW, Lin WL. Sleep hygiene education as a treatment of insomnia: a systematic review and meta-analysis. Fam Pract. 2018;35(4):365–75.

Chapter 7
Sleep Health Promotion in an Individual with Multiple Sclerosis

Catherine F. Siengsukon ⓘ

Introduction

Sleep disturbances are common in individuals with multiple sclerosis (MS), occurring in approximately 70% of individuals [1]. Sleep disturbances in individuals with MS are caused by demyelination or degeneration of sleep/wake centers in the brain [2] and/or by secondary factors such as fatigue, spasticity, bladder dysfunction, mobility impairments, anxiety, depression, and pain [3]. Poor sleep quality has been associated with increased fatigue, depression, and anxiety, and a reduction in physical function, psychological well-being, ability to perform self-care and activities of daily lives, workability, and quality of life in people with MS [4, 5]. Therefore, enhancing sleep health can improve multiple facets of life for individuals with MS.

Sleep medicine focuses on the identification and treatment of sleep disorders, such as insomnia, sleep apnea, and restless legs syndrome. *Sleep health* is a newer term that focuses on sleep as a health behavior along a continuum rather than simply the absence of sleep disorders. Sleep health consists of six dimensions: sleep *regularity, s*atisfaction with sleep, daytime *a*lertness, *t*iming of sleep within a 24-h period, sleep *e*fficiency, and sleep *d*uration (acronym Ru-SATED [6, 7]). Targets to enhance sleep health physiotherapists can glean from the main components of cognitive behavioral therapy for insomnia (CBT-I) and brief behavioral therapy (BBT) to enhance sleep health including entraining circadian rhythm, increasing sleep drive, reducing arousal, and addressing "sleep hygiene education" (SHE) as needed.

The individual presented in this case is a combination of multiple individuals with multiple sclerosis with poor sleep I have worked with over the years. The

C. F. Siengsukon (✉)
Department of Physical Therapy, Rehabilitation Science, and Athletic Training, University of Kansas Medical Center, Kansas City, KS, USA

© The Author(s), under exclusive license to Springer Nature Switzerland AG 2023
C. Frange (ed.), *Clinical Cases in Sleep Physical Therapy*,
https://doi.org/10.1007/978-3-031-38340-3_7

purpose is to illustrate how to conduct a case conceptualization around sleep health, the application of a sleep decision tree, and apply sleep health promotion techniques with an individual with MS.

Patient Information

S.K.L. is a 45-year-old female referred to outpatient physiotherapy following a multiple sclerosis exacerbation. She reports she lives alone in a single-story home. She is experiencing an increase in lower extremity weakness, balance disturbance, and fatigue. She rates her sleep as "fairly bad" and reports she sleeps for 5–8 h "depending on the night." She states she wakes up feeling "groggy" most mornings. She reports she has had difficulty falling back to sleep if she wakes up in the middle of the night since she was diagnosed with MS about 5 years ago due to stress and being anxious about the future, but she says her sleep has gotten worse since her recent MS exacerbation due to the added stress and worry. She said she'll sleep for 5–6 h and then wakes up to use the bathroom and has difficulty getting back to sleep 3-4x/ week because she starts thinking about "things." She typically lays in bed until her alarm goes off at 6:30 am to get ready for work. She says she often dozes off while watching TV and she thinks her tiredness is affecting her work productivity. She does not think she snores and does not have an unpleasant urge to move her legs while resting. She states: "You are the first person [health care provider] to ask me about my sleep since I was diagnosed with MS."

Timeline

- Diagnosed with MS 5 years ago; when sleep disturbance started;
- Recent MS exacerbation; increase in sleep disturbance.

Diagnostic Assessment

No diagnostic testing (i.e., polysomnography, clinical interview) has been conducted to assess for sleep disorders. The physiotherapist uses the sleep decision tree created for physiotherapists [8] to guide their screening process. Based on S.K.L's report of sleeping some nights <7 h, waking up feeling "groggy," and rating her sleep quality as "fairly bad," the physiotherapists moves down the left-hand side of the decision tree (Fig. 7.1).

Based on the S.L.K.'s report that her sleep disturbances started 5 years ago when she was diagnosed with MS and have increased due to the additional stress and worry from her most recent exacerbation, you suspect her sleep issue is NOT due to

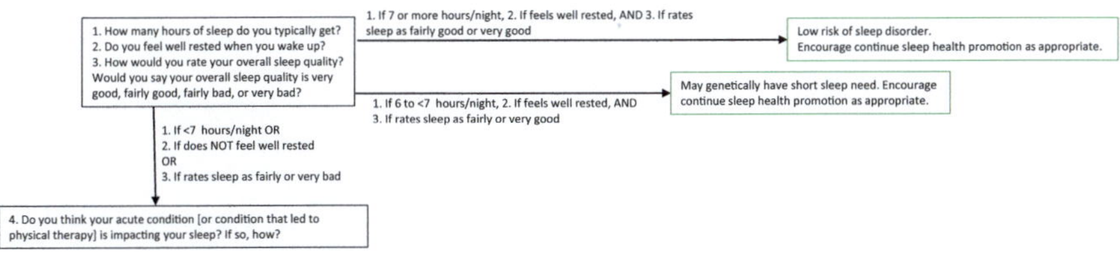

Fig. 7.1 Step 1 of applying the decision tree. (Reprinted with permission from Catherine Siengsukon)

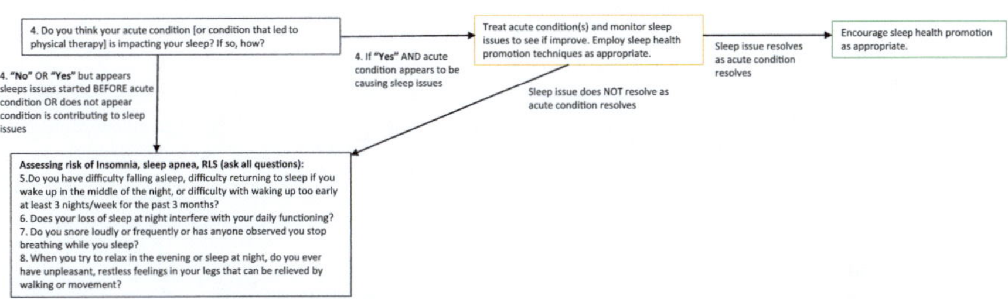

Fig. 7.2 Step 2 of applying the decision tree. (Reprinted with permission from Catherine Siengsukon)

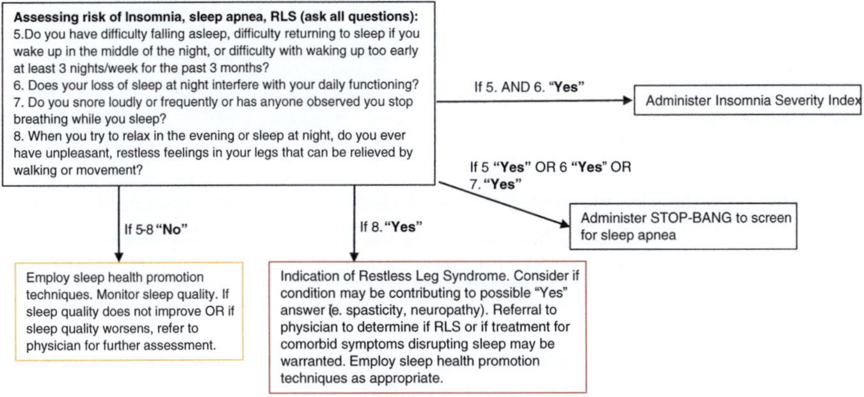

Fig. 7.3 Step 3 of applying decision tree. (Reprinted with permission from Catherine Siengsukon)

solely to her recent MS exacerbation, so the physiotherapists again move down the left-hand side of the decision tree to assess for risk of insomnia, sleep apnea, and restless legs syndrome, (Fig. 7.2) which are the three most common sleep disorders in adults as well as in adults with MS [9, 10].

Based on S.K.L's report that she has difficulty getting back to sleep 3-4x/week after using the bathroom, says she often falls asleep while watching TV and her tiredness is affecting her work productivity, she does not snore, and she does not have an unpleasant urge to move her legs while resting (Fig. 7.3), the

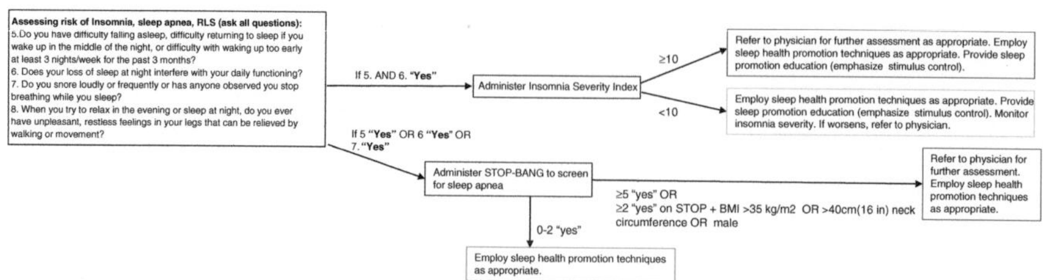

Fig. 7.4 Step 4 of applying decision tree. (Reprinted with permission from Catherine Siengsukon)

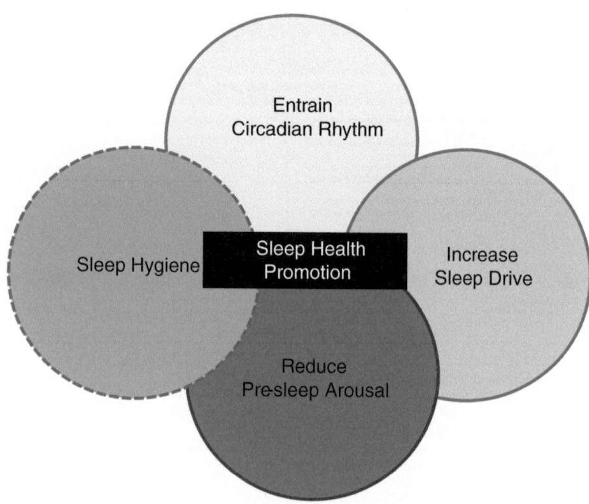

Fig. 7.5 Components of sleep health. Sleep hygiene education is encircled in etched line to indicate it is generally not the focus of sleep health promotion strategies. (Reprinted with permission from Siengsukon C. Physical Therapists' Role in Addressing Acute Insomnia: Could We Prevent Chronic Insomnia- and Chronic Pain? Phys Ther. 2022 Mar 1;102(3):pzab285. doi: 10.1093/ptj/pzab285. PMID: 34939102)

physiotherapist decides to assess for risk of insomnia using the Insomnia Severity Index [11] and obstructive sleep apnea using the STOP-BANG questionnaire [12].

S.K.L scored a 16 on the ISI and answered "yes" to "Do you often feel tired, fatigued, or sleepy during daytime?" and "Do you have or are you being treated for high blood pressure?" Based on the scores on the ISI and STOP-BANG (Fig. 7.4), the physiotherapist decides to refer S.K.L to a psychologist who specializes in treating insomnia using CBT-I (if referral is possible) or a physician for further assessment due to the possible risk of chronic insomnia. The physiotherapist also employs sleep health promotion techniques tailored to the individual.

Physiotherapeutic Intervention

Sleep health promotion techniques that are based on principles of CBT-I and BBT are tailored to the individual. Specially, the sleep health promotion recommendation is based on techniques to entrain circadian rhythm, increase sleep drive, and reduce pre-sleep arousal, as well as general "SHE" recommendations (Fig. 7.5). The SHE recommendations are encircled using an etched line because SHE is generally not sufficient to treat insomnia [13] and is often the control condition in randomized clinical trials. Therefore, SHE is not the focus of sleep health promotion, although studies are needed to determine what interventions are most efficacious to enhance sleep health rather than treat a sleep disorder such as insomnia.

In order to determine which component(s) to emphasize and which sleep health strategies to employ, a more in-depth case conceptualization is needed. Questions to initiate case conceptualization include: (1) On a scale from 0 to 10 with 0 being not important at all and 10 being very important, how important is it to you to improve your sleep? and (2) On a scale from 0 to 10 with 0 being not motivated at all to 10 being very motivated, how motivated are you to improve your sleep? The answers to these questions allow the physiotherapist to consider the individual's readiness to change and coaching strategies to employ to foster behavior change.

To assess if the entraining circadian rhythm is a component warranting emphasis, asking the individual to describe their typical sleep schedule is helpful to determine their typical bedtime and wake time (weekday and weekend if potentially different) to gauge how regular (indicating a well-entrained circadian rhythm so likely not an area of need of emphasis) or variability (indicating circadian rhythm entrainment may need to be emphasized).

To assess the opportunity to increase sleep drive and potential strategies to employ to increase sleep drive, the physiotherapist can ask if the individual takes naps, and if so, for how long and how often. Two other questions to use include asking if they spend time in bed not sleeping (and if so, what they are doing) and what they do for regular exercise. It is also helpful to ask a question such as "Tell me about the schedule of your typical day" because while we often sleep during night-time, what we do during the day can impact our sleep.

To assess opportunities to reduce pre-sleep arousal, the physiotherapist can ask the individual to describe their typical bedtime routine, what they do for relaxation (gauging type, regularity, amount, timing, and if occurs as part of the bedtime routine or, throughout the day as needed), and for this case in particular, what she thinks is contributing to her difficulty falling back to sleep after she gets up to use the restroom. She reported that she thinks about "things" but strategies that are recommended will likely differ depending on what is contributing to her difficulty falling back to sleep. For example, if she is thinking about her to-do list for the upcoming day, suggesting she has a set "planning time" to plan the following day and write a "to-do list" can be helpful; if she is ruminating about past life events, suggesting she works with a therapist or counselor to manage ruminations can be helpful. Also, reducing sympathetic nervous system activity by using relaxation training (i.e., deep breathing, progressive muscle relaxation, and meditation) can reduce somatic and cognitive arousal and promote sleep [14, 15].

The term "sleep hygiene" generally refers to behaviors and environmental factors that impact sleep, such as caffeine and alcohol consumption, nicotine use, as well as the bedroom/household environment. Environmental factors include sleeping alone vs. sharing the bed with a partner or co-sleeping with a child, amount of ambient light, noise, temperature, and perceived comfort of the sleeping environment. Ask the individual to describe their sleep environment (i.e., location, set-up, bed partner, comfort level, restful, and safety) to gauge the environment. Ask the individual if they use caffeine, alcohol, and tobacco products, and if so, how often and how much. Also, ask the individual to describe their water/fluid consumption and the time of day they consume fluids.

The answers given to the above questions and appropriate follow-up questions will allow the therapist to adequately and appropriately determine factors that are likely disrupting as well as promoting sleep health. Furthermore, the answers will provide information regarding areas to focus and tailor sleep health promotion techniques.

For this particular case, the primary sleep issue for S.K.L. appears to be that she has difficulty falling back to sleep after waking up to use the bathroom. The focus of sleep health promotion for S.K.L. should be (Fig. 7.6): (1) stimulus control (while being mindful of fall risk and mobility limitations; part of increasing sleep drive), and (2) stress/worry management (part of reducing pre-sleep arousal). The general recommendation for stimulus control is to get out of bed if unable to fall asleep in what feels like 15–20 min, go somewhere else, and do a mildly pleasant, minimally stimulating, distracting activity (i.e., listen to an audiobook or music) until adequately sleepy [16, 17]. Ideally, light is kept to a minimum except for what is needed to navigate safely to reduce the impact on the circadian system. However,

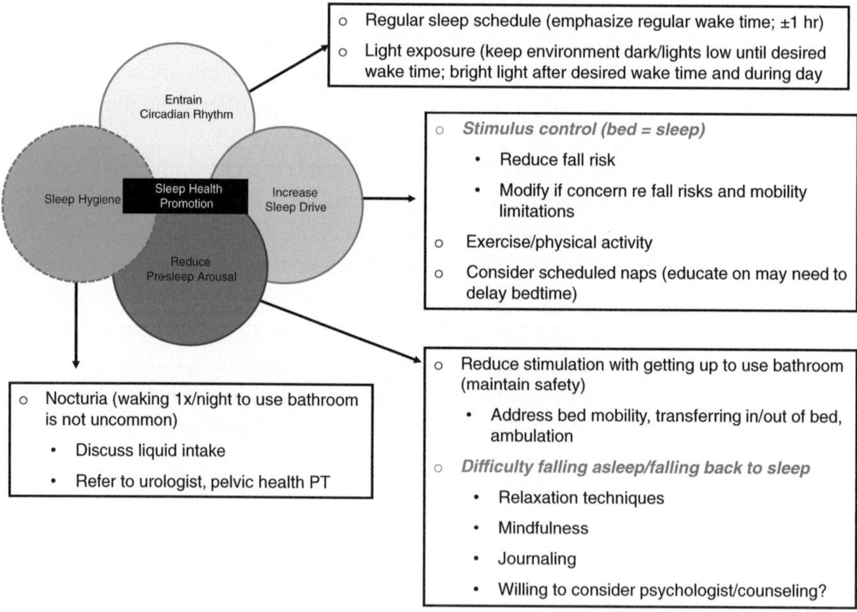

Fig. 7.6 Sleep health promotion strategies. Areas to emphasize are noted in grey italic. (Reprinted with permission from Siengsukon C. Physical Therapists' Role in Addressing Acute Insomnia: Could We Prevent Chronic Insomnia-and Chronic Pain? Phys Ther. 2022 Mar 1;102(3):pzab285. doi: 10.1093/ptj/pzab285. PMID: 34939102)

depending on S.K.L.'s mobility limitations and fall risk, stimulus control may need to be modified so the relaxing, distracting activity is performed in bed for safety purposes. The strategies to address stress/worry will largely depend on the factor(s) that S.K.L thinks is contributing to her stress and worry as discussed previously.

Other opportunities to enhance sleep health are to emphasize exercise to enhance sleep drive and, if a scheduled nap is needed to address fatigue due to MS exacerbation, provide education to S.K.L. that she may need to delay her bedtime until she is adequately sleepy (this supports the concept of stimulus control so the brain learns to associate the bed with sleep). Other opportunities include addressing bed mobility, transferring in/out of bed, and ambulation to reduce stimulation with getting up to use the bathroom and to maintain safety. Because S.K.L. is waking up earlier than her preferred/typical wake time, a recommendation would be to keep the environment dark (or lights as low as needed for safety) until the preferred/typical wake time and then be exposed to bright light at the desired wake time (or upon awakening when she does wake up at the preferred/typical wake time) for 10–20 min to aid in entraining her circadian rhythm. Also, address SHE factors that may interfere with sleep health (i.e., alcohol, nicotine, and caffeine use) that emerged during the case conceptualization process. It is not unusual for an individual to need to use the bathroom during the night; however, a conversation regarding her liquid intake timing and amount might be warranted. Also, a referral to a pelvic health physiotherapist and/or urologist to discuss possible neurogenic bladder may be warranted.

References

1. Siengsukon C, Alshehri M, Aldughmi M. Self-report sleep quality combined with sleep time variability distinguishes differences in fatigue, anxiety, and depression in individuals with multiple sclerosis: a secondary analysis. Mult Scler J Exp Transl Clin. 2018;4(4):205521731881592.
2. Taphoorn M, et al. Fatigue, sleep disturbances and circadian rhythm in multiple sclerosis. J Neurol. 1993;240(7):446–8.
3. Fleming WE, Pollak CP. Sleep disorders in multiple sclerosis. Semin Neurol. 2005;25(1):64–8.
4. Lobentanz IS, et al. Factors influencing quality of life in multiple sclerosis patients: disability, depressive mood, fatigue and sleep quality. Acta Neurol Scand. 2004;110:6–13.
5. Merlino G, et al. Prevalence of 'poor sleep' among patients with multiple sclerosis: an independent predictor of mental and physical status. Sleep Med. 2009;10:26–34.
6. Buysse DJ. Sleep health: can we define it? Does it matter? Sleep. 2014;37(1):9–17.
7. Ravyts SG, et al. Sleep health as measured by RU SATED: a psychometric evaluation. Behav Sleep Med. 2019;19:1–9.
8. Siengsukon CF, et al. Application accuracy of the sleep decision tree to standardized patient cases by physiotherapists: an observational study. Physiother Theory Pract. 2022;38(13):2874–83.
9. Braley TJ, et al. Sleep and cognitive function in multiple sclerosis. Sleep. 2016;39(8):1525–33.
10. Veauthier C. Sleep disorders in multiple sclerosis. Review. Curr Neurol Neurosci Rep. 2015;15(5):21.
11. Morin CM, et al. The insomnia severity index: psychometric indicators to detect insomnia cases and evaluate treatment response. Sleep. 2011;34(5):601–8.
12. Chung F, Abdullah HR, Liao P. STOP-Bang questionnaire: a practical approach to screen for obstructive sleep apnea. Chest. 2016;149(3):631–8.

13. Edinger JD, et al. Behavioral and psychological treatments for chronic insomnia disorder in adults: an American Academy of sleep medicine clinical practice guideline. J Clin Sleep Med. 2021;17(2):255–62.
14. Morgenthaler T, et al. Practice parameters for the psychological and behavioral treatment of insomnia: an update. An american academy of sleep medicine report. Sleep. 2006;29(11):1415–9.
15. Jerath R, Beveridge C, Barnes VA. Self-regulation of breathing as an adjunctive treatment of insomnia. Front Psych. 2018;9:780.
16. Trauer JM, et al. Cognitive behavioral therapy for chronic insomnia: a systematic review and meta-analysis. Ann Intern Med. 2015;163(3):191–204.
17. Medicine, A.A.o.S. Healty Sleep Habits. 2020; http://sleepeducation.org/essentials-in-sleep/healthy-sleep-habits.

Chapter 8
Surgical Menopause, Musculoskeletal Pain, and Insomnia

Cristina Frange ⓘ

Introduction

Insomnia may occur as a result of increased sleep latency (insomnia onset) or sleep fragmentation (maintenance insomnia), or early morning awakening (terminal insomnia), or any of the combinations. The diagnosis of insomnia is clinical (no polysomnography exam is necessary), and consists of sleep history (i.e., sleep habits, sleep environment, work schedules, and circadian factors). Insomnia is often accompanied by pain [1], having a bidirectional relationship. In this cycle, insomnia increases pain sensitivity and pain contributes to the occurrence of sleep fragmentation and disorders such as insomnia [2]. Insomnia and pain are both symptoms of climacteric (i.e., symptoms that may accompany the physiological decline of ovarian function) and during the postmenopausal stage (i.e., the stage after the cessation of menses, indicating the end of the reproductive life) are known with perceived worse sleep by women [3]. These "forced" climacteric symptoms may be even worse when surgical menopause occurs (estrogen and androgen levels are significantly and speedily reduced), as the physiologic changes of menopause occur quickly.

Global Posture Reeducation (GPR) rehabilitation is based on an integrated idea of the muscular system as formed by muscle chains, which can face shortening resulting from constitutional, behavioral, and psychological factors [4]. The rationale of GPR is to stretch the shortened muscles using the property of viscoelastic

C. Frange (✉)
Neurology and Neurosurgery Department, Federal University of São Paulo (UNIFESP), São Paulo, SP, Brazil

C. Frange (ed.), *Clinical Cases in Sleep Physical Therapy*, https://doi.org/10.1007/978-3-031-38340-3_8

tissue and to enhance the contraction of the antagonist's muscles, thus avoiding postural asymmetry and compensations [5]. As an isometric exercise, done individually by a physiotherapist specialized in GPR, the rationale of this clinical case was that GPR could decrease pain and insomnia, therefore, decreasing the postmenopausal symptoms.

Patient Information

S.R.A., a 43-year-old married woman with no children, sought treatment for insomnia prescribed by her gynecologist. At the age of 39, she underwent an oophorectomy, salpingectomy, and hysterectomy due to endometriosis—and all the symptoms started! The patient was at the early surgical postmenopausal stage, facing climacteric symptoms (i.e., insomnia, vasomotor symptoms (hot flashes) vaginal dryness, mood changes, and musculoskeletal pain). She was not in hormonal therapy. She was a schoolteacher but unable to work for the last 4 years because of generalized myalgia. She reported being unable to have a life because of constant pain, including difficulty walking, being sedentary, with a dislike for exercise.

Clinical Findings

Her medical history consisted of dyslipidemia, hypertension, and previous endometriosis. She was in the use of anti-inflammatory, *cimicifuga racemose*, a phytotherapy drug used in the treatment of climacteric symptoms, and antidepressants.

At her first visit, S.R.A. presented with the climacteric syndrome as she complained of insomnia, paresthesia in both arms, nervousness, melancholia, headache, vasomotor symptoms (hot flashes and sweating), arthralgia and myalgia, and reported maximum pain intensity (Table 8.1). The pain was generalized, but mainly in the knee and in the lower back. She complained about her sleep, having poor quality of sleep and never refreshing when waking up, reported sleep latency of 3 h, night sweats and nocturia (average of 5 times per night) that disrupted her sleep. She reported that each time she woke up at night she needed about 1 h to get back to sleep. Her sleep routine was: going to bed at 1:30 and waking up at 9 h. She also complained of daytime somnolence and memory impairments. She denied sleep medications and snoring.

Table 8.1 Before and after GPR intervention measurements

	Before	After
Pain intensity (painVas)	10	1
Insomnia severity (ISI)	28	6
Sleep quality (PSQI)	12	4
Menopausal symptoms (BKI)	29	9
Vasomotor (hot flashes, sweat)	Severe	Mild
Paresthesia	Severe	None
Insomnia	Severe	Mild
Nervousness	Severe	None
Melancholia	Moderate	None
Dizziness/vertigo	None	None
Arthralgia/myalgia	Moderate	Mild
Weakness/fatigue	None	None
Headaches	Mild	Mild
Palpitation	None	None
Formication	None	Mild

PainVAS pain visual analog scale ranges from 0 "no pain" to 10 "worst pain imaginable" [6], *ISI* insomnia severity index evaluates the nature, severity, and impact of insomnia, scores range from 0 to 28, 0–7: absence of insomnia; 8–14: subthreshold insomnia; 15–21: moderate insomnia; and 22–28: severe insomnia [7], *PSQI* pittsburgh sleep quality index assesses sleep quality and disturbances over 1 month, and a PSQI ≤ 5 indicates good sleep quality, while >5 is associated with poor sleep quality, and > 10 indicates sleep disturbances [8], *BKI* Blatt-Kupperman Index includes 11 symptoms and quantifies climacteric symptoms, rating from 0 (none) to 3 (severe), and the final score ranges from ≤ 19: mild, 20–35: moderate, and > 35: severe [9]

Regarding posture, she had pelvic anteversion, lumbar hyperlordosis, thoracic hyperkyphosis, protracted and inwardly rotated shoulders, knees valgus, and right *cavus* foot, resulting in postural dysfunction.

Diagnostic Assessment

Her medical diagnoses were climacteric syndrome and insomnia disorder, specifically the onset and maintenance of insomnia.

The following measures were performed pre- and post-intervention: (1) pain intensity was measured by Visual Analogue Scale (painVAS from 0 to 10) [6]; (2) insomnia severity was assessed by the Insomnia Severity Index (ISI) [7]; (3) sleep quality was assessed by the Pittsburgh Sleep Quality Index (PSQI) [8]; (4) menopausal symptoms were assessed by the Blatt-Kupperman Index (BKI) [9].

Physiotherapeutic Intervention

The patient attended 16 sessions of GPR, weekly, approximately 60 min each, individualized. GPR sessions were focused on stimulating awareness of the body image, balancing muscle function, stabilizing the spine, and correcting posture alterations. At the beginning of each session, 5 min of *Pompage* maneuvers were performed in association with breathing exercises, while the patient lays down on her back with all limbs relaxed, to stretch the *fasciae* that connect the shoulder and cervical spine muscles. As the patient had anterior and posterior impairments, two postures were used, one posture at each session, for about 30 min:

1. to stretch the anterior muscle chain (i.e., diaphragm, pectoralis minor, scalene, sternocleidomastoid, intercostalis, iliopsoas, arm, forearm, and hand flexors), the patient lays in the supine position with flexed, abducted and laterally rotated hips, soles of the feet touching each other, the upper limbs abducted at 30°, the forearms supine and retroversion of the pelvis (lumbar spine stayed stabilized), the lower limbs were extended as much as possible while sustaining the tibiotarsal angle at 90° (Fig. 8.1).

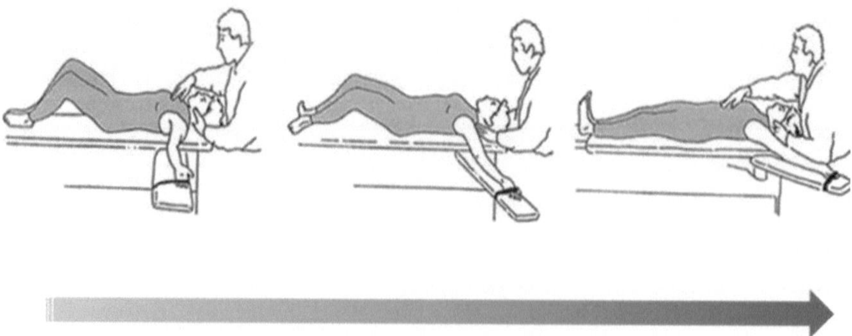

Fig. 8.1 Anterior muscle chain stretching in supine. The arrow indicates the progression of the posture: leg extension progression

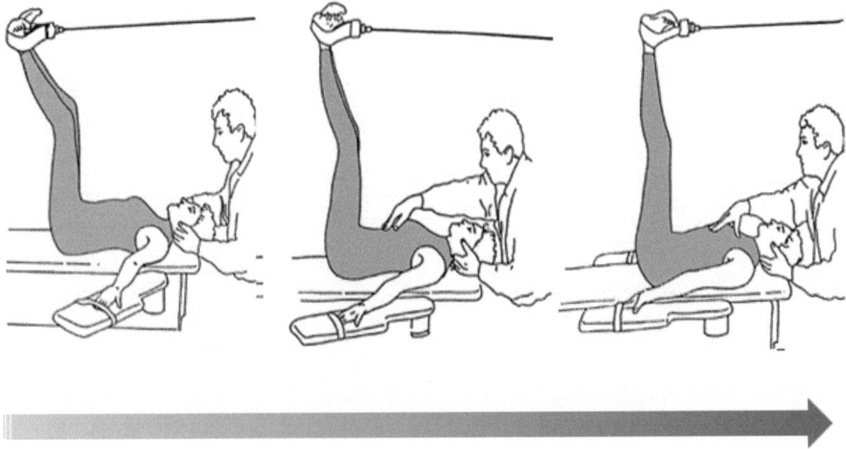

Fig. 8.2 Posterior muscle chain stretching in supine. The arrow indicates the progression of the posture: leg flexion progression

2. to stretch the posterior muscle chain (i.e., upper trapezius, levator scapulae, suboccipital, erector spine, gluteus maximus, ischiotibial, triceps surae, and foot intrinsic muscles), the patient lays in the supine position with the occipital, lumbar, and sacral spine stabilized, with the lower limbs at 90° hip flexion, and performed gradual knee extensions as far as she could (Fig. 8.2).

The PT used verbal commands and manual contact to maintain the alignment and make the necessary postural corrections, to optimize the stretching and avoid compensatory movements. After the GPR posture, techniques integrating static and dynamic functions were engaged for about 10 min to allow the patient to experience and use the recovered flexibility in her functional activities (e.g., walking, bending forward, dressing, or reaching items at the bottom).

Follow-Up and Outcomes

After the 4-month treatment, the patient improved her body posture, especially the position of the shoulders, neck, and head, as well as her *cavus* foot. She reported a decrease in pain intensity (Table 8.1). Her sleep issues were better, she had no longer an insomnia diagnosis as reported by her gynecologist, and presented with no clinically significant insomnia on ISI. Her sleep quality also ameliorated, as she reported having good sleep quality, getting to bed at 23 h, having about 20 min of sleep onset, and waking up at 9 h. Her sleep perception was 8 h. Her climacteric symptoms improved from severe to mild symptoms, mainly due to sleep and pain issues being resolved.

Unexpectedly, we noticed an improvement in weaning medication for pain (e.g., anti-inflammatories), vasomotor symptoms (e.g., *cimicifuga racemose*), and antidepressants, with the constant monitoring of her physician. To maintain her well-being, she started a physical activity routine of walking 5 times a week for about 30 min.

Discussion

In the present study, GPR led to a reduction in pain, improved self-rated sleep quality, and insomnia diagnosis and perception, therefore improving the climacteric symptoms, and unpredictably, the medication dependence. Somehow, GPR dissociated the sleep-pain interaction.

There is plenty of evidence in the literature that postmenopausal women complain of diffuse musculoskeletal pain, combined with poor sleep quality and/or quantity, fatigue, and anxiety [10–12]. This combination of symptoms can be similar to fibromyalgia and has been questioned by some authors as part of the climacteric symptoms [13]. Sleep plays an important role in pain management. Clinical and epidemiological studies demonstrated that individuals with chronic pain have a variety of sleep disorders, including insomnia [14, 15].

GPR induced a hypoalgesic effect, in line with other investigations [4, 5, 16, 17]. Our PT sessions aimed to "normalize" the tone in the muscular chains, providing a neuro-muscular re-education that involved stretching and acting upon the electrical activity of the muscles. The used stretched positions evolved gradually from an initial position with minimum tension to progressive stretching (isometric exercise) until the final tension is reached at the end of the posture. S.R.A. experienced changes in viscoelastic properties of musculotendinous structures, as neural modifications characterized by muscle spindle influence, Golgi tendon organ, and joint receptors [18, 19].

Therefore, postural modifications might not be attributed only to the plasticity of the tissues involved. There might have happened psychomotor and proprioceptive reprogramming, which modified her corporal scheme [20]. The proprioceptive stimuli of this technique produce an overload of the muscles that may have reduced pain. Stretching can promote an amplified joint range of motion due to decreased passive resistance to stretching (e.g., decrease in muscle stiffness or increase in muscle compliance), especially when the duration of stretching is longer, contributing to pain decrease [21].

Despite the few gains in posture, we noticed that the patient weaned from medication to pain and depressive symptoms. The postmenopausal symptoms might have ameliorated because of improvement in pain and insomnia. The medication could have interfered with sleep and contributed to insomnia and poor sleep quality. However, with the PT sessions, the patient herself indicated that she had "forgotten" to take the medication, and her gynecologist prescribed the gradual washout of the medication. Therefore, the literature does not present until now any studies that had the same repercussion regarding medications when treated with GPR.

Initial findings are encouraging but warrant further investigation, especially regarding mechanisms of action and long-term follow-up. GPR seems to be a great nonpharmacological treatment for disentangling the sleep-pain relationship.

References

1. Andersen ML, Araujo P, Frange C, Tufik S. Sleep disturbance and pain: a tale of two common problems. Chest. 2018;154(5):1249–59.
2. Schuh-Hofer S, Wodarski R, Pfau DB, Caspani O, Magerl W, Kennedy JD, Treede RD. One night of total sleep deprivation promotes a state of generalized hyperalgesia: a surrogate pain model to study the relationship between insomnia and pain. Pain. 2013;154:1613–21.
3. Shaver JL, Woods NK. Sleep and menopause: a narrative review. Menopause. 2015;22:1–17.
4. Pillastrini P, Banchelli F, Guccione A, Di Ciaccio E, Violante FS, Brugnettini M, Vanti C. Global postural reeducation in patients with chronic nonspecific neck pain: cross-over analysis of a randomized controlled trial. Med Lav. 2018;109(1):16–30.
5. Castagnoli C, Cecchi F, Del Canto A, Paperini A, Boni R, Pasquini G, Vannetti F, Macchi C. Effects in short and long term of global postural reeducation (GPR) on chronic low back pain: a controlled study with one-year follow-up. ScientificWorldJournal. 2015;2015:271436.
6. Price DD, McGrath PA, Rafii A, Buckingham B. The validation of visual analog scales as ratio scale measures for chronic and experimental pain. Pain. 1983;17:45–56.
7. Bastien CH, Vallières A, Morin CM. Validation of the insomnia severity index as an outcome measure for insomnia research. Sleep Med. 2001;2:297–307.
8. Buysse DJ, Reynolds CF, Monk TH, Berman SR, Kupfer DJ. The Pittsburgh sleep quality index: a new instrument for psychiatric practice and research. Psychiatry Res. 1989;28:193–213.
9. Kupperman HS, Wetchler BB, Blatt MH. Contemporary therapy of the menopausal syndrome. J Am Med Assoc. 1959;171:1627–37.
10. Frange C, Hachul H, Hirotsu C, Tufik S, Andersen ML. Temporal analysis of chronic musculoskeletal pain and sleep in postmenopausal women. J Clin Sleep Med. 2019;15:223.
11. Frange C, Naufel MF, Andersen ML, Ribeiro EB, Girão MJBC, Tufik S, Hachul H. Impact of insomnia on pain in postmenopausal women. Climacteric. 2017;20(3):262–7.
12. Frange C, Hirotsu C, Hachul H, Pires JS, Bittencourt L, Tufik S, Andersen ML. Musculoskeletal pain and the reproductive life stage in women: is there a relationship? Climacteric. 2016;19(3):279–84.
13. Blümel JE, Chedraui P, Baron G, Belzares E, Bencosme A, Calle A, Danckers L, Espinoza MT, Flores D, Gomez G, Hernandez-Bueno JA, Izaguirre H, Leon-Leon P, Lima S, Mezones-Holguin E, Monterrosa A, Mostajo D, Navarro D, Ojeda E, Onatra W, Royer M, Soto E, Tserotas K, Vallejo MS, Collaborative Group for Research of the climacteric in Latin America (REDLINC). Menopausal symptoms appear before menopause and persist 5 years beyond a detailed analysis of a multinational study. Climacteric. 2012;15(6):542–51.
14. Morin CM, Gibson D, Wade J. Self-reported sleep and mood disturbance in chronic pain patients. Clin J Pain. 1998;14:311–4.
15. Sivertsen B, Krokstad S, Overland S, Mykletun A. The epidemiology of insomnia: associations with physical and mental health. The HUNT-2 study. J Psychosom Res. 2009;67:109–16.

16. Bonetti F, Curti S, Mattioli S, Mugnai R, Vanti C, Violante FS, Pillastrini P. Effectiveness of a 'Global postural Reeducation' program for persistent low back pain: a non-randomized controlled trial. BMC Musculoskelet Disord. 2010;11:285.
17. De Lima e Sá Resende F, Vanti C, Banchelli F, Trani Brandao JG, Oliveira Amorim JB, Villafañe JH, Guccione A, Pillastrini P. The effect of global postural reeducation on body weight distribution in sitting posture and on musculoskeletal pain. A pilot study. Med Lav. 2017;108(3):187–96.
18. Avela J, Finni T, Liikavaiinio T, Niemelã E, Komi PV. Neural and mechanical responses of the triceps surae muscle group after 1h of repeated fast passive stretches. J Applied Physiol. 2004;96:2325–32.
19. Weir DE, Tingley J, Elder GCB. Acute passive stretching alters the mechanical properties of human plantar flexors and the optimal angle for maximal voluntary contraction. Eur J Appl Physiol. 2005;93(5–6):614–23.
20. Lapierre A. Cinesiologia reeducação postural: reeducação psicomotora. 6a ed. São Paulo, SP: Manole; 1987.
21. McHugh MP, Cosgrave CH. To stretch or not to stretch: the role of stretching in injury prevention and performance. Scand J Med Sci Sports. 2010;20(2):169–81.

Chapter 9
Fatigue and Sleep Disturbances in a Man with Parkinson's Disease

Mayis Aldughmi ⓘD

Introduction

Parkinson's disease (PD) is a neurodegenerative disease characterized by motor symptoms such as tremors, rigidity, and bradykinesia [1]. Non-motor symptoms such as cognitive dysfunction, fatigue, and sleep disturbances are also common in the PD population that often precedes motor impairments [2, 3]. Sleep disturbances are one of the most common non-motor symptoms in PD with a prevalence that can exceed 80% even at early stages of the disease [4, 5]. REM sleep behavior disorder (RBD), insomnia, restless leg syndrome (RLS), sleep fragmentation, sleep apnea, and excessive daytime sleepiness can all negatively affect the quality-of-life of these individuals [5]. Specifically, sleep fragmentation is common in PD, which is defined as disruption of nocturnal sleep presented as an increased number and lengthy arousals during the sleep-wake cycle [6]. Factors that may influence sleep fragmentation in PD are diverse such as muscle cramps, nocturia, insomnia, sleep apnea, and limb movement sleep disorders [7, 8]. Unfortunately, sleep fragmentation in PD can lead to abnormal changes in sleep parameters such as increase in wake after sleep onset, leading to fatigue and excessive sleepiness in daytime [9]. Evidence suggests that nonpharmacological treatments such as exercise therapy can have positive effects on various sleep disturbances in people with PD [10]. In this clinical case, we discuss the physical therapy (PT) assessment and management of poor sleep in a 62-year-old male with PD.

M. Aldughmi (✉)
Department of Physiotherapy, School of Rehabilitation Sciences, University of Jordan, Amman, Jordan

C. Frange (ed.), *Clinical Cases in Sleep Physical Therapy*,
https://doi.org/10.1007/978-3-031-38340-3_9

"""

Patient Information

A 62-year-old man, F.M.C. with a 9-year history of idiopathic PD (stage 2.5 on the Modified Hoehn and Yahr Scale) presented to the PT clinic after referral from a neurologist for further assessment and to maintain his functional status. The patient is a retired businessman who lives with his wife in a one-story house. He currently takes a low dose of Levodopa and is compliant with his medication and sometimes takes a painkiller for uncomfortable cramping in his legs and feet. He is a non-smoker and drinks one glass of wine in the evening. He enjoys gardening but reported feeling unsteady lately which caused less frequent activities in his home garden. The patient also reported feelings of exhaustion during the day and reported that for almost 1 year, he takes long naps (~ 1.5 h) specially in the afternoon. He also reported having difficulty falling asleep and staying asleep during the night, with frequent arousals from sleep. Regarding the current functional status of the patient, he has no problems in bed mobility, or bathing/toileting, he ambulates independently without any assistive device, only drives if necessary, and reported less confidence in walking outside the house specially in his home garden. Patient does not perform any form of regular exercise.

Clinical Findings

The PT conducted a thorough physical assessment of the patient and identified the following: The patient posture was mildly stooped with a forward head position, his gait was slow (mild bradykinesia), active range of motion (AROM) and passive range of motion (PROM) of upper extremity revealed limited shoulder flexion and abduction (left > right), AROM and PROM of lower extremity revealed limited dorsiflexion bilaterally (left > right) with mild cogwheel rigidity, trunk rotation was also limited bilaterally. There was apparent weakness in antigravity muscles in the neck, hip, and back extensors, as well as hip flexors. Other neurological tests including sensation, reflexes, and tone were normal.

Balance was assessed using the Berg Balance Scale (BBS): 42/56 (standing items had the least scores), standard Timed-Up-Go (TUG) test score was 13.5 s.

Diagnostic Assessment

Upon further investigation by the PT, the patient reported that his neurologist referred him to a sleep specialist a month ago where he undertook a polysomnography (PSG) test. The PT requested to have a look at his sleep report, which confirmed sleep fragmentation indicated by low sleep efficiency (63%), high wake after sleep onset (WASO) (62 min), and high nocturnal arousal index (14 arousals per hour). The patient has a scheduled appointment in 2 months to follow up with the neurologist and sleep specialist.

Based on the symptoms reported by the patient and his current medical condition, the PT used the following self-reported outcome measures: Activities-Specific Balance Confidence Scale (ABC Scale): 65% (indicating moderate confidence in maintaining balance while performing various daily activities),

Parkinson's Disease Questionnaire (PDQ-39) quality-of-life measure: 32% (low dimensions include: mobility, bodily discomfort, and activities of daily living), Fatigue Severity Scale (FSS): 48 (indicating high levels of fatigue), Parkinson's Disease Sleep Scale (PDSS): 84 (indicating disturbed nocturnal sleep, scores on items such as frequent urination at night, painful muscle cramps, and sleepiness during the day were high), Insomnia Severity Index (ISI): 15 (indicating moderate severity insomnia), Epworth Sleepiness Scale (ESS): 16 (indicating excessive daytime sleepiness).

Major clinical findings from the physical objective assessment indicated that the patient may be at increased risk of falls mainly due to poor posture, weak antigravity muscles, dyskinesia, decreased range of motion (ROM), rigidity in lower extremities, poor balance (BSS score less than the cut-off of 45, and TUG score more than the PD cutoff of 12 s), fear of falling and low confidence in performing daily activities. This might explain the unsteadiness the patient reported and the decreased participation in the enjoyable activities he used to do. In addition to that, the PT detected high levels of fatigue and an overall poor sleep quality, specifically a moderate risk for insomnia and excessive daytime sleepiness. These symptoms are highly associated with the confirmed diagnosis of sleep fragmentation, the daily napping, and exhaustion the patient reported.

Another major finding from the diagnostic assessment by the PT was the muscle cramps reported by the patient that are often painful and uncomfortable. The PT discovered that the patient reported these symptoms at night as indicated in the PDSS scale. SF can be influenced by painful muscle cramps among patients with PD.

The patient's overall health has declined as indicated by low scores on the quality-of-life measure (PDQ-39). If the patient's fatigue, physical deconditioning, and poor sleep was not managed, his health may deteriorate more further limiting his quality-of-life. Lifestyle modifications, fatigue management, exercise therapy, and functional management may decrease the patient's sleep fragmentation and other limiting symptoms ultimately improving his health status.

Physiotherapeutic Intervention

F.M.C. worked with the PT for 12 weeks. His treatment is included in the following Table 9.1.

Table 9.1 The physical therapy treatment protocol used with the patient

Treatment	Rationale	Frequency	Intensity
Sleep hygiene education (SHE)	First explained the role of PT in sleep management. SHE to promote sleep health and modify behaviors that interfere with sleep such as: • avoid alcohol and caffeine in the evenings at least 4 h before bedtime • do not drink water right before bedtime to avoid frequent urination during the night • make yourself comfortable in bed (may use pillows) with proper sleep positions to avoid discomfort specially for lower limbs Emphasis on sleep regularity and avoiding long naps late in the day	Started from initial assessment	As appropriate
Education on energy conservation techniques	To manage fatigue patient was instructed to: • prioritize activities: To reduce the overall energy expenditure throughout the day. Identify the essential tasks that need to be done • pace yourself: Break up activities into smaller segments with resting periods in between to conserve energy • modify your environment: For example, use a raised toilet seat to conserve energy while getting ready in the morning • planning daily activities in advance to avoid unnecessary stress and energy expenditure • use assistive devices: Use a cane in outdoor activities to conserve energy • practicing relaxation techniques or meditation, patient was encouraged to join a yoga class • A short nap at noon may conserve energy for the rest of the day Exercise therapy (explained in detail below)	Started from initial assessment	Education as appropriate Nap at noon less than 90 min

Table 9.1 (continued)

Treatment	Rationale	Frequency	Intensity
Gait	Nordic walking with auditory cues using a metronome. Nordic walking improves postural control and coordination. The cues improve gait speed and stride length which boosts confidence	3x/week	Inside and outside PT clinic for a total of 300 m
Balance	Balance training activities focusing on standing items (tandem stance, feet together, eyes closed, turning 360°)	2x/week in clinic and at home	20 min
Muscle cramps	• Stretching to reduce cramps and stiffness and improve flexibility: Static stretches for calf muscles, toes extensors and flexors, and knee extensors. Dynamic stretches for upper and lower extremities (arms and leg swings), and trunk rotations • Therapeutic massage for lower limbs Exercise therapy (explained in detail below)	Stretches 3x/week at the beginning and ending of every session. Patient performed stretching at home every day Therapeutic massage for lower limbs 3x/week	Static stretches 3 repetitions each holding 30 s Dynamic stretches 5 min daily Therapeutic massage for lower limbs as tolerated
Combined exercise program	To manage poor sleep, fatigue, muscle cramps, strengthen weak muscles, and improve balance/gait impairments • Aerobic exercise in clinic on a seated bicycle and as patient improved a treadmill was used. At home patient encouraged to walk, swim, or join a dance class • Resistance training using TheraBand and cuff weights of varying intensities. As well as postural general strengthening exercises	1 h long session 2x/week on separate days from other treatments. 30 min for aerobic exercise and 30 min for resistance training	Aerobic exercise: Moderate intensity program at 60%–80% of maximal heart rate Resistance training: Muscle groups 3 sets of 10 repetitions at 60% 1RM. TheraBand and cuff weights progressed based on patient tolerance and improvements

Follow-Up and Outcomes

After F.M.C's initial assessment and the beginning of the therapy, the patient supervised sessions progressively decreased in number as the patient was progressing. The patient in the first 3 weeks was coming to therapy three times per week, then 2x per week, then once a week for a total of 12 weeks. At 12 weeks, a follow-up assessment was made. The patient presented to the clinic with improved gait, increased

ROM, and increased muscle strength in antigravity muscles. Outcome scores were as follows: ABC: 85%, PDQ-39: 24%, FSS: 38, BBS: 38/56, TUG: 10.5, PDSS: 72, ISI: 11, ESS: 12.

In addition to these measures, adherence to home exercises was measured by giving the patient a home exercise log after the first session. The patient reported daily when and what exercises were performed. The patient also reported in this log any incidence of a fall. After 12 weeks, the patient compliance to the home program was 65% with no reporting of any fall. Also, the patient was given a sleep diary to record the times he goes to bed, falls asleep, and wakes up every night. The PT noticed that the number of times he woke up during the night toward the end of week 12 was less compared to week 1 (6 times vs. 11 times). The patient in general, reported feeling more energetic, he is participating more in the community specially through a yoga class he and his wife joined. He also reported that he has less muscle cramps during the night and only naps if he was feeling tired. The patient was encouraged by the PT to continue following sleep hygiene behaviors, his exercises, and fatigue management. The PT asked the patient to come for follow-up to the clinic once every 3 weeks.

Overall, the patient showed improvements in his sleep quality and other impairments. Symptoms that seemed to minimally resolve were his mild stooped posture and balance impairments, as well as frequent urination during the night. The PT asked the patient to schedule an appointment with his neurologist for a follow-up neurological assessment with an emphasis on nocturia. The PT also recommended the patient to schedule a follow-up PSG assessment with the sleep specialist to investigate any objective improvements in his sleep fragmentation.

Discussion

Sleep disturbances in patients with PD are prevalent and multidimensional associated with various symptoms and factors [5]. Sleep fragmentation was recently reported as an important clinical characteristic of sleep disorders among patients with PD [6]. The pathophysiology of the disease together with frequent motor manifestations increases the incidence of sleep fragmentation in the PD population [5]. Treatment options can be nonpharmacological and can have a significant impact on improving sleep quality in patients with PD [10]. This clinical case highlighted the important role physical therapists can offer to manage sleep disturbances in patients with PD using a holistic approach. The therapist took into consideration the different factors that might influence the patient's sleep fragmentation and tried to manage each one separately and comprehensively. Exercise therapy specially combined programs of endurance, strengthening, and flexibility exercise previously improved various sleep disturbances in patients with PD, but there is no consensus on the optimal type and intensity of exercise to recommend in this population [10].

Limitations in this case do exist. The therapist did not assess a major factor that is highly associated with poor sleep and specifically sleep fragmentation, which is psychological status. Evidence suggests that sleep disturbances including sleep fragmentation are risk factors for conditions such as anxiety, depression, and cognitive impairments [11, 12]. The patient in the case may have symptoms of depression that influenced his recovery, this might explain his frequent long naps, fatigue, and why he was compliant only for 65% of the home exercises. Also, instead of relying only on PSG as an objective measure of sleep, The PT had the ability to use actigraphy, which is a common objective measure of sleep that is highly associated with the gold standard PSG [13]. It is less invasive, portable, and less costly compared to PSG [13]. Actigraphy provides objective scores of various sleep parameters including sleep fragmentation [14].

In conclusion, PT can be an important therapy for managing sleep problems in PD. By incorporating exercise, education, movement strategies, fatigue management, and relaxation techniques, PT can help improve sleep quality and promote overall well-being in patients with PD.

References

1. Radhakrishnan DM, Goyal V. Parkinson's disease: a review. Neurol India. 2018;66(7):26.
2. Frange C, Filho LHP, Aguilar AC, Coelho FMS. Exercise for "sleep rehabilitation" in Parkinson's disease. Mov Disord. 2020;35(7):1285.
3. Schapira AH, Chaudhuri KR, Jenner P. Non-motor features of Parkinson disease. Nat Rev Neurosci. 2017;18(7):435–50.
4. Albers JA, Chand P, Anch AM. Multifactorial sleep disturbance in Parkinson's disease. Sleep Med. 2017;35:41–8.
5. Lajoie AC, Lafontaine A-L, Kaminska M. The spectrum of sleep disorders in Parkinson disease: a review. Chest. 2021;159(2):818–27.
6. Cai G-E, Luo S, Chen L-N, Lu J-P, Huang Y-J, Ye Q-Y. Sleep fragmentation as an important clinical characteristic of sleep disorders in Parkinson's disease: a preliminary study. Chin Med J. 2019;132(15):1788–95.
7. Falup-Pecurariu C, Diaconu Ş. Sleep dysfunction in Parkinson's disease. Int Rev Neurobiol. 2017;133:719–42.
8. Norlinah M, et al. Sleep disturbances in Malaysian patients with Parkinson's disease using polysomnography and PDSS. Parkinsonism Relat Disord. 2009;15(9):670–4.
9. Comella CL. Sleep disorders in Parkinson's disease: an overview. Mov Disord. 2007;22(S17):S367–73.
10. Memon AA, Coleman JJ, Amara AW. Effects of exercise on sleep in neurodegenerative disease. Neurobiol Dis. 2020;140:104859.
11. Sobreira ES, et al. Global cognitive performance is associated with sleep efficiency measured by polysomnography in patients with Parkinson's disease. Psychiatry Clin Neurosci. 2019;73(5):248–53.
12. Junho BT, Kummer A, Cardoso FE, Teixeira AL, Rocha NP. Sleep quality is associated with the severity of clinical symptoms in Parkinson's disease. Acta Neurol Belg. 2018;118:85–91.
13. Ancoli-Israel S, Cole R, Alessi C, Chambers M, Moorcroft W, Pollak CP. The role of actigraphy in the study of sleep and circadian rhythms. Sleep. 2003;26(3):342–92.
14. Luik AI, Zuurbier LA, Hofman A, Van Someren EJ, Tiemeier H. Stability and fragmentation of the activity rhythm across the sleep-wake cycle: the importance of age, lifestyle, and mental health. Chronobiol Int. 2013;30(10):1223–30.

Part IV

Clinical Cases: Restless Legs Syndrome (RLS)/Willis-Ekbom Disease

Chapter 10
Leg Jerks and "Terrible" Sleep

Cristina Frange ⓘ

Introduction

Restless legs syndrome (RLS), also called Willis-Ekbom disease, is a neurological disorder with a very complex pathophysiology, which makes it challenging to treat. RLS is characterized by an urge to move the limbs (usually the legs but can affect the arms) to alleviate the sensation of dysesthesia or hyperesthesia; being partially or totally relieved by movement; with symptoms worsening at rest and inactivity (such as sitting or lying down) and having a circadian component, which means that symptoms appear at evening or night. Patients with RLS have poor quality of sleep (therefore poor quality of life) due to dysesthesia and difficulties in initiating and maintaining sleep due to discomfort in the limbs and fragmented sleep.

Patient Information

At the end of 2017, L.B.P., an 74-year-old woman, artist, sought physiotherapy for leg pain relief and "leg jerks." She was referred to me by the geriatric physician. Her physician suspected of peripheral neuropathy, had ordered blood sample exams and electroneuromyography of both lower limbs.

At anamnesis, she complained of pain in both legs, worse on the left one. In the legs, she felt heaviness, unpleasant sensations, cramps, jerks, and stiffening/

C. Frange (✉)
Neurology and Neurosurgery Department, Federal University of São Paulo (UNIFESP), São Paulo, SP, Brazil

C. Frange (ed.), *Clinical Cases in Sleep Physical Therapy*, https://doi.org/10.1007/978-3-031-38340-3_10

97

hardness of the muscles during the evening. She was vegetarian since the 70' s, and presented with anemia while young. She had a bilateral meniscectomy (20 years ago on the left knee, and 12 on the right knee), and reported cardiac arrhythmia accompanied by the cardiologist. She also referred to low back pain due to mild scoliosis.

She was physically active, eutrophic, and since the meniscectomy, she reported that never stopped physical exercises. She was very attentive to her weight, as she knew that gaining weight could negatively impact her knees. In fact, she reported that she never liked to exercise and, as an intellectual artist, she preferred a good book than exercising. She also reported being sedentary for the most part of her life until the pain in the lower limbs started. She said that she had to start exercises before both surgeries. She was oriented by her physiotherapist's daughter that she would have proper conditions of the muscles for her rehabilitation after the meniscectomy. Prior the surgeries she also had pain in her leg. And the pain accompanied her also after the surgeries. She had aquatic rehabilitation immediately after the surgeries and followed a rehabilitation program for both knees. She told me that she loves Pilates and myofascial release and was performing both twice a week to help with the pain. She also said that she liked to do everything walking by her home (e.g., market, shopping), to maintain a good level of physical activity along with her exercises. But she started feeling so much pain in both lower limbs that she was very upset and worried again.

When we started talking about her pain, she complained of fatigue, diffuse pain burning, aching, cramps, and jerky feeling in both legs, uncontrolled urge to move both legs, worse on the left side, worsening when at rest. There was no report of tingling and burning pain, characteristics of neuropathic pain. During the day there were no complaints. Leg jerks, pain, and an "incredible discomfort" were primarily nocturnal, interfering mainly with sleep initiation. She recorded that once when she traveled to Europe, she felt this pain and discomfort earlier, during the day—so she understood it was not related to the activities she did before sleep.

She mentioned that she slept about 3.5 h/night for a long time and that she never knew "what was to have a good night's sleep." She thought that pain was interfering with her sleep because during the night her pain seemed to get worse and she needed to get out of bed and move around, and walk a little to get better. But she got confused with the earlier symptoms during her travel. She complained of having trouble initiating and to maintain sleep. She felt never restored, never refreshed. She reported no snoring, kept a routine regarding bedtime and wake-up times, and had no feelings of excessive daytime sleepiness. At some time she reported that she was just like her father: having these sleep issues and feeling that bed was a place not to restore because of leg pain, and the terrible feeling that she had in her legs. She told me that her father used to say that his bed was full of needles, and therefore he hated sleep. She was on hormone replacement therapy (estradiol and norethisterone acetate), prescribed by the gynecologist, trazodone hydrochloride for insomnia, and pregabalin for pain, both prescribed by the geriatric physician. She said she was having difficulties with memory, focus, and concentration since she started pregabalin.

Clinical Findings

Physiotherapeutic neurological examination was without alterations. No physical changes were found in the lower limbs, such as muscle atrophy, edema, skin, reflexes, sensation, and motor control changes. She presented with mild idiopathic scoliosis. By this point, many thoughts came to my mind: Misperception of sleep? Insomnia? Medication? Restless legs syndrome? The fact that when she traveled to other time zone and it got better before sleep, indicated to me not a sleep disorder but a circadian one. She was then referred to a physician specialized in sleep medicine and neurology, for an accurate diagnosis and/or adjustment of medication—her sleep and rhythms needed to be evaluated.

She was diagnosed with chronic RLS causing severe distress. The sleep medicine physician changed the medication: instead of pregabalin and trazodone hydrochloride; she was prescribed gabapentin and zolpidem, respectively, for pain and insomnia. Adjunctly to pharmacological we started physiotherapeutic treatment.

Diagnostic Assessment

The blood sample exams were normal (e.g., urea, glucose, TSH, liver enzymes), except for the iron panel, which required intravenous iron supplementation prescribed by the physician. The electroneuromyography of both legs were normal. Neuropathy was dismissed as a diagnosis by the sleep medicine and neurologist physician, who required polysomnography (PSG). PSG was within normal values and showed no respiratory or periodic limb movement events. At the baseline evaluation, the insomnia severity index was severe [1], and the International Scale of Restless Legs was very severe [2].

Physiotherapeutic Intervention

The physiotherapeutic intervention comprised of an intensive approach discussed previously with the patient: (1) sleep hygiene education (SHE), not to exacerbate the RLS symptoms (avoid caffeine and alcohol, avoid sleep deprivation, having a relaxing bedtime routine, maintain a regular schedule and physical activity and exercise [3–5]). Each of the SHE rules was explained to her in one session, along with the rationale and the applicability in her life [6]; (2) hands-on myofascial release therapy [7]; followed by (3) lower limbs stretching exercises [7–9] (Fig. 10.1), performed twice a week; (90 min), and (4) pain control with transcutaneous electrical nerve stimulation (TENS) performed once a week [10] (45 mins), all under supervision. The parameters utilized for TENS were frequency of 75 Hz, pulse duration of 120 µs, for 45 min, electrodes placed at peroneal nerve (one placed

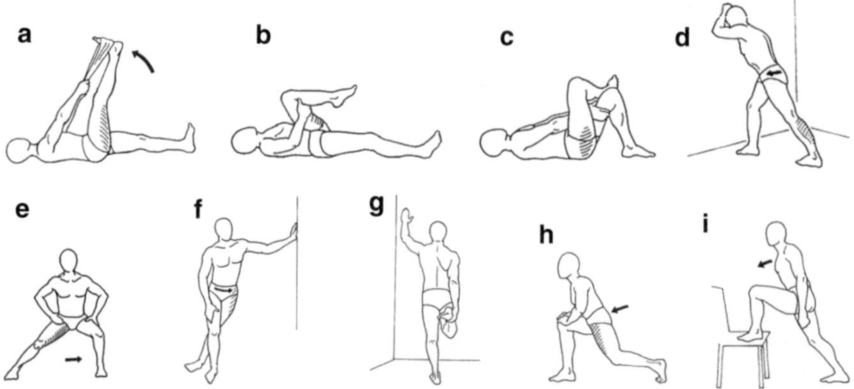

Fig. 10.1 Lower extremity stretching home exercise program. (**a**) Hamstring stretching; (**b**) Low back, buttock stretching; (**c**) Piriformis stretching; (**d**) Gastrocnemius and soleus stretching; (**e**) Hip adductor stretching; (**f**) Iliotibial band stretching; (**g**) Quadriceps stretching; (**h**, **i**). Hip flexor stretching

outside of the fibula just below the knee, and the other one placed up to the lateral malleolus). Exercises were prescribed (30 min) for the weekdays with no PT sessions and she chose to perform them in the morning as it fitted her schedule.

Immediately after PT sessions, the patient reported improvement that lasted for up to 48 h, no more than that. At the beginning, she had a little difficulty in performing the exercises by her own, but we repeated them exhaustively until she felt security to perform them. We changed exercise frequency to almost every day, except for those ones she had PT sessions, including weekends. Six months later, she was performing them daily, even with PT session in the afternoon. For the first time, she reported having slept for 7 h with no awakenings, and taking the medication prescribed.

After 12 months, the patient presented no signs of insomnia (insomnia severity index indicated absence of insomnia (7), and the legs symptoms were mild (11) at the International Scale of Restless Legs. The interdisciplinary work between PT and physician was imperative to the success of this treatment, combining pharmacological and non-pharmacological treatment, as recently reviewed [6].

The patient continues to be treated and lives well without intense pain and discomfort, and with longer sleep time. Pain sometimes appears, but the discomfort of RLS is under control, and she manages her RLS well. She learned to notice that when she doesn't sleep well (for some reason) the pain and leg jerks during the evening are intense, and she tries to relax, stretch, and go to bed early at night to restore herself. She is also aware that when she travels, the timing of the discomfort may change because it will be related to her circadian clock, and not to the local time of sleep or night. She learned to manage all the situations.

Discussion

The PT objectives of L.B.P. treatment were discussed with the patient and the physician, and were to relieve the legs symptoms, decreasing its severity; to promote improved sleep hygiene to avoid aggravating factors for RLS; to educate about RLS treatment and its management as it has no cure; and to perform daily exercises and therefore improve quality of sleep and life [6].

She was provided to avoid behaviors related to RLS exacerbations, such as caffeine and alcohol intake, sleep deprivation, irregular routine, and stress [4–6], and to promote awareness and education about RLS; therefore, L.B.P. would be able to manage her condition. The rationale of SHE is crucial to be understood by the patient, as also the flexibility of the SHE rules. Nowadays we talk a lot about SHE, but in practice, it is one of the most difficult things to achieve, because they need discipline, persistence, and a very close approach. In this case, we did it slowly, each week understanding one rule and having time to practice. We did many of these talking about sleep during the hands-on approach.

The hands-on myofascial release approach was chosen to improve nerve mobility in the lower extremity [11]; to reduce restriction by the fascia due to acute or repetitive stress, preventing muscle damage [12]; to increase neuromuscular efficiency, to reduce muscle pain [13]; and to prepare muscles for progressive stretching. The gentle pressure of hands during this type of myofascial release warrants further investigation, yet it can be seen as a proprioceptive touch that activates skin and muscle receptors and might have a role in decreasing symptoms. Hands-on myofascial release was performed before stretching exercises.

The stretching exercises performed alleviated her symptoms when reached a specific amount: neither much nor little, as too much exercise can worsen the symptoms. There is a lack of evidence on "how much" exercise for RLS, as the type of exercise, in the literature. According to the latest review of the literature and combined with our practice, aerobic and resistance exercise are the best for RLS [6], but L.B.P. was not willing to start them. As she liked Pilates, stretches were chosen, so she could also learn and do them by her own. In fact, some non-pharmacological treatments have very low evidence but are still a promise in the treatment of RLS; some of them evolving isometric exercise and stretching [7–9, 14]. The relief caused by stretching in longer periods, in this case, more than a year of regular practice, induces a chronic adaptation of the neuromusculoskeletal system. This improvement in RLS could be also because that exercise has on beta-endorphin system, promoting the regulation of an "endogenous pharmacy," along with the sensation of well-being, and improvement of cerebral blood flow, which can be related to iron metabolism.

TENS has been used by PTs to control pain [15]. Although there is no robust evidence for RLS specifically, TENS has been investigated in a few studies. The effect of TENS for RLS is to reduce spinal cord excitability [16] of leg discomfort, jerks, cramps, pain, etc.—but have been showing a short-lasting effect [17]. This clinical case experience suggests that relief of RLS symptoms begins during TENS stimulation, persists during stimulation, and persists for at least a brief period afterward. The PT sessions of TENS were performed at the beginning of the evening, closest to bedtime, and it was purposed selected because the circadian timing, the peak of RLS symptoms tends to be in the late evening or night [16]. We decided to give it a try for TENS, expecting the relief from the leg consistent with gate control theory [18]. One possible mechanism of action is that TENS activates sensory nerve fibers in the nerve (in this case peroneal) to suppress pathological neural signals beginning in the peripheral nervous system at the level of the spinal cord. An equal mechanism might explain why maintaining activity, stretching, walking, and stretching, which activates proprioceptive nerve fibers in lower limbs, frequently relieve RLS symptoms, even for short times [19].

This clinical case described the long journey searching for the treatment of pain and discomfort for RLS. Probably RLS was hereditary in this patient and required new habits of managing the condition, including daily stretching, pain relief, maintenance of physical activity (walking) and education about the condition and sleep, as well as knowledge of predisposing factors.

Patient Perspective

"This has been a journey! I didn't know about RLS and I think my father also had it. I learned so much about it. The most important thing is that I need to do the exercises daily. Not a few, and not a lot! At first, it was hard, but today I learned to manage. I do feel pain if I don't exercise and stretch. I'm better, I understand my condition and I think I had it my entire life. I feel secure with the interprofessional care from my physician and my physio'. The 'disease management' requires my discipline, and I am aware I have no cure, but with the treatment, I can live well. My pain and discomfort in both legs decreased a lot—and I mean A LOT! I know I take medications and probably will take them forever, but now I sleep better, and live better."

References

1. Bastien CH, Vallieres A, Morin CM. Validation of the insomnia severity index as an outcome measure for insomnia research. Sleep Med. 2001;2(4):297–307.
2. Walters AS, et al. Validation of the international restless legs syndrome study group rating scale for restless legs syndrome. Sleep Med. 2003;4(2):121–32.
3. Siengsukon CF, Al-Dughmi M, Stevens S. Sleep health promotion: practical information for physical therapists. Phys Ther. 2017;97(8):826–36.
4. Irish LA, et al. The role of sleep hygiene in promoting public health: a review of empirical evidence. Sleep Med Rev. 2015;22:23–36.

5. D'Aurea CVR, Passos GS, Frange C. Insomnia: physiotherapeutic approach. In: Frange C, Coelho FMS, editors. Sleep medicine and physical therapy: a comprehensive guide for practitioners. Cham: Springer International Publishing; 2022. p. 61–73.

6. Frange C, et al. Practice recommendations for the role of physiotherapy in the management of sleep disorders: the 2022 Brazilian sleep association guidelines. Sleep Sci. 2022;15(4):515–73.

7. Harrison EG, Keating JL, Morgan PE. Non-pharmacological interventions for restless legs syndrome: a systematic review of randomised controlled trials. Disabil Rehabil. 2019;41(17):2006–14.

8. Aukerman MM, et al. Exercise and restless legs syndrome: a randomized controlled trial. J Am Board Fam Med. 2006;19(5):487–93.

9. Guay A, et al. Current evidence on diagnostic criteria, relevant outcome measures, and efficacy of nonpharmacologic therapy in the Management of Restless Legs Syndrome (RLS): a scoping review. J Manip Physiol Ther. 2020;43(9):930–41.

10. Johnson MI, et al. Efficacy and safety of transcutaneous electrical nerve stimulation (TENS) for acute and chronic pain in adults: a systematic review and meta-analysis of 381 studies (the meta-TENS study). BMJ Open. 2022;12(2):e051073.

11. Hall T, Beyerlein C, Hansson U, Lim HT, Odermark M, Sainsbury D. Mulligan traction straight leg raise: a pilot study to investigate effects on range of motion in patients with low back pain. J Man Manip Ther. 2006;14(2):95–100.

12. Peacock CA, et al. An acute bout of self-myofascial release in the form of foam rolling improves performance testing. Int J Exerc Sci. 2014;7(3):202–11.

13. Aboodarda SJ, Spence AJ, Button DC. Pain pressure threshold of a muscle tender spot increases following local and non-local rolling massage. BMC Musculoskelet Disord. 2015;16:265.

14. Aliasgharpour M, et al. The effect of stretching exercises on severity of restless legs syndrome in patients on hemodialysis. Asian J Sports Med. 2016;7(2):e31001.

15. Robinson AJ. Transcutaneous electrical nerve stimulation for the control of pain in musculoskeletal disorders. J Orthop Sports Phys Ther. 1996;24(4):208–26.

16. Buchfuhrer MJ, et al. Noninvasive neuromodulation reduces symptoms of restless legs syndrome. J Clin Sleep Med. 2021;17:1685.

17. Heide AC, et al. Effects of transcutaneous spinal direct current stimulation in idiopathic restless legs patients. Brain Stimul. 2014;7(5):636–42.

18. Wall PD. The gate control theory of pain mechanisms. A re-examination and re-statement. Brain. 1978;101(1):1–18.

19. Allen RP, et al. Restless legs syndrome/Willis-Ekbom disease diagnostic criteria: updated International Restless Legs Syndrome Study Group (IRLSSG) consensus criteria—history, rationale, description, and significance. Sleep Med. 2014;15(8):860–73.

Chapter 11
A Man with Multiple Sclerosis Running from Restless Legs Syndrome

Turhan Kahraman and Asiye T. Ozdogar

Introduction

Multiple sclerosis (MS) is an inflammatory, demyelinating, chronic disease of the central nervous system and causes various symptoms. According to cohort studies, restless legs syndrome (RLS) affects between 13.3 and 65.1% of people with MS (pwMS) [1]. Despite the significant occurrence of RLS in pwMS, it is frequently underestimated during neurological examination. Therefore, determining a patient's complaint related to RLS and treating this condition is challenging. So far, medical treatments are in the foreground treatment of RLS. But as the benefits of exercise have become more evident, several forms of exercise are being studied in patients with RLS. On the other hand, research on exercise has not included pwMS with RLS. This case report examined how aerobic exercise affects RLS symptoms in a male with MS with RLS.

Patient Information

T.K.O., man, currently 47 years old, applied to our MS center for the first time in 2012, complaining of blurred vision. Following a confirmed diagnosis of MS, interferon beta 1b was prescribed. In 2016, due to the inefficiency of interferon beta 1b,

T. Kahraman (✉)
Department of Health Professions, Manchester Metropolitan University, Manchester, UK

Department of Physiotherapy and Rehabilitation, Faculty of Health Sciences, Izmir Katip Celebi University, Izmir, Turkey

A. T. Ozdogar
Department of Physiotherapy and Rehabilitation, Faculty of Health Sciences, Van Yuzuncu Yil University, Van, Turkey

C. Frange (ed.), *Clinical Cases in Sleep Physical Therapy*, https://doi.org/10.1007/978-3-031-38340-3_11

106   T. Kahraman and A. T. Ozdogar

the medical treatment was switched to fingolimod (immunomodulating medication). Routine evaluations, which comprise physical, psychosocial, and cognitive measurements, were started to be applied annually after 2015 in our MS center. During the second routine evaluation of this case on June 29, 2016, a senior neurologist diagnosed him with an RLS. The existence of a spinal cord lesion is the most frequently cited pathophysiologic explanation for the RLS in pwMS [2]. Therefore, we retrospectively evaluated previous magnetic resonance imaging (MRI) scans, the first was in 2010. Even though there was no spinal cord lesion in the initial MRI scans, the first spinal cord lesion was discovered in the MRI scan in April 2014.

Clinical Findings

The RLS Rating Scale (RLSRS) was used to assess the severity of the RLS symptoms [3]. At the last routine clinical visit, the patient scored 33 out of 40 on the RLSRS, representing he had very severe RLS symptoms even though he was under medical treatment for the RLS symptoms. Therefore, a further management method was discussed. The patient's pre- and post-treatment RLSRS answers are shown in Fig. 11.1.

a

(a) Restless legs syndrome rating scale	
1. Overall, how would you rate the RLS discomfort in your legs or arms?	6. Overall, how severe is your RLS as a whole?
4) Very severe ✓	4) Very severe ✓
3) Severe	3) Severe
2) Moderate	2) Moderate
1) Mild	1) Mild
0) None	0) None
2. Overall, how would you rate the need to move around because of your RLS symptoms?	7. How often do you get RLS symptoms?
4) Very severe ✓	4) Very severe: 6 to 7 days a week ✓
3) Severe	3) Severe: 4 to 5 days a week
2) Moderate	2) Moderate: 2 to 3 days a week
1) Mild	1) Mild: 1 day a week or less
0) None	0) None
3. Overall, how much relief of your RLS arm or leg discomfort do you get from moving around?	8. When you have RLS symptoms, how severe are they on an average day?
4) No relief	4) Very severe: 8 hours per day or more ✓
3) Slight relief ✓	3) Severe: 3 to 8 hours per day
2) Moderate relief	2) Moderate: 1 to 3 hours per day
1) Complete or almost complete relief	1) Mild: less than 1 hour per day
0) No RLS symptoms	0) None
4. Overall, how severe is your sleep disturbance from your RLS symptoms?	9. Overall, how severe is the impact of your RLS symptoms on your ability to carry out your daily affairs (eg, carrying out a satisfactory family, home, social, school, or work life)?
4) Very severe ✓	4) Very severe ✓
3) Severe	3) Severe
2) Moderate	2) Moderate
1) Mild	1) Mild
0) None	0) None
5. How severe is your tiredness or sleepiness from your RLS symptoms?	10. How severe is your mood disturbance from your RLS symptoms (eg, angry, depressed, sad, anxious, or irritable)?
4) Very severe	4) Very severe
3) Severe	3) Severe
2) Moderate	2) Moderate ✓
1) Mild	1) Mild
0) None ✓	0) None

b

(b) Restless legs syndrome rating scale	
1. Overall, how would you rate the RLS discomfort in your legs or arms?	6. Overall, how severe is your RLS as a whole?
4) Very severe	4) Very severe
3) Severe	3) Severe ✓
2) Moderate ✓	2) Moderate
1) Mild	1) Mild
0) None	0) None
2. Overall, how would you rate the need to move around because of your RLS symptoms?	7. How often do you get RLS symptoms?
4) Very severe	4) Very severe: 6 to 7 days a week
3) Severe ✓	3) Severe: 4 to 5 days a week
2) Moderate	2) Moderate: 2 to 3 days a week ✓
1) Mild	1) Mild: 1 day a week or less
0) None	0) None
3. Overall, how much relief of your RLS arm or leg discomfort do you get from moving around?	8. When you have RLS symptoms, how severe are they on an average day?
4) No relief	4) Very severe: 8 hours per day or more
3) Slight relief	3) Severe: 3 to 8 hours per day
2) Moderate relief ✓	2) Moderate: 1 to 3 hours per day
1) Complete or almost complete relief	1) Mild: less than 1 hour per day ✓
0) No RLS symptoms	0) None
4. Overall, how severe is your sleep disturbance from your RLS symptoms?	9. Overall, how severe is the impact of your RLS symptoms on your ability to carry out your daily affairs (eg, carrying out a satisfactory family, home, social, school, or work life)?
4) Very severe	4) Very severe
3) Severe ✓	3) Severe
2) Moderate	2) Moderate ✓
1) Mild	1) Mild
0) None	0) None
5. How severe is your tiredness or sleepiness from your RLS symptoms?	10. How severe is your mood disturbance from your RLS symptoms (eg, angry, depressed, sad, anxious, or irritable)?
4) Very severe	4) Very severe
3) Severe	3) Severe
2) Moderate ✓	2) Moderate
1) Mild	1) Mild ✓
0) None	0) None

Fig. 11.1 T.K.O.'s answers to each item on Restless Legs Syndrome Rating Scale before (**a**) and after (**b**) the aerobic training. The total score ranges from 0 to 40, being classified as mild (0–10), moderate (11–20), severe (21–30) and very severe (31–40) [3]. (Reprinted with permission from T.K.O)

Timeline

The neurological disability and RLS symptoms severity were measured during the follow-up from June 2016 to May 2022. The Expanded Disability Status Scale (EDSS) [4] was used to assess the neurological disability, and the RLSRS was used to assess the RLS symptoms severity. Figure 11.2 presents the timeline of the changes in RLSRS and EDSS scores. After the RLS symptoms became more severe, even medical treatment (pramipexole, a dopamine agonist), the neurologist and physical therapist together decided to utilize aerobic exercise training in May 2022. Soon after, the baseline assessments were conducted before the aerobic exercise training. The training program was started in the next session following the baseline assessment.

Diagnostic Assessment

Despite the lack of gold standard or objective clinical approaches for diagnosing RLS, the most used method is the RLS diagnostic criteria. The International RLS Working Group created the first version of the RLS diagnostic criteria in 1995 [5]. The neurological examination and anamnesis provide the basis of those four criteria [5]. In 2003 and 2014, there were two revisions made to those criteria. The fifth criterion was included in the most recent revision to increase specificity by excluding pathologies that mimic RLS symptoms [6]. Our patient fulfilled all five criteria and was diagnosed with RLS on June 29, 2016.

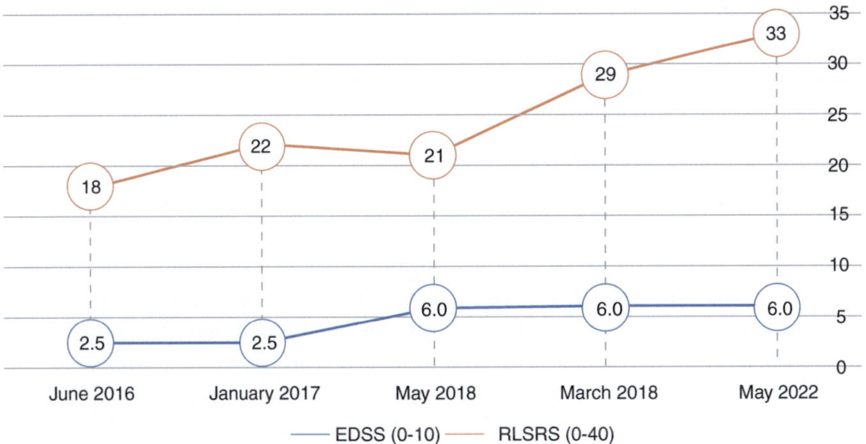

Fig. 11.2 Changes in the EDSS and RLS severity scores. *EDSS* expanded disability status scale, *RLS* restless legs syndrome, *RLSRS* RLS rating scale (the total score ranges from 0 to 40, being classified as mild (0–10), moderate (11–20), severe (21–30) and very severe (31–40) [3]). (Reprinted with permission from T.K.O)

Physiotherapeutic Intervention

After deciding to utilize aerobic exercise, the exercise program was scheduled by a physical therapist in May 2022, following the protocol described in a previous study that investigated the effects of aerobic exercise training in people with RLS [7]. The patient's target exercise heart rate was calculated using the Karvonen formula [((220–age–Resting Heart Rate) × percentage of intensity) + Resting Heart Rate] [8]. Exercise intensity was adjusted from 60 to 75%. Aerobic exercise training was applied twice a week under the supervision of a physical therapist for 12 weeks using a *recumbent exercise bike* starting from 20.05.2022. The sessions started with 20 min, with 2–3 min of warm-up, 15 min of loading, and 2–3 min of cool-down, and reached 30 min at the end of 12 weeks. The heart rate was monitored via Polar H10 Hear Rate Sensors. The last session was performed on August 10, 2022. The patient attended all sessions with high motivation (a total of 24 sessions) and did not report any adverse events.

Follow-Up and Outcomes

Because the RLS symptoms can affect many aspects, such as gait, sleep quality, quality of life, and physical capacity, we chose comprehensive assessment tools which are valid and reliable in pwMS. Before and after the aerobic exercise training, the RLSRS, Epworth Sleepiness Scale (ESS), Pittsburgh Sleep Quality Index (PSQI), Timed 25-Foot Walk (T25FW), Timed Up and Go (TUG), 6-Min Walk Test (6-MWT), Multiple Sclerosis International Quality of Life (MusiQoL) and the estimated VO_2max were performed.

The primary outcome was the RLSRS which was developed to evaluate RLS symptoms severity, and it consists of a 10-item scale scored from 0 (not affected by the symptoms) to 4 (affected very severely by symptoms) [3].

The T25FW, TUG, and 6-MWT were performed for the gait assessment. The T25FW was used to assess the walking speed [9]. The TUG test is a simple test that assesses a person's mobility and requires both static and dynamic balance [10]. The 6-MWT is a submaximal exercise test that entails the measurement of distance walked over 6 min [11].

The ESS was used to assess daytime sleepiness, whose scores range from 0 to 24. A higher score indicates higher daytime sleepiness [12]. The PSQI includes seven subscales that assess subjective sleep quality, sleep latency, duration, habitual sleep efficiency, sleep disturbance, use of sleep medication, and daytime dysfunction. The total PSQI score is calculated from these seven sections and ranges from 0 to 21 [13]. Higher scores indicate worse sleep quality. The MuSiQoL is the MS-specific health-related quality of life questionnaire that comprises 31 items [14]. The total score ranges from 0 to 100, and higher scores indicate a better health-related quality of life.

To calculate VO_2max from submaximal data, the Astrand-Rhyming nomogram approach was used [15]. It is one of the most used indirect VO_2max measurement protocols [16]. The heartbeat rate obtained from the test and the applied workload combined with the Astrand-Rhyming nomogram to calculate the estimated VO_2max.

Table 11.1 presents the baseline and after-aerobic exercise training results. The RLSRS score decreased from 33 to 21, indicating a 36% improvement. Except for the ESS, all outcome measures improved.

Discussion

Several non-pharmacological modalities have been reported to be effective in managing RLS, including exercise, compression devices, infrared therapy, and conventional acupuncture. However, their effectiveness is controversial as the studies lack methodological quality [1]. Therefore, there is a need for evidence-based studies to develop rehabilitation programs that can be applied in this population and to determine their effectiveness and treatment duration. Although there is no strong evidence, most studies investigating the effects of aerobic exercise on RLS symptoms reported that it could decrease RLS severity [7, 17, 18]. Thus, we decided to apply aerobic exercise to this patient with MS and RLS. As a result, our case showed that aerobic exercise might be a promising method for improving RLS severity, sleep quality, gait, and health-related quality of life.

Cederberg and Motl (2021) examined the feasibility and effectiveness of the physical activity behavior modification method to improve RLS severity and sleep outcome measures in pwMS. They showed that the RLS severity, self-report sleep satisfaction, total time spent in bed, and total sleep time had all improved. The authors hypothesized that because the pathological pathways of MS and RLS are

Table 11.1 Baseline and after-aerobic exercise training results of the patient

	Baseline assessment	After-aerobic exercise training assessment (week 12)	Percentage of change from baseline to week 12
RLSRS (0–40)	33	21	36%
ESS (0–24)	9	9	0%
PSQI (0–21)	14	6	57%
T25FW (s)	10.39	7.06	47%
TUG (s)	24.35	17.25	29%
6-MWT (m)	260	327	20%
MusiQoL (0–100)	71.64	77.78	9%
Estimated VO_2max (mL/kg/min)	27.1	32.5	20%

RLSRS RLS rating scale, *ESS* epworth sleepiness scale, *PSQI* pittsburgh sleep quality index, *T25FW* timed 25-foot walk, *TUG* timed up and go, *6-MWT* 6-min walk test, *MusiQoL* multiple sclerosis international quality of life

mutual, the improvement in dopaminergic signaling through physical activity or exercise could positively affect both MS and RLS symptoms [19]. Our results support this hypothesis. In our case, the improvement was observed not only in the RLS severity and sleep-related symptoms but also in physical components such as gait and estimated VO_2max.

This case report examined the effects of a 24-sessions aerobic exercise training for the first time in a male with MS and RLS. Our results showed that aerobic exercise might be a promising method for improving RLS severity, sleep quality, gait, and health-related quality of life. Also, this case report showed that RLS symptoms should not be considered separately from MS symptoms. When deciding both assessment tools and intervention parameters (frequencies, type, intensity, time), thinking about how MS-related symptoms could affect this process may be the best way to manage RLS symptoms. It seems like a full-scale randomized controlled trial investigating aerobic exercise training would be warranted and worthwhile to perform.

Patient Perspective

At the end of the aerobic exercise training program, T.K.O. reported, "My wife and I realized that I could easily fall asleep. Also, the restless feeling in my legs has reduced, so I sleep longer and wake up more energic. Moreover, I can walk longer distances during the day because I feel more energic. At the beginning of the exercise sessions, I was prejudiced about how this kind of activity could reduce my sensory symptoms. However, after 4 or 5 weeks, I noticed I was improving. After this point, I started to feel more and more cravings for each session. It should be considered that I live 90 km from the hospital, where I attend to do aerobic exercise sessions. It was a great experience for me, and even after my sessions are over with my physical therapist, I will continue cycling to keep its' positive effect on me."

References

1. Ozdogar AT, Kalron A. Restless legs syndrome in people with multiple sclerosis: an updated systematic review and meta-analyses. Mult Scler Relat Disord. 2021;56:103275. https://doi.org/10.1016/j.msard.2021.103275.
2. Irkec C, Vuralli D, Karacay Ozkalayci S. Restless legs syndrome as the initial presentation of multiple sclerosis. Case Rep Med. 2013;2013:1–4. https://doi.org/10.1155/2013/290719.
3. Walters AS, LeBrocq C, Dhar A, et al. Validation of the international restless legs syndrome study group rating scale for restless legs syndrome. Sleep Med. 2003;4:121–32. https://doi.org/10.1016/s1389-9457(02)00258-7.
4. Kurtzke JF. Rating neurologic impairment in multiple sclerosis: an expanded disability status scale (EDSS). Neurology. 1983;33:1444–52. https://doi.org/10.1212/wnl.33.11.1444.
5. Walters AS, Aldrich MS, Allen R, et al. Toward a better definition of the restless legs syndrome. Mov Disord. 1995;10:634–42. https://doi.org/10.1002/mds.870100517.

6. Allen RP, Picchietti DL, Garcia-Borreguero D, et al. Restless legs syndrome/Willis-Ekbom disease diagnostic criteria: updated International Restless Legs Syndrome Study Group (IRLSSG) consensus criteria—history, rationale, description, and significance. Sleep Med. 2014;15:860–73. https://doi.org/10.1016/j.sleep.2014.03.025.
7. Aukerman MM, Aukerman D, Bayard M, et al. Exercise and restless legs syndrome: a randomized controlled trial. J Am Board Fam Med. 2006;19:487–93. https://doi.org/10.3122/jabfm.19.5.487.
8. Karvonen MJ, Kentala E, Mustala O. The effects of training on heart rate; a longitudinal study. Ann Med Exp Biol Fenn. 1957;35:307–15.
9. Kieseier BC, Pozzilli C. Assessing walking disability in multiple sclerosis. Mult Scler. 2012;18:914–24. https://doi.org/10.1177/1352458512444498.
10. Sebastião E, Sandroff BM, Learmonth YC, Motl RW. Validity of the timed up and go test as a measure of functional mobility in persons with multiple sclerosis. Arch Phys Med Rehabil. 2016;97:1072–7. https://doi.org/10.1016/j.apmr.2015.12.031.
11. Goldman MD, Marrie RA, Cohen JA. Evaluation of the six-minute walk in multiple sclerosis subjects and healthy controls. Mult Scler. 2008;14:383–90. https://doi.org/10.1177/1352458507082607.
12. Johns MW. A new method for measuring daytime sleepiness: the Epworth sleepiness scale. Sleep. 1991;14:540–5. https://doi.org/10.1093/sleep/14.6.540.
13. Buysse DJ, Reynolds CF, Monk TH, et al. The Pittsburgh sleep quality index: a new instrument for psychiatric practice and research. Psychiatry Res. 1989;28:193–213. https://doi.org/10.1016/0165-1781(89)90047-4.
14. Simeoni M, Auquier P, Fernandez O, et al. Validation of the multiple sclerosis international quality of life questionnaire. Mult Scler. 2008;14:219–30. https://doi.org/10.1177/1352458507080733.
15. Åstrand P-O, Ryhming I. A nomogram for calculation of aerobic capacity (physical fitness) from pulse rate during submaximal work. J Appl Physiol. 1954;7:218–21. https://doi.org/10.1152/jappl.1954.7.2.218.
16. Legge BJ, Banister EW. The Astrand-Ryhming nomogram revisited. J Appl Physiol. 1986;61:1203–9. https://doi.org/10.1152/jappl.1986.61.3.1203.
17. Mortazavi M, Vahdatpour B, Ghasempour A, et al. Aerobic exercise improves signs of restless leg syndrome in end stage renal disease patients suffering chronic hemodialysis. Sci World J. 2013;2013:1–4. https://doi.org/10.1155/2013/628142.
18. Xu X-M, Liu Y, Jia S-Y, et al. Complementary and alternative therapies for restless legs syndrome: an evidence-based systematic review. Sleep Med Rev. 2018;38:158–67. https://doi.org/10.1016/j.smrv.2017.06.003.
19. Cederberg KLJ, Motl RW. Feasibility and efficacy of a physical activity intervention for managing restless legs syndrome in multiple sclerosis: results of a pilot randomized controlled trial. Mult Scler Relat Disord. 2021;50:102836. https://doi.org/10.1016/j.msard.2021.102836.

Part V
Clinical Cases: Circadian Rhythm Sleep Disturbances

Chapter 12
A Truck Driver with an Irregular Sleep Schedule

Melissa A. Ulhôa ⓘ and Mario A. Leocadio-Miguel ⓘ

Introduction

Some truck drivers work irregular hours due to job strains, including long working hours at night. These characteristics may contribute to chronic sleep deprivation, circadian diseases, unhealthy dietary habits, sedentary lifestyle, cardiovascular disease, and obesity.

Long-haul drivers should deliver goods from one city to another on time. Thus, they have time to depart, but the end of the shift is uncertain. This routine schedule can affect biological rhythms, impacting the sleep-wake cycle and disrupting the circadian system [1, 2]. Actually, irregular and long working hours at night may cause circadian desynchronization and stressors. This situation can affect cortisol release, a well-known marker of stress. According to Ulhoa et al. [3], high cortisol levels in irregular-shift workers were correlated with certain stressors, such as short sleep duration, and low job satisfaction, and metabolic parameters, such as total cholesterol. The aim of this chapter is to present a driver who was referred by his physician to physical therapy for sleep treatment. He has sleep complaints and fatigue. This chapter is about a hypothetical patient, and it is based on the true stories of several Investigations we have performed.

M. A. Ulhôa (✉)
Faculty of Medicine, UNIVAÇO - AFYA, Ipatinga, MG, Brazil

M. A. Leocadio-Miguel
Department of Psychology, Northumbria University,
Newcastle upon Tyne, United Kingdom

C. Frange (ed.), *Clinical Cases in Sleep Physical Therapy*,
https://doi.org/10.1007/978-3-031-38340-3_12

Patient's Information

L.R.D., a 45-year-old male truck driver, arrived at the clinic for physical sleep therapy treatment in April/2022. He has been working as a truck driver for the last 15 years. He looked for a physiotherapist specialist in sleep after his doctor's suggestion. The driver is married, non-smoker, and has regular social drinking habits. His family background has a history of blood pressure, hypertension, and diabetes. Nowadays, he doesn't have those diagnoses. No relevant genetic information was informed.

He has been working for 15 years as a long-haul truck driver on an irregular night shift. His ordinary schedule includes arriving at the transportation company at 7 PM., where he waits for the lorry to be set in the truck. Then, he takes the road to deliver the goods on time. He rarely knows when he will arrive at the delivery address because of the traffic and some eventual problems on the road. He likes his job but reported worries about his safety because he has fallen asleep behind the wheel twice.

During the anamnesis, L.R.D. complained about his sleep and that he wakes up feeling tired. We used the visual analogue scale and actigraphy for 1 week to evaluate his sleep quality. The actogram showed that the driver slept about 399 min. Sleep efficiency was 80%. Sleep quality was 7 points (from 0 to 10 points, the greater the score, the more significant subjective level of sleepiness).

He considers his own house environment not suitable for sleeping. According to him, noise from people and telephones are the main reasons that usually disturb his sleep at home. He also reported being unable to fall asleep when going to bed. Considering Karolinska's sleepiness scale [4], there is more sleepiness between 6:00 and in the afternoon (14:00 to 18:00), on working days. During days off, the higher point of sleepiness is early in the day.

Work Schedules and Routine

From information obtained by completing the activities protocol during the week, the average duration of each activity during work was calculated. The average duration of time spent driving was 386.3 min/day. Approximately 2 h, on average, was the delay in releasing the truck. The time waiting for the release was 117.74 min. The nap duration at work was 28.18 min. He sleeps during his routine when arriving home; however on some days, he does some leisure activities and eats before sleeping. We illustrate the actigraphy record showing active and resting moments in Fig. 12.1. The dark bands in the actogram below represent periods of activity. The gray one represents rest.

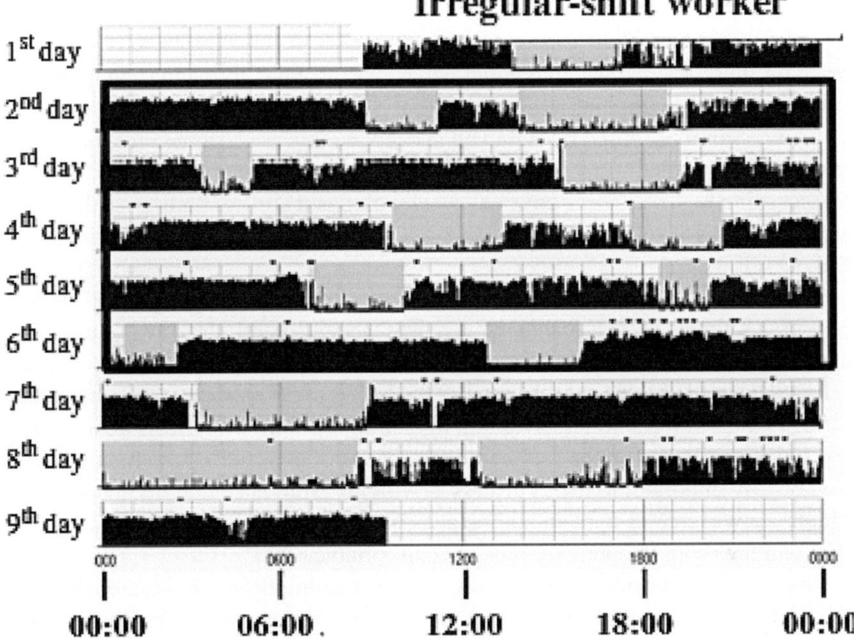

Fig. 12.1 The patient's actigraphy record shows an irregular sleep-wake rhythm disorder. (Reprinted with permission form [3])

Clinical Findings

He is obese, with body mass index of 32 kg/m^2 and blood pressure of 140/90 mmHg. The waist-hip ratio is 1.1. The resting heart rate is 72 bpm. He underwent surgery to remove his appendix 2 years ago. He doesn't complain about sexual dysfunction or other comorbidities. Patient's snoring and probable sleep apnea are under investigation by his physician, who suggested polysomnography, which has not been performed so far.

According to the major complaints of irregular sleep and daytime tiredness, an evaluation and treatment plan were developed [5]. Data from sleep and wake activity extracted from the actogram and from the sleep and activities diary (described in his routine) were used for better evaluation. We identified circadian rhythm alterations. We also investigated his circadian preferences using the chronotype questionnaire [6], characterizing him as intermediate type.

The analysis of the patient's sleep hygiene routine was watching TV or, eventually, using smartphones before going to sleep. He does not drink coffee before sleeping, only when he wakes up. However, eventually, he eats an enormous meal before going to sleep. He usually wakes up to go to the bathroom to urinate during sleep.

Physiotherapeutic Intervention

Based on these results, we elaborated behavioral changes following guidelines on waking up and sleeping times, naps, and lifestyle habits. Furthermore, physiotherapeutic interventions, based on light and chronotherapy, are adequate for the irregular circadian disorder.

According to the patient's physical examination and clinical findings, a therapeutic protocol was developed based on relevant literature [5, 7, 8], with specific objectives, as following:

Objective 1: To promote circadian rhythms alignment using light and dark at appropriate times as a therapeutic resource according to sleep-wake circadian rhythm cycle disorder.

Intervention 1: In this case, Light 1–2 h of 2500 to 5000 lux was recommended, in the first half of the shift and avoiding light after the shift. Moreover, wearing blue light blocking glasses on the way home after the shift ends during the light phase of the day. It is important to avoid drowsy driving to avoid accidents. While sleeping at home, any source of light should be avoided, the room has to be as silent as possible, and the room temperature must be comfortable.

Objective 2: To promote sleep quality and proper duration and to establish sleeping and waking times (chronotherapy) as a strategy to sleep-wake circadian rhythm cycle disorder.

Intervention 2: To reach these goals, chronotherapy was recommended to insert sleeping and waking up routine and low-intensity physical exercises (e.g., walking, cycling) at appropriate times and away from bedtime.

Objective 3: To promote life quality and well-being and to recommend sleep hygiene education to increase efficiency and sleep quality.

Intervention 3: To encourage physical exercise practice to benefit the patient in terms of general health, healthy eating, and other recommendations related below.

Discussion

Physical exercise is a strategy in the way to benefit health and sleep when properly applied. Exercising just before bedtime should be avoided because of the alert it promotes, as there is an activation of the sympathetic autonomous nervous system, with adrenaline release. It is necessary to pay attention to the duration and intensity of the exercises. The duration should be short or intermediary, preferentially (30 min to 1 h). Considering exercise intensity, it is better to practice with low or medium intensity, because long-duration and high-impact exercises can lead to fatigue, pain and sleeping disorders. Mentally exciting activities should be avoided close to sleeping time [7].

Using caffeine and waking may be strategies to mitigate drowsiness among drivers [9].

The organization of work in shifts may mitigate fatigue and drowsiness during working time by limiting long hours of work, avoiding irregular shifts, inserting resting periods, and promoting training to recognize fatigue to avoid work accidents.

Moreno et al. [10] suggest implementing a circadian hygiene program. Besides physical exercise and light with proper intensity and at an appropriate time, guidance can also be provided on proper nutrition. Both caloric content and the time of meals should be taken into consideration. The authors also add the importance of chronobiotics. With that, drugs that act in line with circadian rhythms are highlighted, considering that they potentiate the effects in some hours of the day. Exogenous melatonin is one of the chronobiotics that shows positive effects on sleep duration and consolidation. Finally, the effect of social meetings (school, work) is to adjust (or misalign) biological rhythms. Here, we can highlight how the work commitment has impacted patients´ life in this chapter. There is a mismatch between the demands of irregular work and sleeping needs. Literature shows that working in shifts is associated with a low-duration, irregular sleep pattern, and with an impact on others' circadian rhythms. Nap is used as a strategy during or before the shift to decrease the consequences of shift work on workers´ sleep. Naps help to keep alertness and working performance [8, 10].

Sunlight or electricity interferes with biological rhythms as they reach photosensitive ganglion cells in the retina. Consequently, light may promote alertness, changes in brain activities, and endogenous melatonin levels and, thus, interfere with circadian rhythms. Therefore, prolonged use of electronic equipment close to bedtime should be avoided [10]. Besides, the use of sunglasses after the shift and blue light blocking for electronics is recommended. In addition, exogenous melatonin can be used to help synchronize.

In the specific case of professional drivers, anti-collision technology can be implemented in vehicles, as technologies and system resources are advancing quickly, such as Automated Driving System Technologies (ADS). Besides, early fatigue detection is important, such as a driver monitoring system (it verifies eyelid closure and head position indicating drowsing). Those systems have not been widely incorporated into fleet vehicles until recently, but their use is promising [2].

To conclude, irregular and long working hours at night may cause circadian desynchronization and stressors. It is important to have a specific evaluation with anamneses, actigraphy, diary, Karolinska sleepiness scale, and chronotype questionnaire. Then, it is possible to set the intervention on the patient's routine. The treatment is unique and must to promote circadian rhythms alignment using the application of light and dark at appropriate times; to promote sleep quality and duration; and to promote life quality and well-being. Each patient and intervention are unique. It expects a better sleep parameter, less fatigue, and increased quality of life after these implementations.

References

1. Gentry NW, Ashbrook LH, Fu Y-H, Ptáček LJ. Human circadian variations. J Clin Invest. 2021;131:e148282. https://doi.org/10.1172/JCI148282.
2. Mabry JE, Camden M, Miller A, et al. Unravelling the complexity of irregular shiftwork, fatigue and sleep health for commercial drivers and the associated implications for roadway safety. Int J Environ Res Public Health. 2022;19:14780. https://doi.org/10.3390/ijerph192214780.
3. Ulhôa MAJ, Marqueze EC, Kantermann T, Skene D, Moreno C. When does stress end? Evidence of a prolonged stress reaction in shiftworking truck drivers. Chronobiol Int. 2011;28:810–8.
4. Åkerstedt T, Gillberg M. Subjective and objective sleepiness in the active individual. Int J Neurosci. 1990;52:29–37. https://doi.org/10.3109/00207459008994241.
5. Frange C, Franco AM, Brasil E, et al. Practice recommendations for the role of physiotherapy in the management of sleep disorders: the 2022 Brazilian sleep association guidelines. Sleep Sci. 2022;15:515–73.
6. Benedito-Silva AA, Menna-Barreto L, Marques N, Tenreiro S. A self-assessment questionnaire for the determination of morningness-eveningness types in Brazil. Prog Clin Biol Res. 1990;341B:89–98.
7. Gurubhagavatula I, Barger LK, Barnes CM, et al. Guiding principles for determining work shift duration and addressing the effects of work shift duration on performance, safety, and health: guidance from the American Academy of sleep medicine and the Sleep Research Society. J Clin Sleep Med. 2021;17:2283–306.
8. Wickwire EM, Geiger-Brown J, Scharf SM, Drake CL. Shift work and shift work sleep disorder: clinical and organizational perspectives. Chest. 2017;151:1156–72.
9. Krishnaswamy UM, Chhabria MS, Rao A. Excessive sleepiness, sleep hygiene, and coping strategies among night bus drivers: a cross-sectional study. Indian J Occup Environ Med. 2016;20:84–7.
10. Moreno CRC, Raad R, Gusmão WDP, et al. Are we ready to implement circadian hygiene interventions and programs? Int J Environ Res Public Health. 2022;19:16772. https://doi.org/10.3390/ijerph192416772.

Part VI
Clinical Cases: Sleep Bruxism

Chapter 13
Recurrent Orofacial Pain with Concomitant Diffuse Pain and Sleep Bruxism

Jacqueline T. A. T. Lam ⓘ, Alberto Herrero Babiloni ⓘ, Dany H. Gagnon ⓘ, and Gilles Lavigne ⓘ

Introduction

In this case report, the patient had a longstanding history of orofacial pain. In 2018, she visited with an oral medicine and sleep medicine qualified dentist (GL) who diagnosed her with sleep bruxism (SB). She received a night guard to prevent night-time clenching/grinding. Even though the night guard helped with orofacial pain complaints, the patient has had recurrent bouts of severe acute pain (8/10), once in 2019 and once in 2022 that motivated her to consult twice with physiotherapy. Although jaw exercises and targeted manual treatments have diminished jaw muscle and joint pain, subsequent exercises directed to other areas of her body (i.e., head, neck, and shoulders) further decreased the patient's pain to a more manageable level overtime.

J. T. A. T. Lam (✉) · D. H. Gagnon
School of Rehabilitation, Institut Universitaire sur la Réadaptation en Déficience Physique de Montréal of CIUSSS Centre-sud de Montréal, Université de Montréal, Montreal, QC, Canada

A. Herrero Babiloni
Division of Experimental Medicine, McGill University, Montreal, QC, Canada

G. Lavigne
Faculty of Dental Medicine, Research Center of CIUSSS Nord Ile de Montréal, Sleep and Trauma Unit and CHUM-Stomatology, Université de Montréal, Montreal, QC, Canada

C. Frange (ed.), *Clinical Cases in Sleep Physical Therapy*,
https://doi.org/10.1007/978-3-031-38340-3_13

Patient Information

The first physiotherapy (PT) consultation was in 2019. A.E.C. was an athletic right-handed 29-year-old woman, with a primary complaint of increased pain at bilateral temporomandibular joints (TMJs). The patient reported her temporomandibular disorder (TMD) pain started with removal of her wisdom teeth when she was 16 years old. At the time of consultation, other complaints included pain at her head, neck, shoulders, and spasms in her tongue. Pain was described as a pulling and a tight sensation. In addition, she expressed some occasional right-side numbness of her tongue, and difficulty with mouth opening. Furthermore, she reported occasional tension-type headaches without aura.

Intensity of her symptoms increased with stress and were worst in the fall, at the return of stressful activities (i.e., sedentary work on the computer) as a doctoral student. Intensity of her symptoms decreased with yoga and swimming which she practices regularly. She was a competitive swimmer, rower, and figure skater during her teenage years. She slept on her left side or on her stomach with her head turned left.

Medical history includes asthma and general hyperlaxity. She was not taking any medication except for as needed ibuprofen, an over-the-counter non-steroidal anti-inflammatory. She wore orthodontic braces for 2 years during her teenage period.

As described above, she used a night guard for sleep, most of the time in periods of stress but by this point she was wearing it almost every night. The night guard contributed to reduce her everyday pain especially in mornings. However, in periods of high stress, pain increased, and mouth opening was more difficult. Referral in PT was recommended.

Clinical Findings

Upon evaluation, she presented with forward head posture and a very flat thoracic spine. The patient had pain at bilateral TMJs, predominantly on the right side as well as pain at the tongue, head, neck, and shoulders (Fig. 13.1).

She rated her pain on a 0 to 10 numeric pain scale at 4/10 when it is at its best and 8/10 at its worse. No red flags (i.e., signs of serious pathology) were identified. Her neurological examination with cranial nerves reactivity was within normal limits, excluding the need for a referral in neurology. Her tongue resistance was weaker on the right side in comparison to the left side. Overall, the right side was dominated by pain and muscle spasms, both of intermittent occurrence. Her mouth opening was of 35 mm and a decreased extension and left side flexion of the cervical spine was observed with reports of pain at end of range of motion. Her neck flexion, however, was increased. Her scapular positioning at rest was within normal limits, but her scapular rhythm was unequal between her right and left side as her right scapula presented with a decreased superior rotation with abduction/flexion of her arms.

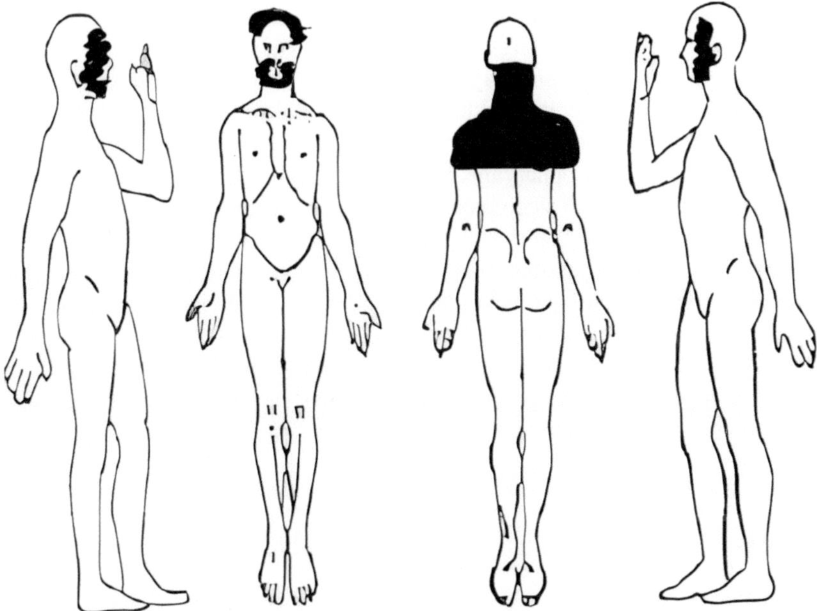

Fig. 13.1 Representation of pain areas as described by the patient. (Original figure. Reprinted with permission from A.E.C.)

Upon palpation, she presented with tightness of bilateral masseter, lateral pterygoid, posterior temporalis, levator scapulae, and sternocleidomastoid muscles. Manual muscle testing (i.e., evaluating the function and strength of muscles against gravity or manual resistance [1]) showed that her right superior trapezius, inferior trapezius, and her deep neck flexors were weak at 3+/5. Finally, assessment of arthrokinematics of her cervical spine showed decreased right rotation at C1–2 and increased opening and closing at bilateral C4–5. At her jaw, bilateral lateral glides and traction were decreased with early capsular end feels.

Diagnostic Assessment

TMD and SB initial diagnosis, as described above, was accomplished in 2018. Based on clinical history and examination, a working diagnosis of myofascial pain into the TMD category with SB was made. For TMD pain, these include objectively reported pain and soreness in jaw muscles and both TMJs upon palpation, based on the TMD diagnostic criteria (DC/TMD) [2]. For SB, muscle tension or discomfort upon awakening, with awareness of jaw clenching during sleep or in mornings, with diurnal activity of jaw bracing and clenching, with occasional tooth grinding confirmed by sleep partner, plus localized shiny spot on tooth and mild bilateral masseter muscle hypertrophy were reported. No complaints or signs and symptoms related to insomnia (i.e., 30 min delay in sleep onset or long duration sleep interruption 3 times a week for 3 months) or sleep apnea (i.e., sleepiness or fatigue, reported cessation of breathing, and upon clinical examination retrognathia, deep palpate, Mallampati or Friedman oropharyngeal high score, high body mass index/obesity) were reported. Therefore, no sleep recording test was ordered.

Relaxation therapy and referral to PT were suggested with use of over-the-counter pain medication (i.e., ibuprofen or acetaminophen with methocarbamol) at bedtime during stressful life periods. Moreover, we suggested she consider having a night guard (bite splint) to be made to manage sleep jaw clenching and tooth grinding to protect teeth and reduce jaw muscle contraction. The night guard was made on the upper jaw since, as listed above, no risk factors of sleep apnea were present, nor snoring was reported.

Diagnosis

PT clinical impression, upon evaluation, was that her TMD and neck pain with concomitant SB may be correlated with right rotation C1-2 hypomobility, bilateral C4-5 hypermobility, combined with weak shoulder blades more prominently on her right side. However, since the patient had other symptoms such as spasms and intermittent numbness in her tongue, a nerve irritation or radiculopathy was considered. However, since cranial nerves examination was within normal limits, including the hypoglossal nerve function, that last hypothesis was eliminated. A radiculopathy of the lower cervical nerves was considered. However, this hypothesis was eliminated due to all upper limb nerve tests (i.e., median, radial, and ulnar nerves), and the spurling test being negative.

Finally, possibility of myofascial pain with disc displacement was also considered. However, since there was no clicking or popping with jaw movement, no deviation with opening, no painful locked episodes and a quick improvement in jaw opening with muscle release (i.e., masseter), this hypothesis was also eliminated.

Prognosis

After working on and off with the patient with bilateral TMJ pain and SB for 3 years, she could be autonomous and cope with the situation most of the time if she was educated on: which exercises to maintain, how to manage her stress, and how to manage her posture. In cases like this, educating and motivating the patient are as important as PT manual therapies to manage overall pain, SB, and stress overlapping conditions.

Physiotherapeutic Intervention

Patient was seen in a private setting; she was seen approximately once a week for 7 follow-ups in 2019 and 5 follow-ups in 2022 (treatment is still ongoing (Fig. 13.2). First session of each period was 1 h, and follow-ups were 45 min. The last three sessions in 2022 were with a physiotherapist that practices dry needling and sessions were 30 min.

Many types of therapeutic intervention were used for the patient. Every session included education about posture (i.e., while sleeping and while working), stress, pain modalities (Table 13.1), and exercises (Fig. 13.3). A combination of manual therapy and myofascial release (i.e., stripping or trigger point release) was used according to what relieved the patient's pain, and what helped increase the mouth opening of the patient (Table 13.1).

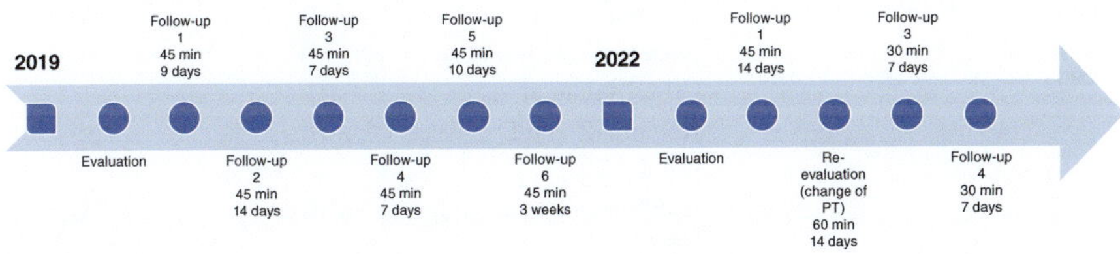

Fig. 13.2 Period with evaluation and follow-up including session lengths and time elapsed between sessions

Table 13.1 Example of one physiotherapeutic session

Categories		Subcategories	Explication/ recommendation	Time in session
Education	Postural education	Forward head posture	Cranio-cervical region -brings into flexion	2 min
		Flat thorax	Tighten the core and bring down the lower ribs closer to pelvis	2 min
		Sleeping positioning	Pillow height, i.e., height of shoulder to ear if sleeps on the side	2 min
	Exercises	Neck strengthening, shoulder blade strengthening, jaw strengthening, automassage	See Fig. 13.3 Demonstrate the exercise and have the patient does them simultaneously	5 min
	Stress management	Cardiorespiratory exercise	1–3 ×/week for 1 h	2 min
		Yoga	1–3 ×/week for 1 h	2 min
	Pain management	Heat and/or ice	15–20 min 1×/day	2 min
		Medication	When needed, to be discussed with the pharmacist	2 min

continued

Table 13.2 (continued)

Categories		Subcategories	Explication/ recommendation	Time in session
Myofascial release	Deep stripping	Paraspinals bilateral	4 × 1 min	4 min
		Sternocleidomastoid bilateral	4 × 1 min	4 min
		Masseter bilateral	3 × 1 min	3 min
		Temporalis bilateral	3 × 1 min	3 min
	Trigger point release	Lateral pterygoid bilateral	3 × 30 s	1 1/2 min
		Masseter bilateral	3 × 30 s	1 1/2 min
		Temporalis bilateral	3 × 30 s	1 1/2 min
Manual therapy	Neck	General neck traction	2 × 10 s	20 s
		Posterior-rotation glide C0-C1 bilateral	2 × 10 s	20 s
		Rotation R and L glide C1–2	2 × 10 s	20 s
		Anterior-posterior glide C4–6	2 × 10 s	20 s
		Posterior-anterior glide C4–6	2 × 10 s	20 s
	Temporomandibular joint	Lateral glide bilateral	2 × 10 s	20 s
		Traction mandible bilat	2 × 15 s	30 s

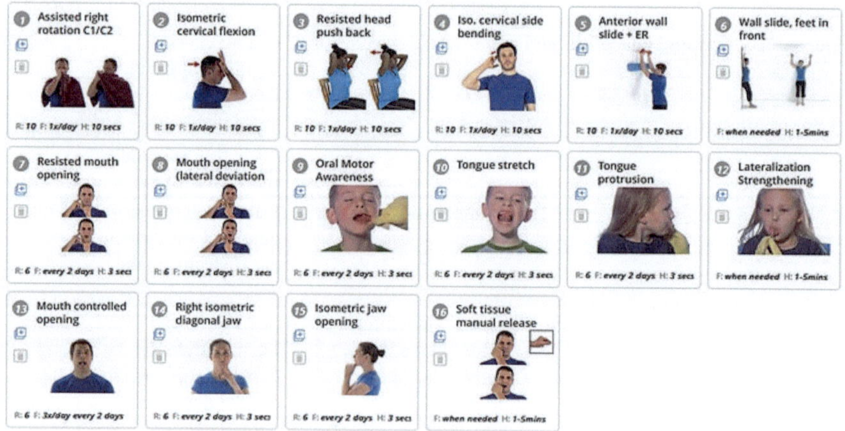

Fig. 13.3 Example of exercise program. (Image courtesy from Dr. J.T.A.T.Lam. Physiotec (https://physiotec.ca/ca/en, 1996–2023 all rights reserved))

Table 13.2 Example of dry needling techniques in one session

Physiotherapeutic puncture with dry needles (PPAS)		
Muscles	Length of needle	Parameters
Masseter	25 mm	Right + left × 1 each side
Lateral pterygoid	40 mm	Right + left × 1 each side
Suboccipital	25 mm	Right + left × 1 each side

Patient was diligent with recommended exercises. She kept on working on her posture during work and adapting to stress to the maximum of her abilities. Therefore, in the second period of PT treatment in 2022, we decided to try a new technique to quickly relieve pain since the patient was considering botulinum toxin injections into her masseters. Dry needling was suggested and done with success (Table 13.2).

Follow-Up and Outcomes

Adherence to exercises was subjectively evaluated by questioning the patient as well as the patient filling-in an exercise journal on the exercise software provided by the clinic. The software allows the patient to record the date when the exercises were accomplished, and its level of difficulty. Pain level was subjectively assessed every PT session with the pain numeric scale. Overtime, her pain slowly decreased and at the end of periods of treatments, pain was more manageable at around 0–2/10. Mouth opening was physically measured with a ruler at every session to monitor her progress. In both 2019 and 2022, the patient presented at the beginning of her treatment sessions with a maximal mouth opening of around 35 mm with pain, and by end of treatment, it was measured approximately at 50 mm without pain.

Discussion

One limitation in this case report is lack of standardized tools used to assess the patient. The reality in many private practices is that there is a lack of time to administer them. Neck Disability Index (NDI) [3] and Jaw Disability Index (JDI) may have been great tools to support neck-jaw function and presence of TMD [4]. The literature suggests that certain physiotherapy interventions can affect sleep quality as measured by the Pittsburgh Sleep Quality index (PSQI) questionnaire which is a validated sleep questionnaire for sleep quality [5]. Therefore, this questionnaire could have been used in this patient to monitor her sleep quality improvement secondary to the different PT interventions.

Another limitation was not addressing the psychological component of her SB diagnosis with a psychologist as it is commonly comorbid to anxiety disorders. However, psychological interventions (i.e., biofeedback, hypnotherapy, cognitive behavioral therapy, stress, and relaxation management) efficacy has not yet been confirmed [6, 7]. Possibly improving the patient's outcome by having a holistic approach should always be considered [8].

One of the strengths of the suggested intervention was the type of exercises chosen for the patient: cranio-cervical mobility, cervical strengthening, postural training, jaw strengthening, relaxing, and eccentric control and tongue strength. Even though the total number of exercises towards the end of the period of treatment was more than what is suggested for adherence (should be a maximum of 2 exercises) and here we had around 10 exercises, patient was still diligent and felt relief with them [9]. Most of the exercises were strengthening exercises, which support the literature which says masticatory muscle stretching for the jaw in SB is not efficient and, in the contrary, could increase SB episodes during sleep [10]. Furthermore, exercises targeting her posture and shoulder blade strength were also added underlying the positive effect that shoulder and neck muscles exercises can affect TMJ pain [11].

Types of chosen technique to treat the patient was also a strength of this case report. Manual therapy, here the specialization that has evolved within the field of PT such as TMJ mobilization and soft tissue mobilization, has been validated many times and is a viable and useful approach towards TMD management [5, 12–14]. In addition, deep-stripping massage has been shown to improve PSQI and jaw mobility of the masticatory muscles compared with trigger-point pressure release massage and traditional treatment techniques in SB patients in a 2022 randomized control study [5].

In PT, clinical recommendations are still being studied. A few recommendations, however, exist and are summarized below according to the Strength of Recommendation Taxonomy (SORT) for evaluating the strength of a recommendation based on a body of evidence and the quality of an individual study [15]. For now, deep muscle stripping of masticatory muscles seems to be a great avenue to improve pain and function in patient with concomitant SB [5, 11]—SORT A. Manual therapy, a subspecialty in PT, is a viable, cost-effective, and reversible technique of conservative treatment [14]—SORT B. Dry needling seems to be a promising avenue to decrease pain and tenderness of masticatory muscles as well as increase maximal jaw opening and function [16]—SORT C. Kinesiotaping, an elastic cotton strip with an adhesive is supported to ease pain and disability, is also an avenue to be explored. Combination of manual therapy and kinesiotaping for management of pain is effective, and more effective than manual therapy alone [17, 18]—SORT A. Stress management is important as there is a link between stress and SB [19]—SORT B.

Interventions made by other professionals are also strongly supported. Oral appliances are the main supported treatment for SB, no matter the type. There is more support for appliances that provide more mandibular advancement [20]—SORT A. Pharmacological approaches (i.e., botulinum toxin, clonazepam, and clonidine) may reduce sleep bruxism by their intrinsic action but placebo effect cannot be excluded [20, 21]—SORT A. Botulinum toxin in itself seems to be an acceptable short-term management technique to minimize symptoms and reducing intensity of muscle contraction (yet not contractions themselves) , although more studies are necessary [22, 23]—SORT A. Management of SB also involves treating any underlying sleep-disordered breathing (e.g., insomnia, snoring, sleep apnea) or other movement disorders (e.g., periodic limb movement). Therefore, polygraphic recordings might be necessary for certain cases [24]—SORT B. Collaboration in presence of comorbid SB with dentists and psychologist with expertise in sleep medicine may contribute to improve patients' outcomes [8]—SORT C. Future avenues are to be explored for SB such as transcranial magnetic stimulation which has shown positive results to decrease pain until now [25]—SORT C. However, more research on larger population and longer periods is needed.

In conclusion, as physiotherapists, we are trained to treat main complaints and its subsequent impacts. Even though a patient arrives to treatment with a prescription for the treatment of a specific condition, here SB, it is very important to question that diagnosis and emit a hypothesis of our own. In this situation, diagnosis was correct, but it was necessary to consider alternative hypotheses that could result in a similar clinical presentation. Furthermore, as physiotherapists, we must consider collaborative management including dentists, psychologists, and sleep specialists in cases such as reported above. By having a multidisciplinary approach, every aspect potentially affecting the patient (i.e., stress, sleep disturbances, insomnia, and snoring) and their chief complaint will be considered, and the patients will be provided with the necessary tools to be manage their pain more successfully.

References

1. Mindova S, Karaganova I. Innovative approach in the study of muscle strength-theoretical analysis. Health Promotion Section of the 2021 Online Scientific Conference; Online: University of Ruse and Union of Scientists - Ruse 2021;8(60):71–72.
2. Schiffman E, Ohrbach R, Truelove E, Look J, Anderson G, Goulet J-P, et al. Diagnostic criteria for temporomandibular disorders (DC/TMD) for clinical and research applications: recommendations of the International RDC/TMD Consortium Network and Orofacial Pain Special Interest Group. J Oral Facial Pain Headache. 2014;28(1):6.
3. Vernon H, Mior S. The Neck Disability Index: a study of reliability and validity. J Manipulative Physiol Ther. 1991;14:409.
4. Olivo SA, Fuentes J, Major P, Warren S, Thie N, Magee DJ. The association between neck disability and jaw disability. J Oral Rehabil. 2010;37(9):670–9.
5. El-Gendy MH, Ibrahim MM, Helmy ES, Neamat Allah N, Alkhamis BA, Koura GM, et al. Effect of manual physical therapy on sleep quality and jaw mobility in patients with bruxism: a biopsychosocial randomized controlled trial. Front Neurol. 2022;13:1041928.
6. Yap AU, Chua AP. Sleep bruxism: current knowledge and contemporary management. J Conserv Dent. 2016;19(5):383.
7. Wang L-F, Long H, Deng M, Xu H, Fang J, Fan Y, et al. Biofeedback treatment for sleep bruxism: a systematic review. Sleep Breath. 2014;18(2):235–42.
8. Herrero Babiloni A, Lam J, Exposto FG, Beetz G, Provost C, Gagnon DH, et al. Interprofessional collaboration in dentistry: role of physiotherapists to improve care and outcomes for chronic pain conditions and sleep disorders. J Oral Pathol Med. 2020;49(6):529–37.
9. Eckard T, Lopez J, Kaus A, Aden J. Home exercise program compliance of service members in the deployed environment: an observational cohort study. Mil Med. 2015;180(2):186–91.
10. Gouw S, de Wijer A, Kalaykova SI, Creugers NHJ. Masticatory muscle stretching for the management of sleep bruxism: a randomised controlled trial. J Oral Rehabil. 2018;45(10):770–6.
11. Calisgan E, Talu B, Altun O, Dedeoglu N, Duman BJM. The effects of proprioceptive neuromuscular facilitation, myofascial releasing maneuvers and home exercises on pain and jaw function in patients with bruxism. Med Sci. 2018;7(3):617–21.
12. Von Piekartz HJ. Kiefer, gesichts-und zervikalregion. Stuttgart: Thieme; 2005. p. 168–225.
13. Rocabado M, Iglarsh Z. Physical modalities and manual techniques used in the treatment of maxillofacial pain. 1st ed. Philadelphia, PA: JB Lippincott; 1991. p. 187–92.
14. Kalamir A, Pollard H, Vitiello AL, Bonello R. Manual therapy for temporomandibular disorders: a review of the literature. J Bodyw Mov Ther. 2007;11(1):84–90.
15. Ebell MH, Siwek J, Weiss BD, Woolf SH, Susman J, Ewigman B, et al. Strength of recommendation taxonomy (SORT): a patient-centered approach to grading evidence in the medical literature. Am Fam Physician. 2004;69(3):548–56.
16. Blasco-Bonora PM, Martín-Pintado-Zugasti A. Effects of myofascial trigger point dry needling in patients with sleep bruxism and temporomandibular disorders: a prospective case series. Acupunct Med. 2017;35(1):69–74.
17. Yazici G, Kafa N, Kolsuz ME, Volkan-Yazici M, Evli C, Orhan K. Evaluation of single session physical therapy methods in bruxism patients using shear wave ultrasonography. Cranio. 2020;1-7:41.
18. Lietz-Kijak D, Kopacz Ł, Ardan R, Grzegocka M, Kijak E. Assessment of the short-term effectiveness of Kinesiotaping and trigger points release used in functional disorders of the masticatory muscles. Pain Res Manag. 2018;2018:5464985.
19. Polmann H, Réus JC, Massignan C, Serra-Negra JM, Dick BD, Flores-Mir C, et al. Association between sleep bruxism and stress symptoms in adults: a systematic review and meta-analysis. J Oral Rehabil. 2021;48(5):621–31.
20. Manfredini D, Ahlberg J, Winocur E, Lobbezoo F. Management of sleep bruxism in adults: a qualitative systematic literature review. J Oral Rehabil. 2015;42(11):862–74.

21. Huynh N, Manzini C, Rompré PH, Lavigne GJ. Weighing the potential effectiveness of various treatments for sleep bruxism. J Can Dent Assoc. 2007;73(8):727–30.
22. De la Torre CG, Câmara-Souza MB, Do Amaral CF, Garcia RCMR, Manfredini D. Is there enough evidence to use botulinum toxin injections for bruxism management? A systematic literature review. Clin Oral Investig. 2017;21(3):727–34.
23. Shim YJ, Lee MK, Kato T, Park HU, Heo K, Kim S. Effects of botulinum toxin on jaw motor events during sleep in sleep bruxism patients: a polysomnographic evaluation. J Clin Sleep Med. 2014;10(3):291–8.
24. Carra MC, Huynh N, Fleury B, Lavigne G. Overview on sleep bruxism for sleep medicine clinicians. Sleep Med Clin. 2015;10(3):375–84, xvi.
25. Herrero Babiloni A, De Beaumont L, Lavigne GJ. Transcranial magnetic stimulation: potential use in obstructive sleep apnea and sleep bruxism. Sleep Med Clin. 2018;13(4):571–82.

Chapter 14
Hands-On Approach for Patients with Pain and Difficulty Opening the Mouth

Elisa Çalisgan ⓘ and Betül Akyol ⓘ

Introduction

Bruxism refers to the unintentional grinding and clenching of teeth that occur during both the day (diurnal) and night (nocturnal) [1]. It is regarded as one of the most significant parafunctional activities of the stomatognathic system. Temporomandibular joint dysfunction (TMD) and sleep bruxism lead to discomfort and trouble with mouth opening. TMD's causes and development involve various factors, including emotional disorders (i.e., anxiety and stress), occlusal factors (i.e., malocclusion and hard bite), the position of sleeping with the face towards mattress or pillow, forward head posture, whiplash syndrome, inflammation resulting from cytokines, hypermobility, female hormonal factors, and parafunctional habits [2, 3]. Symptoms of bruxism and TMD are abnormal tooth wear, pain and difficulty opening the mouth, grinding or clenching of the teeth and their respective sounds, swallowing difficulties, restriction of interincisal opening, decrease in salivary flow, frequent coughing, the feeling of obstruction in the throat, gingival inflammation, headache, ocular pain, limited mouth opening, tinnitus, the sensation of the blocked ear, temporomandibular joint (TMJ) pain, clicking sounds, hypertrophy, and destruction of the masseter and temporal muscles [4]. One of the most common symptoms is jaw clicking when opening the mouth, with oral muscle deviation to one side, pain in the cheek muscles, and uncontrollable movement of the

E. Çalisgan (✉)
Department of Physiotherapy and Rehabilitation, Faculty of Health Science, Kahramanmaras Sutcu Imam University, Kahramanmaras, Turkey

B. Akyol
Department of Physical Education and Sport Malatya, Faculty of Sport Science, Inonu University, Malatya, Turkey

C. Frange (ed.), *Clinical Cases in Sleep Physical Therapy*,
https://doi.org/10.1007/978-3-031-38340-3_14

jaw. Neck problems can develop with pain in the shoulders and back, stiffness, and limited jaw mobility (trismus). Facial changes can also be seen in patients with bruxism, such as facial muscles atrophy or hypertrophy, and drooping of the corners of the mouth [5].

There are different approaches to treating sleep bruxism, such as Botox, oral devices, behavioral therapy, and medication [6–8]. While the occlusal appliance can prevent teeth from wearing down during sleep, it doesn't entirely eliminate the automatic grinding or clenching, and it also doesn't ease any related pain or discomfort [9]. Sometimes it worsens the situation.

Manual treatment options may involve using mouthguards, dental restorations, or occlusal splints combined with massage or physical therapy to ease muscle tension [10, 11], and to increase proprioception. Nonetheless, the most successful sleep bruxism treatment relies on the cause and should be individualized. To date, there are physiotherapeutic treatments focusing on sleep bruxism symptoms [12]. Physiotherapy and rehabilitation provide facial muscle control and restoration of functionality and proprioception, being important in sleep bruxism treatment, with time and cost advantages [13].

In this case report, we evaluated the effects of a hands-on approach (proprioceptive neuromuscular facilitation exercises (PNF), myofascial release techniques, Rocabado's 6 × 6 exercises, home exercises) for a 28-year-old patient with neck, back, and TMJ pain and difficulty opening the mouth.

Patient Information

E.S.C., a woman, 28-year-old, diagnosed with bruxism at the Department of Maxillofacial Radiology, Faculty of Dentistry, Inonu University, sought for treatment for her sleep bruxism, neck and back pain, and difficulty opening the mouth. Her body mass index (BMI) was 23 kg/m^2.

Clinical Findings

During the initial examination, E.S.C. reported a resting pain score of 4.3, an activity pain score of 7.3, and a night pain score of 7.0. She was having pain at the masticatory, neck, trapezius, and back muscles, postural disorders (forward head, thoracic kyphosis), facial asymmetry, and crepitation in TMJ during the past month and denied systemic rheumatic disease or fibromyalgia, dental issues, or orofacial pain disorders, TMJ disc displacement, osteoarthritis, cervical structural problems, was not taking over-the-counter analgesics or using narcotics, hypnotic drugs, sedatives, or muscle relaxants.

Diagnostic Assessment

E.S.C.'s progress was assessed at the beginning and end of the 8 weeks using: measures for pain intensity, limitations of jaw movement, and oral behavior. The intensity of pain was assessed utilizing a Visual analog scale (VAS), which measures pain on a scale of 0 (no pain) to 10 (unbearable pain) [14]. Limitations of jaw movement were measured by Jaw Restriction Scale, which include 8 items related to typical mouth functions like chewing, yawning, swallowing, and smiling. Each item is scored on a scale from 0 to 10, with 0 indicating no restrictions and 10 indicating high restrictions. The total score on this scale ranges from 0 to 80. A score of 0 shows that no jaw restriction and a very good condition, while a score of 80 indicates complete jaw limitation [4]. The Oral Behaviour Checklist (OBC) comprises 21 questions that inquire about harmful oral/parafunctional habits that can contribute to TMJ degeneration, hypertrophy of specific muscles, headaches, and other issues like loss of muscle strength and pain in cervical vertebrae muscles such as long colli, splenius, and scalenus. The checklist utilizes a 5-point Likert scale, where respondents select one of the five responses ranging from never to always. The total score for the checklist ranges from 0 to 84 [15].

Physiotherapeutic Intervention

PNF exercises, myofascial relaxation, Rocabado's 6 × 6 exercises, and home exercises including self-care program were performed for 6 days a week for 8 weeks. In this protocol, a combination of isotonic techniques was employed, involving the use of both concentric and stabilizing contractions.

The proprioceptive neuromuscular facilitation (PNF) technique began with a concentric contraction of the targeted muscle, followed by maintaining the end position for 6 s (isometric) while resisting against any movement (stabilizing contractions) (Fig. 14.1). PNF therapy is a treatment method used for patients with sleep bruxism that applies equal and symmetrical stimulation to all muscle groups, using specific points of the muscles on the mouth, nose, and eyes. The goal is to alleviate movement restrictions on the affected side by providing resistance with forceful movements. This technique helps to distribute muscle strength. Bruxism primarily affects the buccinator muscle and tongue movements, so coordinated movements are applied to these specific areas using techniques like tongue depressors and exercises that mimic laughing or sucking [16].

Massage therapy techniques used to release myofascial tension involved sliding and kneading movements applied to the masseter and temporal muscles, as well as the neck and upper trapezius muscles. The sliding and kneading maneuvers were performed using hand and finger movements to help relax muscles that were co-contracted [17, 18]. To alleviate myofascial tension, massage therapy techniques

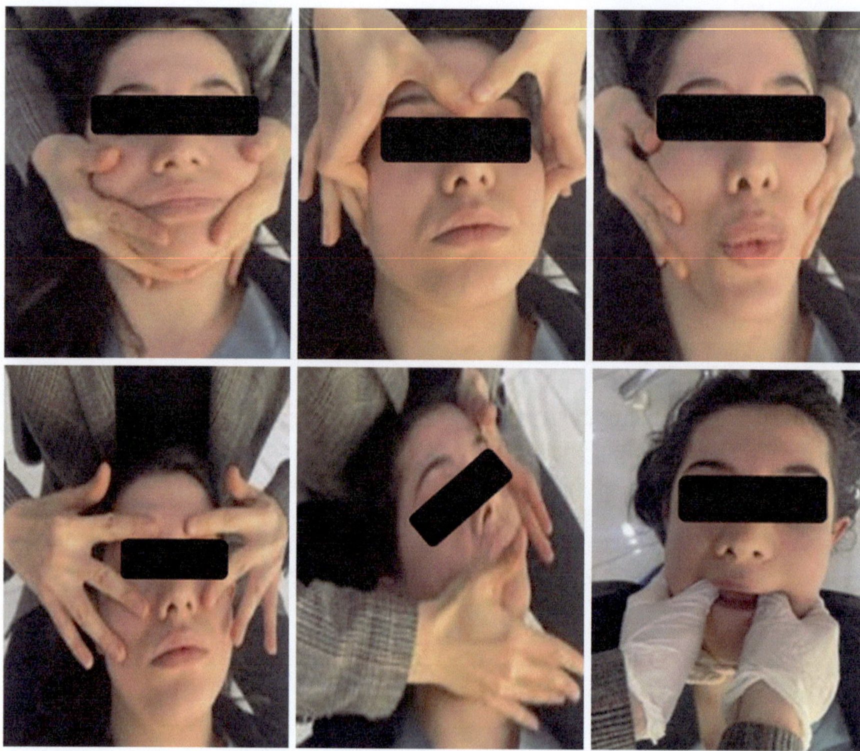

Fig. 14.1 Proprioceptive Neuromuscular Facilitation being applied on selected muscles of the face. (Reprinted with permission from E.S.C.)

were employed, which involved the use of sliding and kneading movements on the masseter, temporal muscles, as well as upper trapezius muscles, and neck area (Fig. 14.2). These sliding and kneading techniques were carried out using hand and finger movements, aimed at relaxing the muscles that were co-contracted. This was followed by 6 sets of 6 repetitions at home under the guidance of a physiotherapist.

E.S.C. experienced pain and difficulty with mouth opening. Therefore, Rocabado's 6 × 6 exercises and self-care exercises to alleviate pain and address various muscles, including the masseter, lateral and medial pterygoid, buccinator, temporalis, orbicularis oris, orbicularis oculi, the upper side of the trapezius muscle, splenius, scalenus, and cervical extensor muscle, were performed [19, 20]. Rocabado's 6 × 6 exercises were administered for 6 days per week for a total of 8 weeks. This program included 6 exercises, each with 6 repetitions, to be performed 6 times a day. The content of Rocabado's 6 × 6 exercises is: (1) rest position for the tongue: to rest the tongue and jaw and to promote diaphragmatic breathing in order to decrease activity of the accessory muscles; (2) shoulder posture: shoulder girdle retraction to correct abnormal scapular protraction; (3) stabilized head flexion: distraction of the upper cervical spine to alleviate mechanical

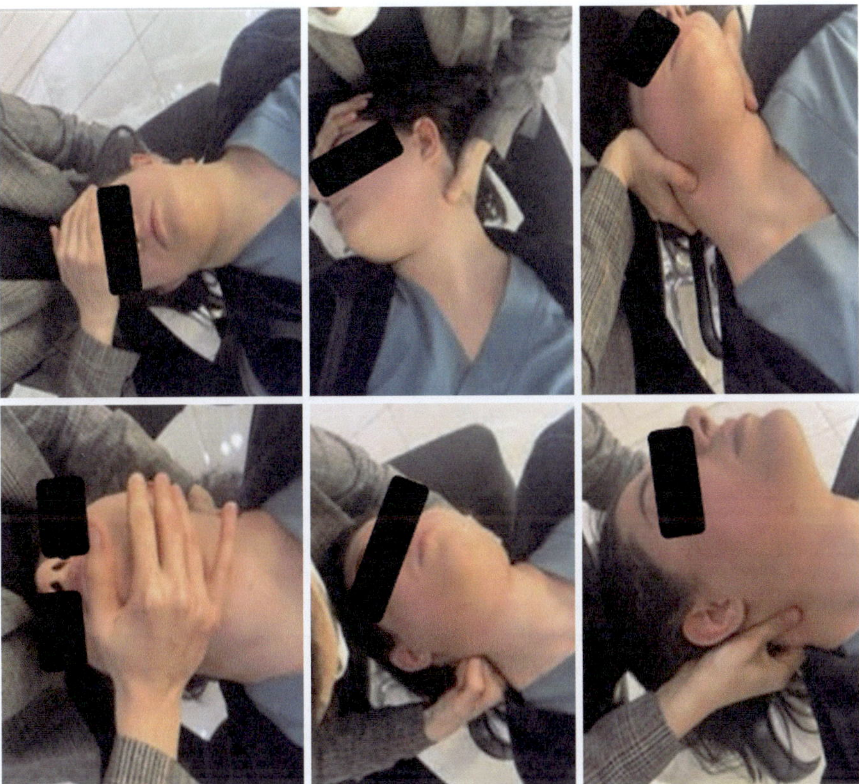

Fig. 14.2 Myofascial release applications maneuvers for the upper side of the trapezius muscle, splenius, scalenus, cervical flexor, and extensor muscles. (Reprinted with permission from E.S.C.)

compressions—this leads to the elongation of the posterior cervical muscles; (4) axial extension of the neck: distraction of the cervical spine—this leads to tension reduction in the supra and infrahyoid muscles and enhances the ability of the chewing muscles to relax. This exercise helps the sternocleidomastoid muscle take a normal posterior angulation, thus reducing unnecessary muscle activity to maintain the position; (5) control of TMJ rotation: reducing translatory component when initiating jaw movements (i.e., protrusive movement in mouth opening, talking, or chewing), which leads to a reduction in masticatory muscle activity and joint overload; and (6) rhythmic stabilization technique, inducing muscle relaxation based on the principle of reciprocal inhibition. When a muscle is actively contracted, its antagonists are consequently relaxed. Rhythmic stabilization also enhances the proper jaw rest position through proprioception [19].

Home exercises such as practicing facial expressions in front of a mirror, such as blowing up a balloon, sending a kiss, raising eyebrows, and tightly closing eyes, as well as self-care practices such as not chewing only on one side, avoiding exerting force on teeth [21] and TMJ with hard objects, and not sleeping on one lateral side [22] were recommended.

Follow-Up and Outcomes

After implementing PNF, myofascial release, and home exercises, significant improvements were observed in E.S.C. pain scores, jaw movements, and oral/parafunctional habits. Specifically, there were significant differences in the patient's resting, active, and night pain scores, which decreased to 1.0, 1.3, and 2.0 points, respectively. The patient's jaw restriction score was significantly reduced from 47 points during the initial evaluation to 24 points after the rehabilitation program. Furthermore, there was a significant improvement in the oral/parafunctional behavior measurements, with a decrease from 61 points to 23 points over the two-month period.

Discussion

The objective of this case report was to explore the impact of PNF, myofascial release, Rocabado, and home exercises on pain, jaw restriction, and oral/parafunctional habits in a woman with sleep bruxism.

Earlier research has examined how the amount of myofascial exercise and home exercise is linked to the sleep bruxism threshold. To improve sleep bruxism symptoms, a physical exercise involving moderate intensity and 3–4 sessions per week, each lasting at least 30 min, has been recommended [8]. Based on the findings of the present study, PNF, myofascial relaxation, and home exercise lead to a reduction in TMJ crepitation, pain, restricted jaw movement, and bad oral/parafunctional habits. The use of PNF and myofascial relaxation is associated with increased local blood flow and the normalization of muscle conditions, leading to a decrease in pain and hypertrophy of the masseter, lateral, and medial pterygoid muscles [16, 20].

Exercises often require warm-up and cool-down phases, but in this case, they were not emphasized. While experts recommend warm-up and cool-down periods for exercises, they can be minimized for bruxism. Studies have revealed that exercise affects the adrenocortical system, increases epinephrine transmission between neurons, and boosts serotonin levels. As a result, exercise is considered a new biological approach to reducing the negative effects of bruxism [23, 24].

Myofascial relaxation and PNF have been shown to enhance the strength of weight-bearing bilateral face muscles, including the temporalis, masseter, buccinator, and lateral and medial pterygoid muscles [20]. PNF, Rocabado's exercises, myofascial relaxation, and home exercises decreased pain, restriction of jaw movement, muscle hypertrophy, and increased strength of the facial muscles, upper trapezius and extensor muscle of the neck, therefore increasing the well-being of our patient.

In an investigation comparing the effects of massage therapy and occlusal splint in patients with sleep bruxism, the participants were allocated into four groups: massage, which included sliding and kneading hand and finger maneuvers on the masseter and temporal muscles; occlusal splint; a combined, with massage + occlusal splint; and a control group. The combined treatment approach was found to provide the most significant pain reduction [25].

Rocabado's 6 × 6 exercises were investigated for myofascial jaw pain in a previous study. The Rocabado's exercises were added to a self-care program and provided additional benefits in reducing myofascial jaw pain and improving forward head posture [21]. The study involved 45 participants who were randomly assigned to either self-care alone or self-care plus the Rocabado's exercises. The primary outcome measure was the intensity of jaw pain, while the secondary outcome measures included neck pain and changes in head posture. Both groups showed significant improvement in jaw and neck pain, but with no significant differences between the groups. Additionally, no significant improvements in head posture were observed in either group within the 4-week study period. Therefore, the study concluded that the Rocabado's exercises did not provide any significant additional benefits in reducing jaw and neck pain or improving head posture beyond self-care alone [21]. Therefore, in our case, Rocabado's combined with PNF and myofascial release played a significant role in decreasing pain and enhancing jaw mobility for E.S.C., contrary to the aforementioned investigation. More studies are warranted.

In conclusion, this case demonstrated that combined techniques of physiotherapy (i.e., PNF, Rocabado's 6 × 6 exercises, myofascial release and home exercise) effectively decreased TMJ, neck and back pain, restriction of jaw movement, and bad/parafunctional oral habits.

References

1. Lavigne GJ, et al. Bruxism physiology and pathology: an overview for clinicians. J Oral Rehabil. 2008;35:476–94.
2. Aguilera SB, Brown L, Perico VA. Aesthetic treatment of bruxism. J Clin Aesthet Dermatol. 2017;10(5):49.
3. Abe S, Kawano F, Matsuka Y, Masuda T, Okawa T, Tanaka E. Relationship between oral parafunctional and postural habits and the symptoms of temporomandibular disorders: a survey-based cross-sectional cohort study using propensity score matching analysis. J Clin Med. 2022;11(21):6396.
4. Ohrbach R. Diagnostic criteria for temporomandibular disorders: assessment instruments. Amsterdam: Department of Oral Health Sciences; 2016.
5. Minervini G, Fiorillo L, Russo D, Minervini G, Fiorillo L, Russo D, Lanza A, D'Amico C, Cervino G, Di Francesco F, et al. Prosthodontic treatment in patients with temporomandibular disorders and orofacial pain and/or bruxism: a review of the literature. PRO. 2022;4(2):253–62.
6. Kim NH, Park RH, Park JB. Botulinum toxin type a for the treatment of hypertrophy of the masseter muscle. Plast Reconstr Surg. 2010;125(6):1693–705.
7. Yu CC, Chen PKT, Chen YR. Botulinum toxin a for lower facial contouring: a prospective study. Aesthetic Plast Surg. 2007;31:445–51.
8. Lobbezoo F, Van Der Zaag J, Van Selms MKA, Hamburger HL, Naeije M. Principles for the management of bruxism. J Oral Rehabil. 2008;35(7):509–23.
9. van der Zaag J, Lobbezoo F, Wicks DJ, Visscher CM, Hamburger HL, Naeije M. Controlled assessment of the efficacy of occlusal stabilization splints on sleep bruxism. J Orofac Pain. 2005;19(2):151.

10. Michelotti A, Steenks MH, Farella M, Parisini F. Short-term effects of physiotherapy versus counselling for the treatment of myofascial pain of the jaw muscles. J Oral Rehabil. 2002;29(9):874.

11. Lang R, White PJ, Machalicek W, Rispoli M, Kang S, Aquilar J, Didden R, et al. Treatment of bruxism in individuals with developmental disabilities: a systematic review. Res Dev Disabil. 2009;30(5):809–18.

12. Frange C, Franco AM, Brasil E, Hirata RP, Lino JA, Mortari DM, Ykeda DS, Leocádio-Miguel MA, D'Aurea CVR, Silva LOE, Telles SCL, Furlan SF, Peruchi BB, Leite CF, Yagihara FT, Campos LD, Ulhôa MA, Cruz MGDR, Beidacki R, Santos RB, de Queiroz SS, Barreto S, Piccin VS, Coelho FMS, Studart L, Assis M, Drager LF. Practice recommendations for the role of physiotherapy in the management of sleep disorders: the 2022 Brazilian sleep association guidelines. Sleep Sci. 2022;15(4):515–73.

13. Kaur J, Masaun M, Bhatia MS. Role of physiotherapy in mental health disorders. Delhi Psychiatry J. 2013;16:404–8.

14. Ferreira-Valente MA, Pais-Ribeiro JL, Jensen MP. Validity of four pain intensity rating scales. Pain. 2011;152(10):2399–404.

15. Ohrbach R, Beneduce C, Markiewicz M, McCall WD Jr. Psychometric properties of the oral behaviors checklist: preliminary findings. J Dent Res. 2004;83(1):1194.

16. Livanelioğlu A, Erden Z, Günel MK. Proprioseptif Nöromusküler Fasilitasyon Teknikleri. 1. Baskı. Ankara: Ankamat Matbaacılık; 2014. p. 87–90.

17. Park MY, Ahn KY, Jung DS. Botulinum toxin type a treatment for contouring of the lower face. Dermatol Surg. 2003;29(5):477–83.

18. Valiente López M, Van Selms MKA, Van Der Zaag J, Hamburger HL, Lobbezoo F. Do sleep hygiene measures and progressive muscle relaxation influence sleep bruxism? Report of a randomised controlled trial. J Oral Rehabil. 2015;42(4):259–65.

19. Uçar İ, Kararti C, Dadali Y, Özüdoğru A, Okçu M. Masseter muscle thickness and elasticity in bruxism after exercise treatment: a comparison trial. J Manipulative Physiol Ther. 2022;45(4):282–9.

20. Kurt A, Turhan B. Physiotherapy management of migraine pain: facial proprioceptive neuromuscular facilitation technique versus connective tissue massage. J Craniofac Surg. 2022;33(8):2328–32.

21. Mulet M, Decker KL, Look JO, Lenton PA, Schiffman EL. A randomized clinical trial assessing the efficacy of adding 6 x 6 exercises to self-care for the treatment of masticatory myofascial pain. J Orofac Pain. 2007;21(4):318–28.

22. Ferrillo M, Nucci L, Giudice A, Calafiore D, Marotta N, Minervini G, de Sire A, et al. Efficacy of conservative approaches on pain relief in patients with temporomandibular joint disorders: a systematic review with network meta-analysis. Cranio. 2022:1–17.

23. Visser A, McCarroll RS, Naeije M. Masticatory muscle activity in different jaw relations during submaximal clenching efforts. J Dent Res. 1992;71(2):372–9.

24. Harness DM, Peltier B. Comparison of MMPI scores with self-report of sleep disturbance and bruxism in the facial pain population. Headache. 1994;34(6):383.

25. de Paula Gomes CAF, El-Hage Y, Amaral AP, Herpich CM, Politti F, Kalil-Bussadori S, Biasotto-Gonzalez DA, et al. Effects of massage therapy and occlusal splint usage on quality of life and pain in individuals with sleep bruxism: a randomized controlled trial. J Jpn Phys Therapy Assoc. 2015;18(1):1–6.

Part VII

Clinical Cases: Obstructive Sleep Apnea

Chapter 15
Only Apnea-Hypopnea Index? What Else to Look For?

Daiana M. Mortari (ID)

Introduction

In this chapter, we will discuss the importance of a detailed analysis of the diagnostic sleep study of a patient with obstructive sleep apnea (OSA) with hypoxemia. The presentation of this case will emphasize the proper interpretation of polysomnographic variables in order to optimize the proposed treatment.

Patient Information

L.A.N. is a woman, 70 years old, who sought for a sleep physician due to loud snoring, witnessed apneas, morning headache, daily sleepiness and fatigue. She used to go to sleep at 10 pm and wake up at 7:30 am. When asked, she reported that her father, mother, and brothers used to complain of snoring as well. The snore symptom used to be eventual and started to increase around the age of 60 years. The tiredness got worse since 67 years of age. Besides that, the patient was having lack of attention at work. In the past 10 years, she gained 15 kg. In addition to snoring and apneas, her daughter also observes irritability and memory loss.

D. M. Mortari (✉)
Federal University of Rio Grande do Sul, Porto Alegre, RS, Brazil

C. Frange (ed.), *Clinical Cases in Sleep Physical Therapy*,
https://doi.org/10.1007/978-3-031-38340-3_15

Clinical Findings

Physical examination showed a body mass index (BMI) of 30.9 kg/m^2, neck circumference of 36 cm, and modified Malampatti [1] grade 3, indicating a higher risk of OSA. Epworth Sleepiness Scale [2] score was 11 points indicating excessive daytime sleepiness and STOP-BANG [3] score was 5 indicating a higher risk of OSA. The patient was already in treatment for hypertension, dyslipidemia, and arrhythmia.

Diagnostic Assessment

As the sleep specialist suspected of OSA, L.A.N. underwent a type I sleep study. She considered the night of the exam similar to her daily nights at home. Table 15.1 and Fig. 15.1 show the relevant data resulting from the polysomnography exam:

Table 15.1 Polysomnographic data

Sleep latency	67 min
Rapid eye movement (REM) latency	86.5 min
N1 sleep stage	13.5%
N2 sleep stage	51.2%
N3 sleep stage	20.1%
REM sleep stage	15.2%
Arousal index	17.7 per hour of sleep
Wake after sleep onset (WASO)	97.2 min
Apnea-hypopnea index (AHI)	40.8 events per hour of sleep
Obstructive apneas	70
Mixed apneas	5
Central apneas	0
Hypopneas	104
Oxygen desaturation index (ODI)	17.9 per hour of sleep
Mean and nadir SpO$_2$	94% e 58%
Time with SpO$_2$ < 90%	51.2 min, 20% of sleep time
Periodic leg movement index	1.3 per hour of sleep

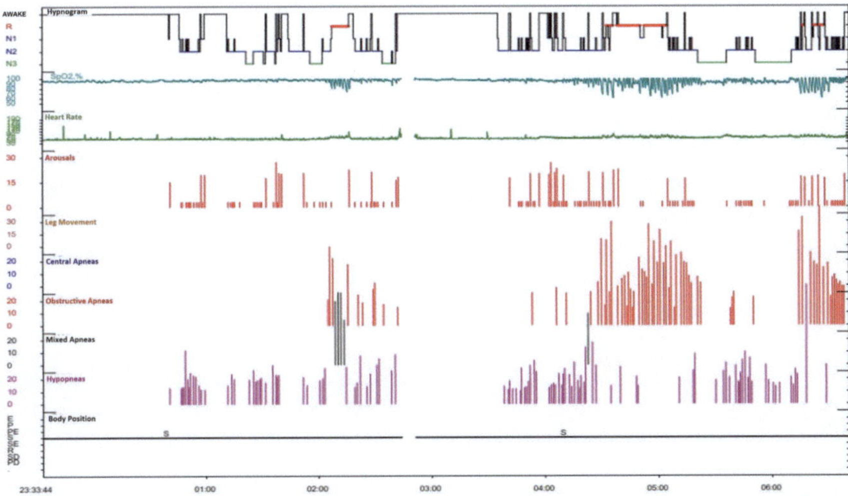

Fig. 15.1 Polysomnography graphic data. (With permission from L.A.N.) Sleep latency and wake after sleep onset (WASO) are increased. REM sleep stage is diminished, and NREM N1 sleep stage is increased. High number of obstructive apneas and hypopneas associated with significant desaturation while in REM sleep stage and arousals while in NREM sleep stages are presented. (Original Figure)

Physiotherapeutic Intervention

Before establishing the appropriate therapeutic approaches for a patient with sleep disorders, a careful analysis of the diagnostic exam is essential. Observing the statistical data is possible to notice an increase in sleep latency (time from lights out until the first epoch of any stage of sleep), and in wake after sleep onset (WASO), and a decrease in the percentage of REM sleep. To exclude a possible laboratory effect, it is essential the patient evaluation certifying that the night of the exam is compatible with the nights at home.

Once increased sleep latency and increased WASO may suggest insomnia, which can be an obstacle to positive pressure adherence and demand interdisciplinary treatment, we proceed to the analysis of the respiratory variables. By looking only at the AHI, we are limited to the information that this is a patient with severe OSA. However, the perception of possible different endotypes and phenotypes in

Compliance Statistics

Start Date - End Date	10/17/2022- 1/14/2023				
Total Days Device Used	6	day(s)	(100%)		
Total Days Device Not Used	0	day(s)	(0%)		
Days Device Used > = 4 hrs	6	day(s)	(100%)		
Average Used (Days on Therapy)	08	hr(s)	25	min(s)	
Average Used (All Days)	08	hr(s)	25	min(s)	
Total Run Time	50	hr(s)	30	min(s)	

Efficacy Statistics

(All efficacy statistics are averages over the report period.)

AHI	1.8	
CAI	0.1	
Apnea Length	12	s
Average Pressure	4.0	cmH2O
90th Percentile Pressure	5.0	cmH2O
% Time at Maximum Set Pressure	0	%
System Leak	28.0	L/min
90th Percentile System Leak	37.0	L/min
% Time with Excessive Leak	2	%

Fig. 15.2 Home titration data. (With permission from L.A.N., Original Figure)

the same patient is essential. In the above case, we only have hypopnea events, mostly validated by arousal, when the patient is in NREM sleep, suggesting a low arousal threshold. In REM sleep, most of the obstructive events are obstructive apneas accompanied by significant drops in oxyhemoglobin saturation, suggesting low muscle responsiveness endotype. These important changes are reflected by the discrepancy between the AHI, ODI, and arousal index.

From these understandings, we can formulate a clinical reasoning focused on a treatment plan for this patient. The low arousal threshold, seen in NREM sleep, could impact the patient adherence once continuous positive airway pressure (CPAP) higher pressures may be needed to open the airway when in REM sleep. After ergonomic instructions, it was agreed with the patient that lateral decubitus, which was not documented on the night of the exam, would be the posture to be adopted whenever possible. So, we would increase the possibility of controlling respiratory events, especially in REM, with lower therapeutic pressures. The patient underwent home automatic titration with a PAP device, with automatic mode activated, minimum pressure of 4.0 cmH$_2$O and maximum pressure of 12.0 cmH$_2$O, and nasal mask. Expiratory pressure relief was off and a pressure relief guided by awake was on. Figure 15.2 shows the statistical data of the titration nights.

As can be seen, the AHI was normalized with CPAP of 5.0 cmH$_2$O. The patient used the device all night from the first night of use with good adaptation to the nasal mask. The association of positional therapy and positive pressure therapy allowed that possible discomfort arising from the different pathophysiological mechanisms involved in this patient's respiratory disorder (i.e., low awakening threshold in NREM and low muscle responsiveness in REM endotypes) to be annulled.

Discussion

Until a few years ago, the AHI was the most important variable to be considered when a polysomnography was analyzed by the respiratory point of view. This variable, which represents the number of apnea and hypopnea events that occur per hour of sleep, determines the OSA severity and, consequently, the most appropriate therapeutic interventions. In recent years, other variables proved to be equally important to better conduct the treatment of patients with OSA. The percentage of time during sleep with an oxygen saturation below 90% established its clinical importance as a better cardiovascular risk marker when compared to the AHI [4]. The determination of the different phenotypes and endotypes of OSA, described by authors such as Subramani et al., allowed a better understanding of the pathophysiology of the disease that affects each of the patients and, therefore, the personalization of conducts and therapeutic objectives [5]. Recently, the development of variables such as hypoxic load tends to further optimize precision medicine [6].

A retrospective study compared patients who underwent manual titration combining positional therapy to CPAP versus CPAP only [7]. Patients titrated with combined therapies had higher BMI, higher neck and waist circumference, lower nadir SpO_2, and spent more time with $SpO_2 < 90\%$. The authors concluded that positional therapy plus CPAP was an effective solution for difficult to treat patients, such as the one in our case report.

It is of fundamental importance that the sleep physiotherapist follows the updates of scientific knowledge that allow greater precision in the adoption of therapies and, consequently, greater effectiveness and adherence by the patient.

Patient Perspective

L.A.N. reported that she felt better since the first night of CPAP usage. She was not sleepy anymore and the tiredness was solved as well. Her daughter mentioned that L.A.N. was not snoring anymore and even her face seemed more rested.

References

1. Friedman M, Salapatas AM, Bonzelaar LB. Updated friedman staging system for obstructive sleep apnea. Adv Otorhinolaryngol. 2017;80:41–8. https://doi.org/10.1159/000470859.
2. Bertolazi AN, Fagondes SC, Hoff LS, Pedro VD, Menna Barreto SS, Johns MW. Portuguese-language version of the Epworth sleepiness scale: validation for use in Brazil. J Bras Pneumol. 2009;35(9):877–83. https://doi.org/10.1590/s1806-37132009000900009.

3. Chung F, Abdullah HR, Liao P. STOP-bang questionnaire: a practical approach to screen for obstructive sleep apnea. Chest. 2016;149(3):631–8. https://doi.org/10.1378/chest.15-0903.
4. Oldenburg O, Wellmann B, Buchholz A, Bitter T, Fox H, Thiem U, Horstkotte D, Wegscheider K. Nocturnal hypoxaemia is associated with increased mortality in stable heart failure patients. Eur Heart J. 2016;37:1695–703.
5. Subramani Y, Singh M, Wong J, Kushida CA, Malhotra A, Chung F. Understanding phenotypes of obstructive sleep apnea: applications in anesthesia, surgery, and perioperative medicine. Anesth Analg. 2017;124(1):179–91. PMID: 27861433; PMCID: PMC5429962. https://doi.org/10.1213/ANE.0000000000001546.
6. Azarbarzin A, Sands SA, Stone KL, Taranto-Montemurro L, Messineo L, Terrill PI, Ancoli-Israel S, Ensrud K, Purcell S, White DP, Redline S, Wellman A. The hypoxic burden of sleep apnoea predicts cardiovascular disease-related mortality: the osteoporotic fractures in men study and the sleep heart health study. Eur Heart J. 2019;40(14):1149–57.
7. Goyal A, Pakhare A, Subhedar R, Khurana A, Chaudhary P. Combination of positional therapy with positive airway pressure for titration in patients with difficult to treat obstructive sleep apnea. Sleep Breath. 2021;25(4):1867–73. Epub 2021 Jan 23. https://doi.org/10.1007/s11325-021-02291-6.

Chapter 16
Be Aware or You Will Be Mistaken: It Is Not Only CPAP!

Flávia B. Nerbass (iD) and Liliane P. S. Mendes (iD)

Introduction

An average of 56% of patients with obstructive sleep apnea (OSA) have position-dependent obstructive respiratory events (POSA), mainly in the supine position [1]. POSA is commonly defined as a difference of 50% or more in apnea-hypopnea index between supine and non-supine positions [2] showed in polysomnography (PSG) report [3]. However, the OSA severity in different body positions is sometimes ignored by the by clinicians, because it can be masked by an elevated overall apnea-hypopnea index (AHI) (indicating globally moderate or severe OSA), mainly when the patient complains of tiredness, loud snoring, daytime sleepiness, etc. Moreover, these variables are not always available in PSG report. However, for those patients with POSA, positional therapy becomes an additional viable treatment option [3]. This chapter reports the case of a patient with severe symptomatic OSA showed by overall AHI on PSG, which was effectively resolved with positional therapy.

F. B. Nerbass (✉)
Sleep Laboratory, Pulmonary Division, University of Sao Paulo School of Medicine, Sao Paulo, SP, Brazil

L. P. S. Mendes
Physiotherapy Department, Federal University of Minas Gerais, Belo Horizonte, MG, Brazil

C. Frange (ed.), *Clinical Cases in Sleep Physical Therapy*, https://doi.org/10.1007/978-3-031-38340-3_16

Patient Information

A 63-year-old, obese (body mass index [BMI] 30.1 kg/m^2), hypertensive, woman presented with hyperglycemia and osteoporosis. She complained of snoring (mainly in the supine position), waking up coughing, choking, and sometimes presenting nocturia. She reported fragmented sleep, maintenance insomnia, waking up tired, daytime sleepiness, sleep bruxism, nocturnal gastroesophageal reflux, memory impairment, and mood swings (mainly irritability and discouragement).

Diagnostic Assessment

Her baseline PSG showed fragmented sleep (arousals 50.5 ev/h), mainly in the first 2 h after sleep onset, and reduced rapid eye movement (REM) sleep time, as shown on the hypnogram (Fig. 16.1). The patient was diagnosed with severe obstructive sleep apnea (overall AHI = 72.3 ev/h), presented mean oxygen saturation (SatO$_2$) of 93%, time of saturation <90% of 11.6 min, and lowest SatO$_2$ of 83%.

She came to our service to adapt the continuous positive airway pressure (CPAP) therapy, but was very uncomfortable with the possibility of long-term CPAP use. However, in our assessment, we identified in her baseline PSG, a higher AHI only in the supine position. She remained almost the entire time of sleep in supine position, when she turned to the right side decubitus; she promptly reached REM sleep

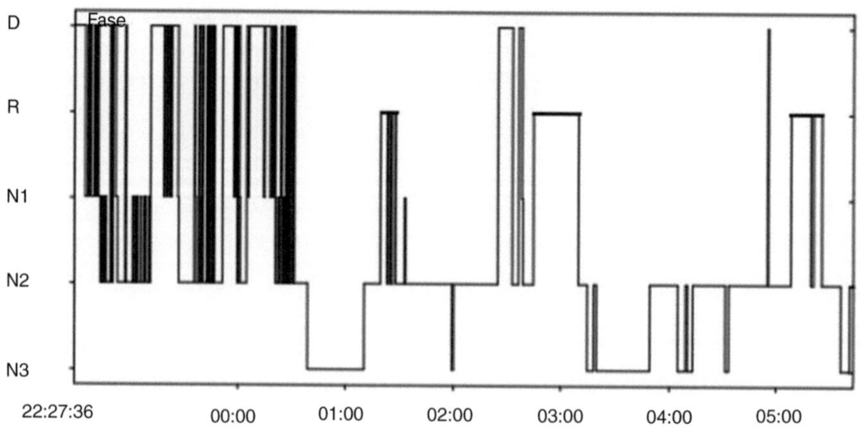

Fig. 16.1 Baseline PSG hypnogram showing successive awakenings and sleep stages shifts, mainly between N1 and N2 in the first 2 h after sleep onset. In addition, we observe few opportunities to reach REM sleep stage, and NREM N3 sleep stage. (*D* awake, *N1* NREM N1 sleep stage, *N2* NREM N2 sleep stage, *N3* NREM N3sleep stage or slow wave sleep, *R* REM sleep stage). (Original figure)

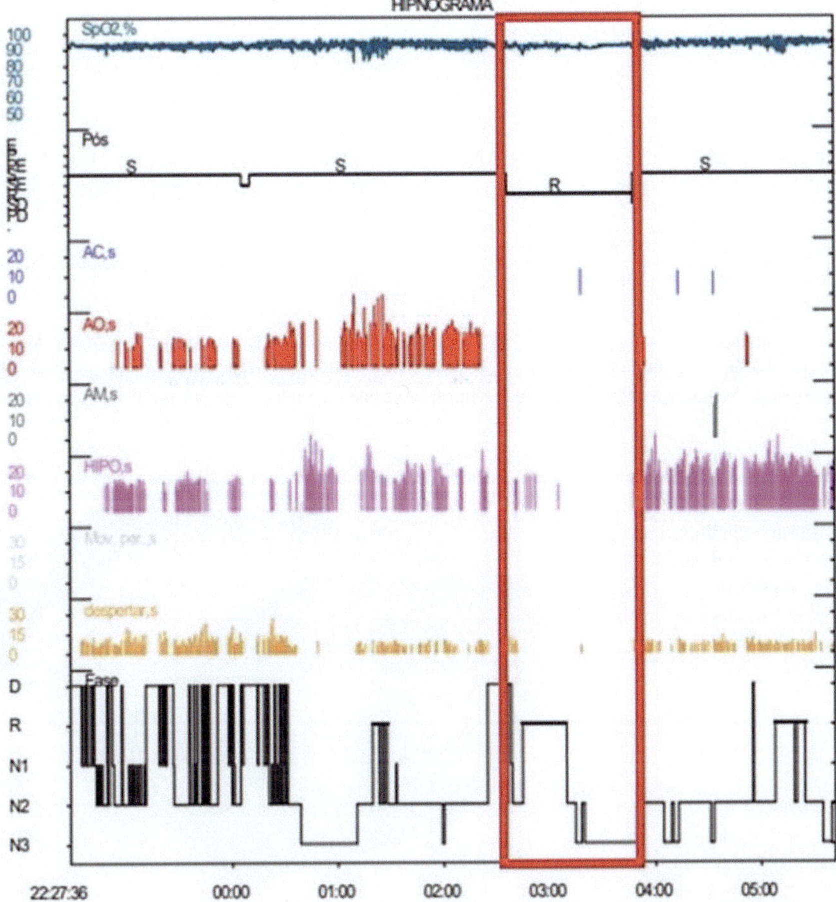

Fig. 16.2 Data from baseline polysomnography showing from top to bottom: SatO$_2$, body position, central events, obstructive events, mixed events, hypopnea events, limb movements, arousals, and hypnogram. The red box shows when the patient turns to the lateral decubitus (right), achieving REM sleep stage and slow wave sleep stage, with very few respiratory hypopnea events. *S* supine, *R* right, *ACs* central sleep apnea, *Aos* obstructive sleep apnea, *AMs* mixed sleep apnea, *Hipos* hypopnea, *Mov per* periodic limb movement, *despertares* arousals, *D* awake, *N1* NREM N1 sleep stage, *N2* NREM N2 sleep stage, *N3* NREM N3 sleep stage, *R* REM sleep stage. (Original figure)

stage (which commonly manifests more obstructive events, due to muscle atony), and NREM N3 sleep stage, as shown in the red box (Fig. 16.2). Additionally, in the right side decubitus, her AHI reduced to 6 ev/h as compared to 87.8 ev/h in the supine position (Table 16.1).

Table 16.1 Data from baseline PSG comparing sleep parameters according to the body position

Body position	Time (min)	Sleep (%)	REM (%)	SWS (%)	CA (#)	OA (#)	MA (#)	Hyp (#)	AHI (ev/h)	Desaturation (#)
Left	–	–	–	–	–	–	–	–	–	–
Prone	–	–	–	–	–	–	–	–	–	–
Supine	352.4	85.4	6.2	13.7	2	175	3	260	87.8	372
Supine left	4.8	0.0	0.0	0.0	0	0	0	0	0.0	0
Right	71.7	97.8	34.9	44.8	1	0	0	6	6.0	7
Supine right	0.1	100.0	0.0	100.0	0	0	0	0	0.0	0

Min minutes, *Sleep* total sleep time, *REM* rapid eye movements, *SWS* slow wave sleep (N3 NREM sleep stages), *CA* central apnea events, *OA* obstructive apnea events, *MA* mixed apnea events, *Hyp* hypopnea, *AHI* apnea-hypopnea index, *#* number of events, *ev/h* events per hour

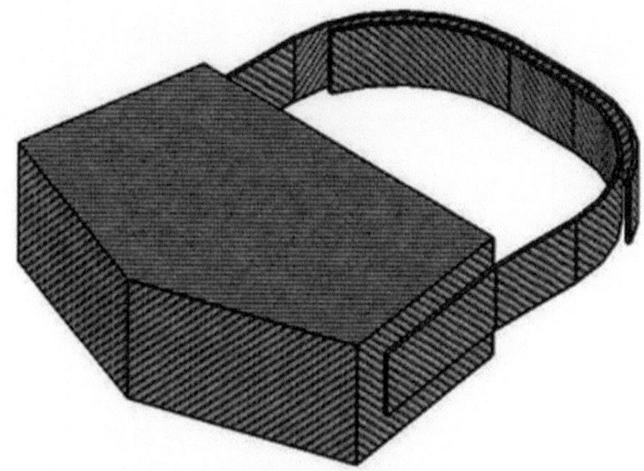

Fig. 16.3 Illustrative image of the homemade positioning pad used to treat positional apnea, and also to perform polysomnography. (Original Figure)

Physiotherapeutic Intervention

After detailed anamnesis and baseline PSG evaluation, and after considering her symptoms, and comorbidities, we explained to the patient that CPAP is the first-line treatment, but that her PSG data were very consistent with POSA. In this way, there was the possibility of testing a positional therapy device, mainly because she achieved REM sleep, and slow wave sleep, with respiratory events correction when she assumed the lateral decubitus (right). Therefore, she agreed to test the positional treatment. Thus, we recommended her to wear a positioning cushion (Fig. 16.3), and suggested that she sleep in lateral decubitus for 30 consecutive days to adapt. A new PSG wearing the positional therapy device (PTD-PSG) was performed after this period.

Follow-Up and Outcomes

The patient followed our instructions and performed a new PTD-PSG, in right lateral decubitus 1 month after PTD training started. The comparative results are shown below in Table 16.2. After PTD device treatment, there was a significant reduction in arousals events and in the percentage of time in light sleep (N1). In addition, there was an increase in the percentage of slow-wave sleep (N3) with small changes in REM sleep.

Table 16.3 shows respiratory-related data from baseline PSG and PTD-PSG. Wearing a positional device resulted in a normal overall AHI (1.4 ev/h) as well as during REM (4.3 ev/h), and NREM sleep (1.0 ev/h). The lowest saturation increased from 85% on baseline PSG to 92% on PTD-PSG, and the time saturation <90% reduced from 11.6% on baseline to 0.1% of total sleep time on PTD-PSG.

Comparative scenario between basal PSG and PDT-PSG is depicted in Fig. 16.4. The change from supine to lateral decubitus normalized respiratory events, stabilized oxygen saturation, and promoted improvement in sleep architecture, with fewer awakenings, less time spent in light sleep, and more time spent in slow wave sleep stage.

After 30 days wearing the PTD, the patient reported improvement in symptoms of snoring, waking up coughing, choking, and nocturia. She improved the quality of her sleep, still had insomnia, but woke up less tired, and reduced the daytime sleepiness. There were no more episodes of nocturnal gastroesophageal reflux; she maintained complaints of memory impairment, and her mood was more stable.

Table 16.2 Sleep architecture according to baseline PSG and PTD-PSG

	N1 NREM (%)	N2 NREM (%)	N3 NREM (%)	REM Sleep (%)	Arousals (ev/h)
Baseline PSG	6.5	59.6	21.7	12.7	50.5
PTD-PSG	1.5	58.4	29.3	10.8	6.5

PSG polysomnography, *PTD-PSG* positional therapy device polysomnography

Table 16.3 The respiratory-related data from baseline and PTD-PSG

	Baseline PSG	PTD-PSG
Overall AHI (ev/h)	72.3	1.4
AHI REM (ev/h)	49.8	4.3
AHI NREM (ev/h)	75.6	1.0
AHI supine (ev/h)	87.8	0.0
AHI nonsupine (ev/h)	6.0	1.4
Medium SatO$_2$ (%)	93	93
Lowest SatO$_2$ (%)	83	92
Time SatO$_2$ < 90% (%)	11.6	0.1

AHI apnea-hypopnea index, *PSG* polysomnography, *PTD-PSG* positional therapy device polysomnography, *SatO$_2$* oxygen saturation

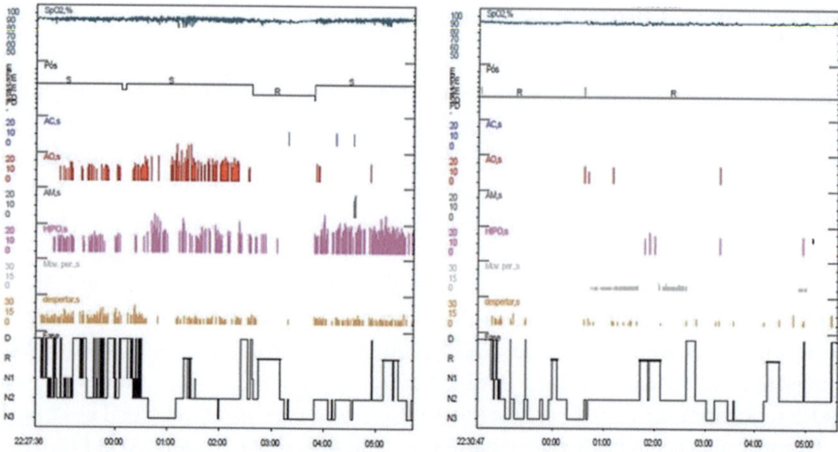

Fig. 16.4 The box on the left side shows the summary from baseline PSG, and the box on the right side shows the summary from PT-PSG. We can observe in the PT-PSG, that the patient remained the entire time sleeping in the right body position, presenting very few respiratory events and reaching slow wave sleep (N3) and REM sleep earlier compared to baseline PSG. (*S* supine, *R* right, *ACs* central sleep apnea, *AOs* obstructive sleep apnea, *AMs* mixed sleep apnea, *Hipos* hypopnea, *Mov per* limb movement, *despertares* arousals, *D* awake, *R* REM, *N1* NREM N1 sleep stage, *N2* NREM N2 sleep stage, *N3* NREM N3 sleep stage. (Original Figure)

Discussion

This interesting case report shows a patient with very symptomatic severe OSA identified on baseline PSG, who was referred for CPAP treatment. However, the severe OSA was resolved with PTD avoiding supine position. Existing evidence points to POSA being attributable to gravity action, unfavorable airway geometry, reduced lung volume, and inability of airway dilator muscles to adequately compensates the airway collapse [4]. It is reasonable to understand that in supine position, the airway is more prone to collapse due do the action of the gravity. Moreover, flow-field computation analysis demonstrated that changes in soft palate displacement and sidewall deformation, when assuming supine position, may generate altered pressured gradients in the velopharynx, and therefore increase the propensity to collapse [5]. Lung volume is another important variable in sleep apnea as it influences upper airway stability, via caudal tracheal displacement, causing changes in upper airway tissue pressure [6]. It is known that supine position reduces functional residual capacity, total lung capacity, expiratory reserve volume, and vital capacity [7]. It was also demonstrated that move from supine to lateral position, increases functional residual capacity, expiratory reserve volume, and lung compliance [8, 9]. Therefore, the supine position may reduce tracheal traction, making the airway more collapsible. Finally, the activity of genioglossus is increased in the supine position, when tongue position secondary to genioglossus contraction will maximally enhance upper airway caliber [10]. However, the magnitude of this response has not been yet quantified in patients with POSA [4].

In this specific case, we used a simple homemade PTD cushion, and our great results are in line with previous studies, and metanalysis recommending various PTD techniques [1], as well as new generation of PTD [11]. It is important to emphasize that the possibility of PTD was raised after detailed observation of her baseline PSG, identifying a short period without events, even in the presence of REM sleep and slow wave sleep, when patient turned to lateral decubitus. An important precaution is to check by PSG whether the proposed treatment has been effective in correcting respiratory events, hypoxemia, and improving sleep quality, and symptoms both acutely and in a long-term follow-up.

A follow-up was carried out to ensure that the patient was still compliant with the treatment and that treatment remained effective. Our team recommended the patient to maintain the PTD use, because in its absence, turning in the supine position the respiratory events and symptoms would return. Additionally, as sleep apnea is a condition that can increase with age, a control PSG to check whether the treatment remains adequate should be performed periodically, especially if the patient presents weight gain, introduction of some sedative or hypnotic medication, and if there is worsening of symptoms. Our patient continues to undergo semiannual follow-up, and continues to be clinically stable, and well-treated with PTD.

In conclusion, this case demonstrates that the detailed observation of the PSG allows other effective treatment possibility, and the periodic follow-up of the patient made all the difference in the successful outcomes and treatment compliance.

References

1. Ravesloot MJ, van Maanen JP, Dun L, de Vries N. The undervalued potential of positional therapy in position-dependent snoring and obstructive sleep apnea-a review of the literature. Sleep Breath. 2013;17(1):39–49.
2. Cartwright RD. Effect of sleep position on sleep apnea severity. Sleep. 1984;7(2):110–4.
3. Yingjuan M, Siang WH, Leong Alvin TK, Poh HP. Positional therapy for positional obstructive sleep apnea. Sleep Med Clin. 2020;15(2):261–75.
4. Joosten SA, O'Driscoll DM, Berger PJ, Hamilton GS. Supine position related obstructive sleep apnea in adults: pathogenesis and treatment. Sleep Med Rev. 2014;18(1):7–17.
5. Lucey AD, King AJ, Tetlow GA, Wang J, Armstrong JJ, Leigh MS, et al. Measurement, reconstruction, and flow-field computation of the human pharynx with application to sleep apnea. IEEE Trans Biomed Eng. 2010;57(10):2535–48.
6. Rowley JA, Permutt S, Willey S, Smith PL, Schwartz AR. Effect of tracheal and tongue displacement on upper airway airflow dynamics. J Appl Physiol (1985). 1996;80(6):2171–8.
7. Behrakis PK, Baydur A, Jaeger MJ, Milic-Emili J. Lung mechanics in sitting and horizontal body positions. Chest. 1983;83(4):643–6.
8. Barnas GM, Green MD, Mackenzie CF, Fletcher SJ, Campbell DN, Runcie C, et al. Effect of posture on lung and regional chest wall mechanics. Anesthesiology. 1993;78(2):251–9.
9. Tanskanen P, Kyttä J, Randell T. The effect of patient positioning on dynamic lung compliance. Acta Anaesthesiol Scand. 1997;41(5):602–6.

10. Douglas NJ, Jan MA, Yildirim N, Warren PM, Drummond GB. Effect of posture and breathing route on genioglossal electromyogram activity in normal subjects and in patients with the sleep apnea/hypopnea syndrome. Am Rev Respir Dis. 1993;148(5):1341–5.
11. Ravesloot MJL, White D, Heinzer R, Oksenberg A, Pépin JL. Efficacy of the new generation of devices for positional therapy for patients with positional obstructive sleep apnea: a systematic review of the literature and meta-analysis. J Clin Sleep Med. 2017;13(6):813–24.

Chapter 17
Nocturia, Enuresis, Sleep Fragmentation, and Embarrassment

Cristina Frange ⓘ

Introduction

Both nocturia and nocturnal enuresis are symptoms of obstructive sleep apnea (OSA) in adults [1]. Pathological nocturia is defined as the need to wake at night to void (≥ 2 times), with each void preceded and followed by sleep [2], and is commonly reported as a cause of sleep disturbance. The effect of nocturia on sleep is harmful, as it increases the risk of falls [3]. Some argue that nocturia is comparable to snoring in screening for OSA, with high sensitivity (>80%) and positive predictive value (>80%) [4]. It is also known that the prevalence of nocturia increases with the severity of obstructive sleep apnea (OSA) [5].

Nocturnal enuresis is an involuntary urinary incontinence happening during sleep [6] and can also be triggered by OSA. Hypoxia, hypercapnia, acidosis, negative pressure breathing, and episodic bursts of sympathetic stimulation are conditions created by OSA [7] that negatively impact on the pathophysiology of pathological nocturia and nocturnal enuresis.

Those urinary symptoms are extremely bothersome. Nevertheless, evidence points out that more than half of the women did not seek help, while more than a third would like to be inquired about urinary symptoms by their health care provider [8]. The difficulties of reporting those symptoms include embarrassment, shame, stigma, the thinking that nocturia is usual and increases with aging, and the thoughts that there is no treatment for nocturia and enuresis [9, 10]. The purpose of this case report is to raise awareness of nocturia and nocturnal enuresis as being potential symptoms of OSA, particularly in women.

C. Frange (✉)
Neurology and Neurosurgery Department, Federal University of São Paulo (UNIFESP), São Paulo, SP, Brazil

C. Frange (ed.), *Clinical Cases in Sleep Physical Therapy*, https://doi.org/10.1007/978-3-031-38340-3_17

Patient Information

D.S.V., a 64-year-old woman, was referred for sleep physiotherapy by her sleep medicine physician with severe OSA for positive airway pressure (PAP) titration and treatment. She sat in front of me with her polysomnography (PSG) and looking very anxious. She had just discovered that she had OSA. She had an appointment with a sleep medicine physician, indicated by a friend of her, searching for help for an embarrassing situation and found OSA. She was concerned about her what was happening during her sleep, not about OSA. During the past 6 months, she started voiding during sleep and used to wake up wet. Her primary concern was that her new boyfriend would notice the bed was wet. Her boyfriend was waiting for her at the reception, and she was speaking very quietly and softly. She was at the post-menopausal stage (menopause happened at 50-year-old, and she denied hormonal therapy). She reported going to the *toilet* about 4 times each night, even having her last ingestion of water at 18:00. She said she went to bed at midnight and woke up at 8:00. But she was so afraid of sleeping and voiding that she has been waking up every time to check if the bed was wet, having a lot of sleep fragmentation (symptom that she denied before this worry). She started crying and claimed for help. She was using levothyroxine for her hypothyroidism, and a vitamin supplement to replace calcium and vitamin D, prescribed by her gynecologist. She was sedentary at the time and had four grown-up children. She didn't tell anyone about nocturia and enuresis episodes—not even the physician! She denied medical problems (no report of hypertension, diabetes, dyslipidemia, no urinary urgency, and daytime incontinence), and past interventions, except plastic surgeries. She was asymptomatic for her severe OSA, except for nocturia and tiredness during the wake period. Indeed, the physician referred to physiotherapy treatment, as OSA rarely occurs in isolation.

Clinical Findings

She reported poor sleep quality, waking up not feeling refreshed, not rested, with a dry mouth, and having the feeling that she did not sleep the entire night for the past month. The enuresis happened twice last month—but she managed her boyfriend didn't notice it (she even did laundry during the night so he would not see her night-dress wet. She denied diurnal somnolence. At physical examinations, she presented with normal neck circumference, no leg edema, and eutrophic, with Mallampati classification of I (soft palate, uvula, and pillars were visible) [11].

Diagnostic Assessment

D.S.V.'s basal PSG showed—total sleep time (TST): 339 min (reference values for TST is variable); sleep efficiency: 87.8% (the ratio of total sleep time to the total amount of time spent in bed in percentage, reference value >85% of TST [12]), sleep onset latency: 10.5 min (the length of time in minutes it takes to transits from wake to sleep, <30 min [12]), rapid eye movement (REM) sleep latency: 83 min (the length of time in minutes to enter REM sleep stage, 90–120 min [12]), wake after sleep onset: 36.5 min (the amount of time in minutes spent awaking after sleep has been initiated, sleep fragmentation, up to 30 min [12]), stage NREM N1 sleep: 14.2% of TST (up to 5% of TST [12]), stage NREM N2 sleep: 48.1% of TST (45–55% of TST [12]), stage NREM N3 sleep: 26.6% of TST (up to 23% of TST [12]), stage REM sleep: 17.1% of TST (20–25% of TST [12]), arousal index: 26 events/hour (the number of awakenings per hour), periodic limb movements index (PLM): 0 (number per hour of involuntary movement of limbs during sleep (<15 ev/h [12]), apnea-hypopnea index (AHI): 58.4 ev/h (mean number of apneas and hypopneas per hour of sleep (<5/h [12]), being central apneas: 5.5 ev/h, obstructive apneas: 6.2 ev/h, obstructive hypopneas: 46.4 ev/h, with maximum duration of 22 s, 30 s and 41.5 s, respectively. Percutaneous oxygen desaturation (SpO_2 < 90%): 81%, with greater desaturations in NREM (293 events) compared to REM sleep stage (72 events). The respiratory events were related to supine position, as she slept only in supine during PSG examination due to discomfort with the electrodes, wires, etc. Snoring was presented for about 30% of PSG examination.

She was referred to her gynecologist and an urogynecology physiotherapist for the investigation of probable other causes of nocturia and enuresis (i.e., urologic disorders, aging of the bladder). After some examinations such as voiding diary and electromyographic evaluation, she presented no signs of incontinence. Her subjective perineal contraction was presented, as grade 2 diaphragmatic hypertonia. The exams found dyssynergia between pelvic floor muscles and abdominal muscles, positive reflexes with no apparent prolapse, and the capability of sustaining contraction time of perineal muscles of 5 s, presenting muscle fibrillation after that.

Physiotherapeutic Intervention

We performed at home PAP titration investigation for 17 days, with adhesion of 88%, meaning that D.S.V. used PAP with automatic pressure (APAP) for more than 4 h/night, for at least 70% of these 17 nights. Before the APAP titration, she had a long consultation explaining the objectives of the treatment and education about sleep, OSA, and PAP therapy. After this education, she tried 2 masks, individually chosen, and felt comfortable with the tube-up pillow mask. We then tried the PAP for the first time, with the lowest pressure of the device (4 cmH_2O) and humidification on, beginning with desensitization strategies (i.e., having the pressure in each hand at a time, each finger and letting the patient understand the pressure (even with no scientific evidence, some argue that this desensitization strategy happens because in the somatosensory areas of the cortex, according to the Penfield homunculus, the lips, mouth, and noose representation areas are closer to the hand and finger representation areas—but this information warrant scientific confirmation). Then D.S.V. tried the pressure closer to her nose but without the mask, and only when she felt confident and ready, we tried the mask with the device pressure on a sitting position. At that time, I was explaining to her the sensation of the pressure with that specific mask in her nose, her throat. I showed the lack of noise of the device, and the humidification and when she felt comfortable, I asked her to lie down. After a few minutes, she was asked to adopt her sleeping position. She stayed there for about 20 min, as I was talking about the benefits of the OSA treatment and explaining how nocturia and enuresis might be a symptom of her untreated severe OSA. Lastly, the pressure was increased by 1 cmH_2O, and let her try for a few minutes until it reached 11 cmH_2O. She felt the increase but tolerated it well.

The PAP titration was done with an automatic pressure between 4 and 11 cmH_2O, with humidification, but with no respiratory relief and no ramp (because of her PSG central sleep apneas, as we expected them to increase with the automatic pressure). Home titration was accompanied via telemonitoring every day. During this titration period, we were also in contact almost daily (via phone calls or messages through a mobile phone app) to solve any problems that may have happened and to encourage D.S.V. for using it. The APAP titration results can be seen in Table 17.1. After APAP titration and with its results, the pressure was fixed at 6.4 cmH_2O, with no ramp and no expiratory relief not to increase central sleep apneas, as mentioned. An overnight pulse oximetry examination was performed, attached to the PAP device, and presented with $SpO_2 \geq 90\%$ during sleep time with CPAP.

Table 17.1 Respiratory data from basal polysomnography exam, APAP titration (session 1), and evolution of PAP treatment for the first 2 years

	Basal PSG	Session 1 APAP titration	Session 2 3 weeks	Session 3 third month	Session 4 fourth month	Session 5 tenth month	Session 6 22nd month
Date	10/ Feb/2021	19/Mar–04/Apr/21	22/Apr/2021	10/Jul/2021	08/Sept/2021	30/March/2022	28/March/2023
Device pressure (cmH$_2$O)		4–11 mean: 6.7; 95thP: 8.9; maximum: 10	6.4	6.4	6.4	6.4	6.4
Apnea-hypopnea index (events/hour)	58.4	8.0	4.8	4.9	4.6	2.9	3.3
Obstructive apneas index (events/hour)	6.2	0.7	0.4	0.1	0.2	0.9	0.2
Obstructive hypopnea index (events/hour)	46.4	1.0	1.4	1.5	1.5	0.1	1.0
Central apneas index (events/hour)	5.5	5.8	2.7	3.1	2.8	1.7	0.2
Respiratory efforts related arousal (RERA, events/hour)	–	0.2	0.1	0	0.1	0.1	0.3
Leak (L/min)	–	Mean = 15.9; 95thP =36.7	Mean = 10.8; 95thP = 28.8	Mean = 6.2; 95thP =32.7	Mean = 4.7; 95thP = 28.9	Mean = 3.6; 95thP = 24.4	Mean = 5.4; 95thP = 25.2

PSG polysomnography, *APAP* automatic positive airway pressure, *95thP* 95th percentile. Normal leakage for the chosen device and mask was 24 L/min

Follow-Up and Outcomes

We faced some situations during the APAP titration and the beginning of the treatment, such as worsening of her dry mouth complaints due to air leakage from the mouth (solved with a small surgical tape to seal the lips), the uncomfortable "cold" she felt with the pressure (she stated having a cold nose, we changed to a heated circuit), and air leakage from the mask, solved adjusting the mask at a nighttime hour, and new pillow, all solved with a video call. After all these were addressed, she was expected to have her first session at 1 month interval from the ending of APAP titration and the "official" beginning of treatment with fixed pressure (continuous PAP, CPAP). She had no dayitime symptoms and no residual AHI.

After 3 weeks of treatment, she called after waking up and came into my office at the first time in the afternoon, desperate and complaining of another episode of sleep enuresis—feeling very embarrassed and ashamed—but she managed not to wake up her boyfriend. As her examinations were all normal, with no symptoms except enuresis, even nocturia ameliorated from 4 times per night, to once each night, no residual AHI (Table 17.1), and O_2 saturation within normal parameters, flow curve analysis was within normal parameters, she was explained that CPAP was still working, that it could take some time for her body to reach proper homeostasis again, with no OSA and its consequences. I wanted to see her within 3 months, but if she needed me, I was there before the scheduled date.

I saw her after 3 months, and she said she was sleeping much better, enuresis episodes did not happen during this time, and nocturia disappeared. She denied sleep fragmentation. We adjusted the leakage of the mask by regulating the mask, by tying her long hair in a ponytail, and then letting her hair down. We did a fourth session in 1 month time because she wanted to tell me that she was getting married and was worried about enuresis happening again. We checked all the data of OSA treatment with PAP, and as there were no daytime symptoms or complaints, and everything was under normal values, she was comforted that she was treated. She was then explained about the importance of physical exercise and asked to join hydrotherapy, which she said to like it. She was explained that physical exercise would help the treatment of OSA, and would help with strengthening the muscles for well-being and health.

The fifth session happened after 6 months, and she was with no AHI residual events, and no leaks or any other troubles to solve. The physiotherapeutic session was scheduled for 1 year time, and she presented with the same pattern, except for a slight increase of leakage of the mask, worn out—we changed it to a new one of the same type. She did not have any episodes of both, nocturia or enuresis for the entire year. And got married meanwhile—although her boyfriend, now husband, still doesn't know about those bothersome episodes of her life. During the treatment period, the physician received the reports and participated in her treatment.

Discussion

The nocturnal enuresis and nocturia presented by D.S.V., in this case, were an evoked response to conditions of negative intrathoracic pressure, due to inspiratory effort against a closed or obstructed airway. This case was an interesting one since D.S.V. presented with no OSA symptoms but was suspected of any sleep-related disease, because of symptoms happening during sleep. That was the main reason she searched for help, but at her physician consultation, she was not able to speak, embarrassed and ashamed of her bothersome condition. The physician without knowing the symptoms ordered a PSG and found a severe OSA and referred her to sleep physiotherapy.

One of the features of airway obstruction is paradoxical breathing, when there is a reversal of the movements of the chest and abdomen caused by the diaphragmatic effort presented against a closed glottis or an obstruction. This is seen when, in an inspiratory effort, the chest is depressed, and the abdomen is inflated. An event of OSA starts with narrowing or occlusion of the upper airway and ends with the opening of the upper airway, after sleep arousal [13]. Throughout one obstructive apnea event, various diaphragmatic contractions can happen, without air exchange. These intrathoracic changes lead to an increased systolic transmural pressure, accompanied by a left ventricular overload [14]. Venous return to the right atrium is then increased, triggering distention of the right ventricle. This distention produces a shift toward the left side of the interventricular septum, impairing left ventricular diastolic and reducing stroke volume [14]. These intrathoracic changes lead to the secretion of atrial natriuretic peptide (ANP), by the right atrium, followed by a high nocturnal urine output due to natriuresis [3, 15]. The mechanism for this natriuretic response is the release of ANP due to cardiac distension caused by the negative pressure environment. This cardiac hormone, ANP, increases sodium and water excretion and inhibits hormone systems that regulate fluid volume, vasopressin, and the rennin-angiotensin-aldosterone complex.

Left ventricular afterload also happens because of hypoxia and hypercapnia through stimulation of the sympathetic nervous system. Besides this disturbance in body water homeostasis, OSA can affect bladder function directly, as the intermittent, exaggerated, and rapid changes in intrathoracic pressures may transmit these changes to fluid-filled abdominal organs, such as the bladder. Investigations of these acute urodynamic changes found correspondence with respiratory efforts during OSA episodes [16].

Treatment of OSA has been shown to reduce or eliminate nocturia and enuresis. An individualized treatment, active listening, daily follow-up, and quick resolution of all issues that arose during the CPAP treatment created a friendship between us. Furthermore, the resolution of these bothersome symptoms after CPAP treatment can provide patient satisfaction and reinforce treatment compliance.

References

1. Pressman MR, et al. Nocturia. A rarely recognized symptom of sleep apnea and other occult sleep disorders. Arch Intern Med. 1996;156(5):545–50.
2. Goessaert AS, et al. Nocturnal enuresis and nocturia, differences and similarities—lessons to learn? Acta Clin Belg. 2015;70(2):81–6.
3. Asplund R. Hip fractures, nocturia, and nocturnal polyuria in the elderly. Arch Gerontol Geriatr. 2006;43(3):319–26.
4. Romero E, et al. Nocturia and snoring: predictive symptoms for obstructive sleep apnea. Sleep Breath. 2010;14(4):337–43.
5. Oztura I, Kaynak D, Kaynak HC. Nocturia in sleep-disordered breathing. Sleep Med. 2006;7(4):362–7.
6. Koo P, et al. Association of obstructive sleep apnea risk factors with nocturnal enuresis in postmenopausal women. Menopause. 2016;23(2):175–82.
7. Umlauf MG, Chasens ER. Sleep disordered breathing and nocturnal polyuria: nocturia and enuresis. Sleep Med Rev. 2003;7(5):403–11.
8. MacDiarmid S, Rosenberg M. Overactive bladder in women: symptom impact and treatment expectations. Curr Med Res Opin. 2005;21(9):1413–21.
9. Weiss JP. Nocturia: focus on etiology and consequences. Rev Urol. 2012;14(3–4):48–55.
10. Bosch JL, Weiss JP. The prevalence and causes of nocturia. J Urol. 2013;189(1 Suppl):S86–92.
11. Mallampati SR, et al. A clinical sign to predict difficult tracheal intubation: a prospective study. Can Anaesth Soc J. 1985;32(4):429–34.
12. Berry RB, Quan SF, Abreu AR, et al. The AASM manual for the scoring of sleep and associated events: rules, terminology and technical specifications. Darien: American Academy of Sleep Medicine; 2020.
13. Sullivan CE, Issa FG. Pathophysiological mechanisms in obstructive sleep apnea. Sleep. 1980;3(3–4):235–46.
14. Shiomi T, et al. Leftward shift of the interventricular septum and pulsus paradoxus in obstructive sleep apnea syndrome. Chest. 1991;100(4):894–902.
15. Krieger J, et al. Atrial natriuretic peptide release during sleep in patients with obstructive sleep apnoea before and during treatment with nasal continuous positive airway pressure. Clin Sci (Lond). 1989;77(4):407–11.
16. Arai H, et al. Polysomnographic and urodynamic changes in a case of obstructive sleep apnea syndrome with enuresis. Psychiatry Clin Neurosci. 1999;53(2):319–20.

Chapter 18
Sleep Attack During Marriage: Narcolepsy? Apnea? Or Both?

Sofia F. Furlan (iD)

Introduction

Screening for excessive daytime sleepiness (EDS) in patients is not a common clinical practice within health professionals, except for sleep specialists. EDS is a common symptom of many diseases, linked mainly with obstructive sleep apnea (OSA) or hypersomnias, such as hypersomnolence syndrome or narcolepsy [1]. Around 50% of patients with OSA present EDS as a main symptom [2]. It is well established that EDS increases the risk for car accidents and accidents at work [3]. Concomitantly, OSA can lead to the development of long-term cardiovascular diseases when left untreated.

This is a peculiar case of a patient who could have his diagnosis of OSA misleading or overlapped by hypersomnias (i.e., narcolepsy or hypersomnolence disorder) due to an EDS far above the normal range, associated with episodes of sleep attack during the day—and even during his marriage! Here, we highlight the importance of a speedy and accurate diagnosis, associated with a non-invasive treatment (continuous positive airway pressure, CPAP) [4]. The CPAP prescription, adherence, and compliance avoided pharmacological treatments that could have side effects and further impair the patient's health and quality of life.

S. F. Furlan (✉)
Sleep Laboratory, Faculty of Medicine, Heart Institute, University of São Paulo, São Paulo, SP, Brazil

© The Author(s), under exclusive license to Springer Nature Switzerland AG 2023
C. Frange (ed.), *Clinical Cases in Sleep Physical Therapy*,
https://doi.org/10.1007/978-3-031-38340-3_18

Patient Information

J.P.W., 37 years-old, male, married. The patient was admitted to the sleep laboratory with complaints of EDS associated with involuntary and sudden unconscious sleep attack episodes many times per day and every day. These episodes occurred during traffic and everyday routine activities. He even had a sleep attack episode during his wedding (Fig. 18.1). He also presented with loud and constant snoring, witnessed respiratory pauses, slowed reasoning, and headache. J.P.W. had to park his car to sleep several times at the traffic light with passengers inside. At the very moment when the priest was taking the oath and he was supposed to say yes, the patient suddenly fell asleep, kept standing, and had to be awakened by the guests.

He was sedentary and without previously diagnosed cardiovascular history such as hypertension, diabetes, dyslipidemia, heart diseases, and stroke. He used to be a former smoker for a year. At that time, he was not in use of any medication.

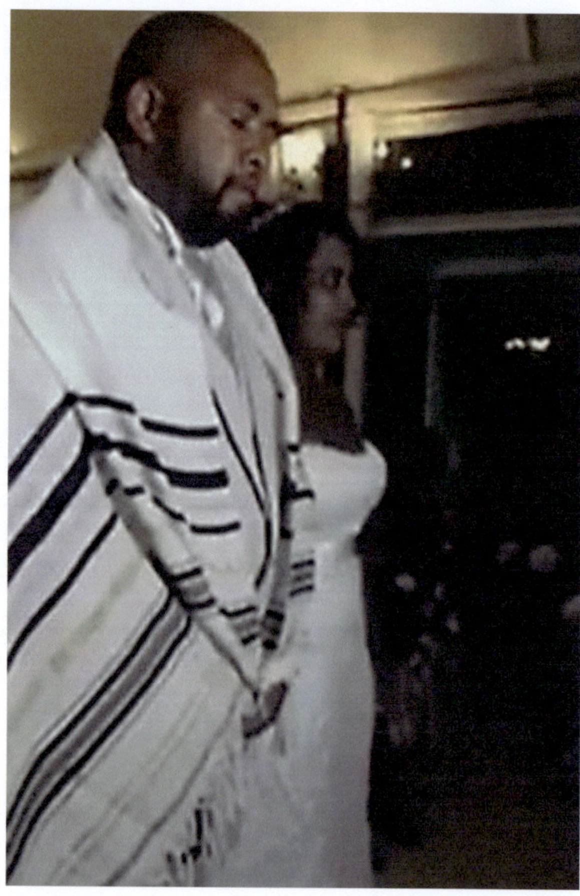

Fig. 18.1 Patient J.P.W. fell asleep during his marriage, in upright position. (Original figure. Courtesy from reprinted with permission from J.P.W.)

Clinical Findings

In the clinical examination, he presented weight of 149.25 kg, height 1.97 m, and body mass index (BMI) 38 kg/m^2; neck circumference: 50.5 cm; waist circumference:125 cm, systolic blood pressure: 140 mmHg, and diastolic blood pressure: 83 mmHg. During the appointment, J.P.W. couldn't be awake for 1 min, and dozed off with eyes open. His wife, who was accompanying him, showed a video of the J.P.W. sleeping at the altar at their wedding at the time of the "yes."

Diagnostic Assessment

The objective and subjective diagnostic assessment of J.P.W. can be seen in Table 18.1.

Even though he was diagnosed with OSA, there was still a clinical suspicion of other sleep disorder overlapping OSA such as hypersomnolence syndrome or narcolepsy.

There was an urge to treat J.P for OSA. If untreated, the patient could develop long-term cardiovascular diseases, and short-term may engage in traffic accidents during his work or day-to-day accidents due to his severe hypersomnolence. By treating OSA, we expected to improve and maybe to abolish his daytime hypersomnolence. In case of residual symptoms, we would further conduct investigation for possible hypersomnias.

Table 18.1 Baseline sleep data

Variables	Findings	Variables	Findings
Polysomnography			
Time of registration (min)	436.9	Minimum SpO$_2$ (%)	63
Total sleep time (TST, min)	397	Average SpO$_2$ (%)	85.1
Sleep efficiency (%)	90.9	Total time SpO$_2$ < 90% (% TST)	71.26
Sleep onset latency (min)	10.9	Total time SpO$_2$ < 80% (% TST)	25.1
Rapid eye movement (REM) sleep latency (min)	13	Number of obstructive apneas	445
Awakening index (events/h)	118.6	Number of mixed apneas	275
Apnea and hypopnea index (AHI) (events/h)	118.2	Number of central apneas	20
Baseline SpO$_2$ (%)	96	Number of hypopneas	42
Snoring	Intense		
Sleep questionnaires			
Epworth sleepiness scale	24 points		
Berlin questionnaire	High risk for OSA		

Physiotherapeutic Intervention

It was decided by the sleep health team to initiate treatment with CPAP immediately and as a matter of urgency, with the aim of maintain upper airways open and promoting adequate repositioning of throat and tongue muscles, preventing them from falling due to excessive muscle relaxation during sleep; increase SpO_2 to levels within normal ranges during the sleep period; decrease/abolish excessive daytime sleepiness and abolish snoring; restore mood in activities of daily living; eliminate the risk of traffic accidents and prevent cardiovascular events in the long term [5], and, after the response of this treatment to evaluate the residual symptoms.

The CPAP adaptation and home titration were performed by a sleep physiotherapist. J.P.W. received education about sleep and OSA, its long-term risks when untreated, as well as the effectiveness of CPAP treatment, the importance of its use and proper cleaning of device and mask. He tried different types of nasal masks, and we defined a comfortable one according to his reports, of adequate size and which did not present unexpected leakage. The patient received an automatic CPAP A-flex for 1 week (automatic CPAP A-flex—This modality is set up to vary the pressure of the CPAP machine during the nigh—always seeking to eliminate apnea events, besides, present an expiratory relief technology during the expiration to improve the comfort, if necessary). Although he was very sleepy, when were asked about how long he took to fall asleep after lying down to sleep, he reported around 30 min, showing a misperception of sleep (please, verify sleep onset time in Table 18.1). The initial CPAP setup was automatic mode, pressure varying between 6 and 14 cmH_2O, expiratory relief was off, the ramp was adjusted in 30 min in this first week to make the patient's adaptation more comfortable, starting at 4 cmH_2O of pressure and the humidifier was turned off.

After 1 week with automatic CPAP, J.P.W. showed excellent adherence to treatment (hours of use: 7 h 8 min, days of use: 7 days with residual AHI within normal ranges: 1.4 events/h, and no leaks). He mentioned an important and significant improvement in EDS and improvement in headache and disposition for day-to-day activities and work. He also reported not feeling sleepy during his work in traffic, and at any time during the day.

In the second visit, J.P.W. referred dryness in the mouth and throat—the humidifier was added to the treatment. Automatic CPAP A-flex was replaced by the CPAP plus C-flex (this is the patient's own CPAP, fixed mode and did not store data such as residual AHI). From the usage report, 90% pressure was used to set the fixed pressure of 14 cmH_2O. This time, J.P.W. reported taking around 15 min to initiate sleep and reported less drowsiness and better perception of his sleep. The ramp was set at 15 min with an initial pressure of 6 cmH_2O. Expiratory relief continued turned off and the humidifier was set on 3.

Table 18.2 Sleep data after 6-month of CPAP treatment

Variables	Findings	Variables	Findings
Polysomnography with CPAP at fixed pressure of 14 cmH$_2$O			
Time of registration (min)	460	Minimum SpO$_2$ (%)	89
Total sleep time (min)	438	Average SpO$_2$ (%)	94.1
Sleep efficiency (%)	95.2	Total time SpO$_2$ < 90% (min)	0.01
Sleep onset latency (min)	7.4	Total time SpO$_2$ < 80% (min)	0
REM sleep latency (min)	95	Number of obstructive apneas	0
Awakening index (events/h)	9.9	Number of mixed apneas	0
AHI (events/h)	2.7	Number of central apneas	5
Baseline SpO$_2$ (%)	96	Number of hypopneas	15
Snoring	Mild		
Sleep questionnaires			
Epworth sleepiness scale	06 points		
Berlin questionnaire	Low risk for OSA		
CPAP treatment (6 months data)			
Average CPAP use (h)	06:33		

Follow-Up and Outcomes

After 1 month of good adherence to CPAP, J.P.W. presented an excellent adaptation to the treatment, abolition of EDS, and good manage of work properly with much higher performance. The humidifier solved the problems regarding to dry mouth and throat, ensuring the consolidation of the adherence without any side effects. As the patient's fixed CPAP model did not allow the visualization of residual AHI, a polysomnography with CPAP was performed to verify the effectiveness of the treatment after 6 months. See polysomnography, sleep questionnaires and CPAP data below (Table 18.2). After physical examination: BMI: 38.8 kg/m^2, neck circumference: 50.5 cm, waist circumference: 123.5 cm, SBP: 130 mmHg SBP:80 mmHg.

Discussion

OSA can trigger a variety of physical and psychological symptoms. This case drew our attention to the unusual presentation of hypersomnolence with several episodes of sudden sleep attack many times per day that were solely related to OSA.

The rapid decrease/abolition of EDS, associated with sudden episodes of sleep attacks during day-to-day situations, was due to the effectiveness of the treatment, the commitment of J.P.W. with the treatment showing excellent hours of CPAP use since the beginning. It is widely recognized that at least 50% of patients with OSA present any symptom of OSA [1].

An interesting fact of this case is that J.P.W., although not hypertensive, had a borderline pressure when measured (140 vs. 80 mmHg) and after 6 months of treatment with excellent adherence, he presented a drop of one point in SBP (130 vs. 83), as described by literature [6].

It is already established that sleep disorders can be presented with overlapping conditions (e.g., OSA + insomnia (COMISA), OSA + narcolepsy). In this case due to the huge hypersomnolence associated with sleep attack episodes, there was a suspicion of hypersomnia or narcolepsy overlapped with OSA, but OSA was chosen to be treated first. The correct treatment in this case, and with a very objective approach to OSA, showed us that one sleep treatment had to be performed at a time, to measure the findings and then, keep investigating if any residual effect remained. The lack of treatment in this case could have contributed to a negative outcome such as traffic accident or the development of cardiovascular disease.

We particularly emphasize the importance of patients with a diagnosis of severe OSA and with suspicion of other associated sleep disorders that treatment of OSA should be immediately initiated, allowing future investigations of other comorbid sleep disorders, in order to avoiding unnecessary hyper medication. Finally, it is worth mentioning that we need to encourage all health professionals to ask about EDS and other symptoms of OSA during their appointment/consultation.

This is an unusual case of a patient who presented with sudden sleep attacks episodes during the day. This patient's symptoms were so intense that the diagnosis could be mistaken for hypersomnias. The quick decision to start this patient's treatment with CPAP and only then to investigate the residual symptoms was a key success to this treatment.

Patient Perspective

"I had an exaggerated drowsiness that interfered not only with my work but also with my day-to-day life. In my mobile driver profession, before the start of treatment, I used to fall asleep several times at the traffic even when there was a passenger in my car and when I woke up he was no longer there. Also, my wife complained a lot about my loud snoring.

I came to the appointment very sleepy and with a lot of expectations. I have gained explanation about the treatment, and told that if I used it correctly, in a week I would already see a new J.P.W.—and I didn't really believe it! When I returned to the appointment a week later, I was moved to tell how my life had already changed for the better in such a short time. We had a 6-month follow-up with monthly appointments in person and via digital medias whenever necessary. I'm still very well adapted to my CPAP and haven't stopped using it for a day since!"

References

1. Gandhi KD, Mansukhani MP, Silber MH, Kolla BP. Excessive daytime sleepiness: a clinical review. Mayo Clin Proc. 2021;96(5):1288–301. Epub 2021 Apr 9. Erratum in: Mayo Clin Proc. 2021 Oct;96(10):2729. https://doi.org/10.1016/j.mayocp.2020.08.033.
2. Lal C, Weaver TE, Bae CJ, Strohl KP. Excessive daytime sleepiness in obstructive sleep apnea. mechanisms and clinical management. Ann Am Thorac Soc. 2021;18(5):757–68. PMID: 33621163; PMCID: PMC8086534. https://doi.org/10.1513/AnnalsATS.202006-696FR.
3. Moreno CR, Carvalho FA, Lorenzi C, Matuzaki LS, Prezotti S, Bighetti P, Louzada FM, Lorenzi-Filho G. High risk for obstructive sleep apnea in truck drivers estimated by the Berlin questionnaire: prevalence and associated factors. Chronobiol Int. 2004;21(6):871–9. https://doi.org/10.1081/cbi-200036880.
4. Patil SP, Ayappa IA, Caples SM, Kimoff RJ, Patel SR, Harrod CG. Treatment of adult obstructive sleep apnea with positive airway pressure: an American Academy of Sleep Medicine clinical practice guideline. J Clin Sleep Med. 2019;15(2):335–43. PMID: 30736887; PMCID: PMC6374094. https://doi.org/10.5664/jcsm.7640.
5. Labarca G, Dreyse J, Drake L, Jorquera J, Barbe F. Efficacy of continuous positive airway pressure (CPAP) in the prevention of cardiovascular events in patients with obstructive sleep apnea: systematic review and meta-analysis. Sleep Med Rev. 2020;52:101312. Epub 2020 Mar 14. https://doi.org/10.1016/j.smrv.2020.101312.
6. Labarca G, Schmidt A, Dreyse J, Jorquera J, Enos D, Torres G, Barbe F. Efficacy of continuous positive airway pressure (CPAP) in patients with obstructive sleep apnea (OSA) and resistant hypertension (RH): systematic review and meta-analysis. Sleep Med Rev. 2021;58:101446. Epub 2021 Jan 28. https://doi.org/10.1016/j.smrv.2021.101446.

Chapter 19
Velumount: A Solution for Uvulo-Palato-Pharyngeal Problems

Cristina Staub

Introduction

The Velumount device (Fig. 19.1) was developed and patented by Arthur Wyss of Switzerland for the treatment of snoring and obstructive sleep apnea (OSA) caused by the soft palate (the velum). Other anatomical structures can also cause obstruction (e.g., tongue, nasal polyps), which require different treatments. To make

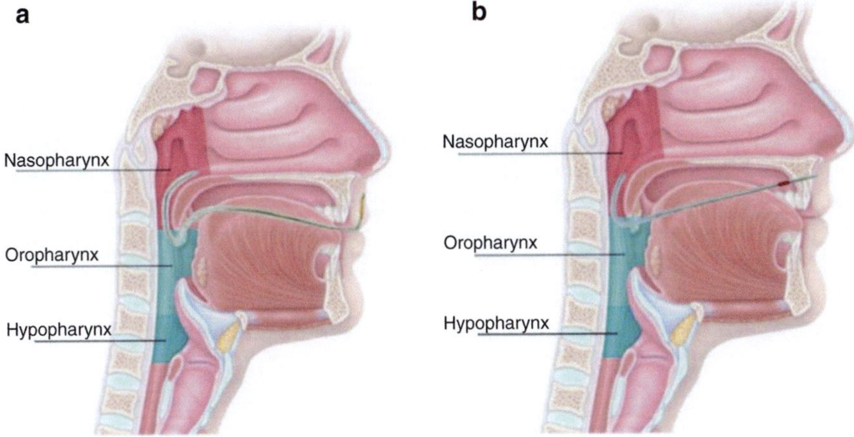

Fig. 19.1 Placement of the Velumount Original (**a**) and the Velumount Intro (**b**) palatal device. (Original figure)

C. Staub (✉)
Ausgeschlafen.ch and Pro Dormo, Zürich, Switzerland

C. Frange (ed.), *Clinical Cases in Sleep Physical Therapy*,
https://doi.org/10.1007/978-3-031-38340-3_19

this simple aid available to others, it was medically certified. It has been fitted to thousands of patients and its effectiveness has been proven in studies [1, 2].

Patient Information

The inventor (slim, athletic and 45 years old at the time) suffered from obstructive sleep apnea including daytime sleepiness. Positive airway pressure (PAP) ventilation was not an option for him because he was in developing countries for very long periods of time where there was not adequate electrical power supply, and surgery (a uvulo-palato-pharyngo-plasty and septoplasty) was not successful.

Clinical Findings

Because of his long, floppy soft palate, the Mallampati score was 3 [3]. The body mass index (BMI) was 23.7 kg/m^2.

Timeline

To improve his overall health, the patient sought further treatment after the PAP adjustment and surgery.

To stabilize the soft palate, he inserted a suction catheter into his nose each evening, pulled the anterior end out of his mouth, and fixed the two ends under his nose. The number of apneas reduced significantly. After a few months of self-experimentation, he made a more comfortable prototype from a plasticized wire, which is inserted only through the mouth, and its bow is placed behind the soft palate. In the years that followed, he continued to tinker with different materials and shapes, so that two effective and comfortable models are now available.

Diagnostic Assessment

The score on the Epworth Sleepiness Scale (ESS) [4] was 11 out of 24 before and after the operation. The patient scored the numeric rating scale (NRS) regarding snoring 8 out of 10 before and 7 after the operation. Two out of 3 categories of the Berlin Questionnaire [5] were positive before and after the operation. Sleep quality NRS was 3 out of 10 points. The overall satisfaction NRS with the therapy was 5 out of 10 points.

The initial apnea-hypopnea index (AHI) on polysomnography was 25 ev/h and blood pressure was 115/65 mmHg.

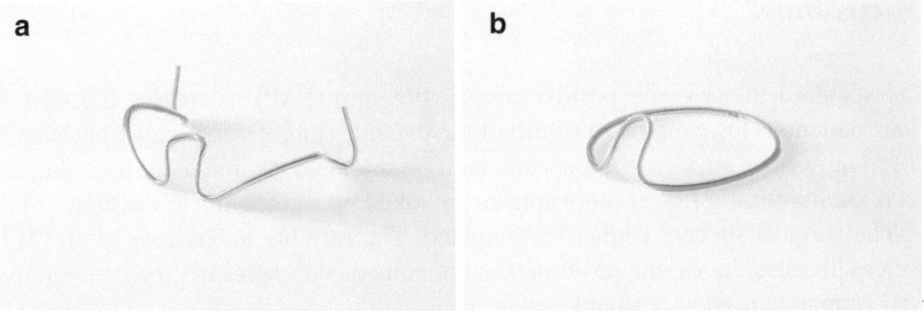

Fig. 19.2 The two shapes of the Velumount palatal device: the Velumount Original (**a**) and the Velumount Intro (**b**) palatal device. (Original figure)

Physiotherapeutic Intervention

Basically, the Velumount Original and the Velumount Intro have an archwire that is pushed behind the velum to stabilize it and keep the airway open (Fig. 19.2). The Velumount Original is open at the front and the two ends of the wire are visible on the left and right sides of the mouth. The Velumount Intro is a closed circle with the front part placed between the upper teeth and the upper lip.

When fitting a Velumount, the size and shape of the mouth are first examined and a suitable palatal device is bent based on specific criteria. The first few times, the Velumount is inserted by the therapist. As soon as the patient feels where to place the bow, he can insert the device himself. Often the Velumount is well tolerated immediately. If there is a gagging sensation, a desensitization period is needed, which may take a few hours in some patients and a few days in other patients. Sometimes a readjustment is needed after a few nights, because there may be small pressure points that are not visible from the outside. The inventor has now been sleeping with a palatal device for 20 years.

Follow-Up and Outcomes

The ESS score with Velumount shows 2 points and the NRS regarding snoring shows 3 points. No category of the Berlin Questionnaire is positive. Sleep quality NRS with Velumount is 8 points and the therapy satisfaction 9 out of 10 points. He no longer feels any side effects, even the gagging sensation when inserting the device disappeared.

The AHI decreased to 4 ev/h. His compliance is 100%: He inserts the device every night before sleeping and takes it out only when he gets up.

Discussion

The standard therapy, the positive airway pressure (PAP), decreases the AHI in some patients. However, up to a third of the patients cannot sleep with it because of different reasons such as compression pain on the face, insomnia, chronic rhinitis, decrease in intimity [2], or more apneas provoked by Bernoulli's law of flow [6].

The surgical success cannot be predicted. The formula in Tschopp et al. [7] is useless because the supine position was not considered, therefore, the preoperative AHI cannot be used as a reliable value.

To reduce the risk factors regarding cardiovascular disease, metabolic dysfunction, reduced physical and neuropsychological performance, immunodeficiency or mental illness, and the risk of accidents [8], an efficient and tolerable treatment must be sought.

In about half of the patients with OSA, positioning (preventing supine position or elevating the head section) can significantly reduce the AHI [9, 10]. In many patients, however, individualized solutions are needed. One of these is the Velumount palatal device [1, 2].

A strength of this story is that it demonstrates how, with persistence, tenacity and will, any patient can be helped to sleep better. The limiting factor is that the patient had to invent the solution himself. Velumount is the best invention for many patients.

Patient Perspective

PAP is a real lifeline for many patients. In order to gradually eliminate the known side effects of using this therapy, great efforts are still being made. Fortunately, uvulo-palato-pharyngoplasty is replaced today by many alternative surgical procedures. Before making a surgical decision of this magnitude, second opinions should always be sought. Velumount was inspired by the Sutra Neti. For me, it was a gift straight from heaven! When lemur families were playing in the rainforest of Madagascar not far above my hammock, it was a clear sign for me that my therapy against loud snoring was successful.

References

1. Tschopp K, Thomaser EG, Staub C. Therapy of snoring and obstructive sleep apnea using the Velumount® palatal device. ORL J Otorhinolaryngol Relat Spec. 2009;71:148–52.
2. Staub C. First comparison of the Velumount® palatal device with continuous positive airway pressure (CPAP), repetition effect in neuropsychological tests, and comparative study factors. Neuropsychol Trends. 2011;9:7–29.
3. Mallampati SR, Gatt SP, Gugion LD, Desai SP, Waraksa B, Freiberger D, Liu PL. A clinical sign to predict difficult tracheal intubation: a prospective study. Can Anaesth Soc J. 1985;32(4):429–34.

4. Johns MW. A new method for measuring daytime sleepiness: the Epworth sleepiness scale. Sleep. 1991;14(6):540–5.
5. Netzer NC, Stoohs RA, Netzer CM, Clark K, Strohl KP. Using the Berlin questionnaire to identify patients at risk for the sleep apnoea syndrome. Ann Intern Med. 1999;131(7):485–91.
6. Staub C. Zusammenhänge zwischen physiologischen und neuropsychologischen Parametern bei gesunden Personen und bei Patienten mit obstruktivem Schlafapnoe-Syndrom (correlations between physiological and neuropsychological parameters in healthy persons and patients with obstructive sleep apnea syndrome). Dissertation. University of Zurich; 2008.
7. Tschopp K, Zumbrunn T, Knaus C, Thomaser E, Fabbro T. Statistical model for postoperative apnea-hypopnea index after multilevel surgery for sleep-disordered breathing. Eur Arch Otorhinolaryngol. 2011;268:1679–85.
8. Staub C. In collaboration with Droth B and Vanderlinden J. Daytime behavior & sleep. Healthy lifestyle book. Ausgeschlafen.ch; 2021.
9. Troester N, Palfner M, Dominco M, Wohlkoenig C, Schmidberger E, Trinker M, Avian A. Positional therapy in sleep apnoea—one fits all? What determines success in positional therapy in sleep apnoea syndrome. PloS One. 2017;12:e0174468.
10. de Barros Souza FJF, Genta PR, de Souza Filho AJ, de Souza Filho AJ, Wellmann A, Lorenzi-Filho G. The influence of head-of-bed elevation in patients with obstructive sleep apnea. Sleep Breath. 2017;21:815–20.

Chapter 20
To Exercise or Not to Exercise?

Rodrigo Torres-Castro and Luis Vasconcello-Castillo

Introduction

Exercise has been shown to have numerous benefits for individuals with obstructive sleep apnea (OSA). Research suggests that exercise can help to reduce the severity and frequency of sleep apnea episodes, improve oxygenation during sleep, and promote overall cardiovascular health [1, 2]. In addition, exercise has been shown to improve daytime sleepiness and quality of life in people with OSA [1]. These benefits are likely since exercise can help to improve muscle tone, reduce inflammation, and promote weight loss, all of which can contribute to improved respiratory function during sleep [1, 3, 4]. In this clinical case, we describe a man with moderate OSA, with continuous positive airway pressure (CPAP) prescribed but not used. Instead, he performed a 2-month exercise program.

Patient Information

We present a young man, 45 years-old, worker in a law office. During the last 6 months, he has noticed unrefreshing sleep, with morning fatigue and excessive daytime sleepiness. These symptoms coincide with a weight gain of 10 kg in the same period. However, he has no significant comorbidities.

R. Torres-Castro (✉) · L. Vasconcello-Castillo
Department of Physical Therapy, University of Chile, Santiago, Chile

C. Frange (ed.), *Clinical Cases in Sleep Physical Therapy*,
https://doi.org/10.1007/978-3-031-38340-3_20

He has no reported health problems in his family history, except for his mother, who has controlled arterial hypertension. From the point of view of his mental health, he only reported having an excessive workload, which has increased his anxiety and job stress, and he felt it has influenced his weight gain and difficulty in falling asleep.

Clinical Findings

We found him calm and collaborative. He had a height of 1.75 m and a weight of 90 kg (body mass index [BMI]: 29.4 kg/m^2). His blood pressure was 126/84 mmHg, and his SpO$_2$ was 96%. His neck, waist, and hip circumferences were 41, 97, and 104 cm, respectively. Usually, he went to bed close to 24 h and woke up at between 7 and 7:30. His wife had complained about his snoring. He reported taking a nap for up to 30 min every day after lunch.

Diagnostic Assessments

A home respiratory polygraphy was performed (Table 20.1).

The patient scored 8 points on the Epworth sleepiness scale (ESS), score between 0 (best) and 24 (worst), indicating mild daytime sleepiness [5]; 5.9 points on the Quebec sleep questionnaire (QSQ), score between 1 (worst) and 7 (best), with most important impact on daytime symptoms, nocturnal symptoms and limitation of activities [6]; and 10 on the Hospital Anxiety and Depression Scale (8 on HADS anxiety and 2 on HADS depression), score between 0 (best) and 21 (worst) of each dimension, indicating mild levels of anxiety and normal level of depression [7].

Table 20.1 Respiratory polygraphy or type III polysomnography

	Index (events/h)	Total events (number)	Mean duration (s)	Maximum duration (s)
Central sleep apneas	1.1	9	13.4	30.5
Obstructive sleep apneas	18.3	150	10.6	21
Mixed apneas	1.2	10	12.9	21.5
Hypopneas	5.7	47	19.4	35.5
Total	26.3	216	13.4	35.5

Physiotherapeutic Intervention

The participant followed a comprehensive community program, including general physical activity and oropharyngeal exercises [8]. The physical activity consisted of 30 min of walking along publicly accessible urban park tracks designed and standardized for chronic obstructive pulmonary disease patients. The participant was encouraged to maintain a high walking intensity by achieving 60–80% of the theoretical maximal heart rate controlled by a heart rate monitor. The intervention program lasted 8 weeks, with 3 walking sessions/per week. A physiotherapist supervised all sessions during the first 2 weeks and 1 session/week from the third until the last week of the program (i.e., 12 supervised sessions, 24 sessions in total). In unsupervised sessions, the physiotherapist called by phone each patient to ask if there was any inconvenience in carrying out the protocol of general exercise. If the patient could not train, a new session was rescheduled.

Oropharyngeal exercises were based on previous studies [9, 10]. The selected oropharyngeal exercises were used to treat speech-language pathologies and include soft palate, tongue, and facial muscle exercises and stomatognathic function exercises (Fig. 20.1). The patient was instructed to practice four exercises daily, (10 times each exercise), at least 5 days per week. A video of each exercise was provided to ensure proper task realization. The physiotherapist in charge of the program weekly asked the patients about the exercise's accomplishments, difficulties, doubts, etc. High session attendance was defined as attending at least 80% of the sessions. The patients completed a compliance chart every day. If they could not perform the exercises 1 day, they would recover on a weekend day. Additionally, the patients received dietary recommendations based on promoting a low-carbohydrate diet, compliance with meal times, and eliminating foods that affect sleep conciliation (e.g., coffee, cola drinks, alcohol). Sleep hygiene education recommendations included, among others, avoiding the use of screens before sleep, avoiding carrying out intense physical exercise before sleep, and avoid heavy meals.

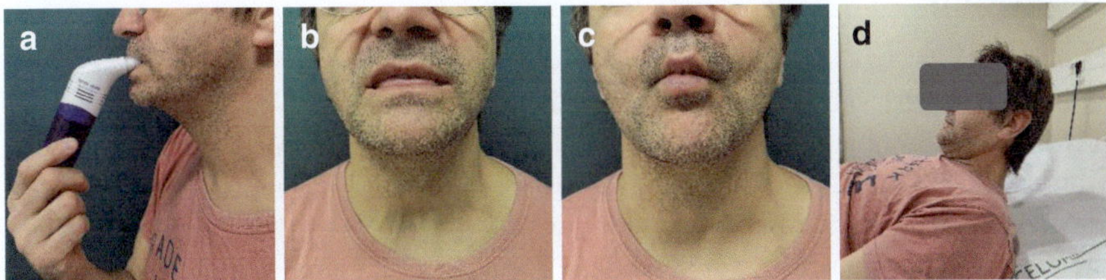

Fig. 20.1 (**a**) Blowing against a resistance of 10 cmH$_2$O; (**b**) Biting the tip of the tongue and swallowing; (**c**) Kissing and generating a negative pressure with cheeks; (**d**) Raising the head and holding it for 10 s (isometric head flexion). (Original figure. Courtesy from Dr. Torres-Castro)

Table 20.2 Pre- and post-intervention measurements

Variable	Pre-intervention	Post-intervention
Anthropometrics		
Weight (kg)	90	86
BMI (kg/m^2)	29.4	28.1
Neck circumference (cm)	41	40
Waist circumference (cm)	97	86
Hip circumference (cm)	104	99
Physical capacity and activity		
6MWD, m	643	693
Steps/day	7985	9662
Objective sleep parameters		
AHI (events/h)	26.3	8.1
CT90%	4	1
Subjective sleep parameters		
ESS	8	4
Quebec sleep questionnaire	199	189
HADS anxiety	8	2
HADS depression	2	0
HADS total	10	2

BMI body mass index, *6MWD* six-minute walking distance, *AHI* apnea-hypopnea index, *CT90* cumulative time spent with oxygen saturation <90% during sleep, *ESS* Epworth sleepiness scale, *HADS* hospital anxiety and depression scale

Follow-Up and Outcomes

The patient was evaluated pre- and post-interventions (Table 20.2).

Discussion

This case report showed that a comprehensive community program combining physical and oropharyngeal exercises reduced AHI scores in one patient with moderate OSA syndrome already indicated to use CPAP. The exercise protocol was carried out in the period between the indication of CPAP treatment and the moment the company takes to deliver it at home. Finally, he did not use it since his AHI and symptoms decreased.

The present report is in line with previously published evidence. Indeed, most studies in patients with OSA reported a significant decrease in the AHI after completing a rehabilitation program based on aerobic exercise [11, 12]. Similarly, results obtained in studies implementing oropharyngeal exercises also observed significant improvements in the AHI [9, 13, 14] thus reducing OSA severity. Our patient had major physical changes with the rehabilitation program, led by a decrease of 4-kilogram in body weight, and 0.7 in BMI. It is known that weight loss has not been related to significant AHI reductions, and the improvements are likely due to changes in body composition (especially reduction in fat mass) [15, 16]. Several mechanisms may explain these improvements. Physical exercise could reduce AHI by reducing fat deposition in the anatomical structures surrounding upper airway and tongue [17]. Additionally, exercise may cause significant abdominal adiposity reductions independently of weight loss [18]. This fact is essential, because abdominal visceral fat accumulation impairs diaphragmatic excursion, and chest wall obesity impairs rib cage expansion [19].

It has been shown that fluid accumulated in the legs during the day (due to gravity and the diminution of the muscular pump activity when lying down at night) is redistributed rostrally while in recumbent posture for sleep [20, 21]. The redistribution of fluid in the neck can increase pressure on tissues surrounding the upper airway, reducing its size and increasing its collapsibility, which is a predisposition toward OSA [20]. Therefore, interventions that reduce fluid accumulation in the legs, such as exercise, diuretics, and wearing compression stockings can attenuate OSA [22–24].

On the other hand, we carried out a protocol of oropharyngeal exercises based especially on the use of positive pressure device with $10cmH_2O$, and on the use of exercises that act directly on the affected muscles, particularly the glossopharyngeal muscle, whose dysfunction is one of the main problems in OSA. Although we did not use respiratory muscle training, the literature has shown a beneficial effect of inspiratory muscle training on improving sleep quality, and of expiratory muscle training on decreasing AHI [25].

Another critical aspect to consider is the applied setting and monitoring program. Most prior studies required subjects to participate in highly supervised exercise programs at hospitals or rehabilitation centers [12, 26]. Conversely, the presently applied protocol supervised a maximum of 50% of exercise sessions (i.e., 1 day per week supervision). Another relevant aspect of this case report is that training was performed outside the hospital, using existing resources within urban park tracks [8]. These urban park tracks were previously validated for chronic respiratory disease to set different exercise intensities [27]. Using urban park tracks could promote program adherence by ensuring that every patient can go to a park near home, thereby preventing an unnecessary avoidance of time and cost consumption while promoting physical activity. From a clinical point of view, this could help to reduce costs and involve patients to a greater degree in their self-care, especially when health-system resources are limited. Our patient reported 100% of accomplishment in the prescribed exercise sessions, oropharyngeal and walking training. Finally, this training methodology should be interesting because it can induce long-term effects and help change patient perspectives towards a healthier lifestyle.

Patient Perspective

The greatest motivation to perform the exercise program for the patient was to avoid the use of CPAP. That motivated him to have a 100% adherence to the exercise protocol. On the other hand, he was very happy because he was able to lose weight and improve his sleep quality.

References

1. Peng J, Yuan Y, Zhao Y, Ren H. Effects of exercise on patients with obstructive sleep apnea: a systematic review and meta-analysis. Int J Environ Res Public Health. 2022;19(17):10845.
2. Van Offenwert E, Vrijsen B, Belge C, Troosters T, Buyse B, Testelmans D. Physical activity and exercise in obstructive sleep apnea. Acta Clin Belg. 2019;74(2):92–101.
3. de Andrade FMD, Pedrosa RP. The role of physical exercise in obstructive sleep apnea. J Bras Pneumol publicacao Of da Soc Bras Pneumol e Tisilogia. 2016;42(6):457–64.
4. Alves ES, Ackel-D'Elia C, Luz GP, Cunha TCA, Carneiro G, Tufik S, et al. Does physical exercise reduce excessive daytime sleepiness by improving inflammatory profiles in obstructive sleep apnea patients? Sleep Breath. 2013;17(2):505–10.
5. Jiménez-Correa U, Haro R, González-Robles RO, Velázquez-Moctezuma J. How is the Epworth sleepiness scale related with subjective sleep quality and polysomnographic features in patients with sleep-disordered breathing? Sleep Breath. 2011;15(3):513–8.
6. Catalán P, Martínez A, Herrejón A, Chiner E, Martínez-García MÁ, Sancho-Chust JN, et al. Consistencia interna y validez de la versión española del cuestionario de calidad de vida específico para el síndrome de apneas-hipopneas del sueño Quebec Sleep Questionnaire. Arch Bronconeumol. 2012;48(4):107–13.
7. Pais-Ribeiro JL, Martins da Silva A, Vilhena E, Moreira I, Santos E, Mendonça D. The hospital anxiety and depression scale, in patients with multiple sclerosis. Neuropsychiatr Dis Treat. 2018;14:3193–7.
8. Torres-Castro R, Vilaró J, Martí J-D, Garmendia O, Gimeno-Santos E, Romano-Andrioni B, et al. Effects of a combined community exercise program in obstructive sleep apnea syndrome: a randomized clinical trial. J Clin Med. 2019;8(3):361.
9. Guimarães KC, Drager LF, Genta PR, Marcondes BF, Lorenzi-Filhoy G. Effects of oropharyngeal exercises on patients with moderate obstructive sleep apnea syndrome. Am J Respir Crit Care Med. 2009;179(10):962–6.
10. Burkhead LM, Sapienza CM, Rosenbek JC. Strength-training exercise in dysphagia rehabilitation: principles, procedures, and directions for future research. Dysphagia. 2007;22(3):251–65.
11. Desplan M, Mercier J, Sabaté M, Ninot G, Prefaut C, Dauvilliers Y. A comprehensive rehabilitation program improves disease severity in patients with obstructive sleep apnea syndrome: a pilot randomized controlled study. Sleep Med. 2014;15(8):906–12.
12. Kline CE, Crowley EP, Ewing GB, Burch JB, Blair SN, Durstine JL, et al. The effect of exercise training on obstructive sleep apnea and sleep quality: a randomized controlled trial. Sleep. 2011;34(12):1631.
13. Ieto V, Kayamori F, Montes MI, Hirata RP, Gregório MG, Alencar AM, et al. Effects of oropharyngeal exercises on snoring: a randomized trial. Chest. 2015;148(3):683–91.
14. Tang S, Qing J, Wang Y, Chai L, Zhang W, Ye X, et al. Clinical analysis of pharyngeal musculature and genioglossus exercising to treat obstructive sleep apnea and hypopnea syndrome. J Zhejiang Univ Sci B. 2015;16(11):931–9.
15. Mendelson M, Bailly S, Marillier M, Flore P, Borel JC, Vivodtzev I, et al. Obstructive sleep apnea syndrome, objectively measured physical activity and exercise training interventions: a systematic review and meta-analysis. Front Neurol. 2018;9:73.
16. Lindberg E, Gislason T. Epidemiology of sleep-related obstructive breathing. Sleep Med Rev. 2000;4(5):411–33.
17. Kim AM, Keenan BT, Jackson N, Chan EL, Staley B, Poptani H, et al. Tongue fat and its relationship to obstructive sleep apnea. Sleep. 2014;37(10):1639–48.
18. Irwin ML, Yasui Y, Ulrich CM, Bowen D, Rudolph RE, Schwartz RS, et al. Effect of exercise on total and intra-abdominal body fat in postmenopausal women: a randomized controlled trial. JAMA. 2003;289(3):323–30.
19. Barnes M, Goldsworthy UR, Cary BA, Hill CJ. A diet and exercise program to improve clinical outcomes in patients with obstructive sleep apnea—a feasibility study. J Clin Sleep Med JCSM. 2009;5(5):409–15.

20. Redolfi S, Yumino D, Ruttanaumpawan P, Yau B, Su M-C, Lam J, et al. Relationship between overnight rostral fluid shift and obstructive sleep apnea in nonobese men. Am J Respir Crit Care Med. 2009;179(3):241–6.
21. Torres-Castro R, Vasconcello-Castillo L, Puppo H, Cabrera-Aguilera I, Otto-Yáñez M, Rosales-Fuentes J, et al. Effects of exercise in patients with obstructive sleep apnoea. Clocks Sleep. 2021;3(1):227–35.
22. Redolfi S, Arnulf I, Pottier M, Bradley TD, Similowski T. Effects of venous compression of the legs on overnight rostral fluid shift and obstructive sleep apnea. Respir Physiol Neurobiol. 2011;175(3):390–3.
23. Redolfi S, Bettinzoli M, Venturoli N, Ravanelli M, Pedroni L, Taranto-Montemurro L, et al. Attenuation of obstructive sleep apnea and overnight rostral fluid shift by physical activity. Am J Respir Crit Care Med. 2015;191(7):856–8.
24. Kasai T, Bradley TD, Friedman O, Logan AG. Effect of intensified diuretic therapy on overnight rostral fluid shift and obstructive sleep apnoea in patients with uncontrolled hypertension. J Hypertens. 2014;32(3):673–80.
25. Torres-Castro R, Solis-Navarro L, Puppo H, Alcaraz-Serrano V, Vasconcello-Castillo L, Vilaró J, et al. Respiratory muscle training in patients with obstructive sleep apnoea: a systematic review and meta-analysis. Clocks Sleep. 2022;4(2):219–29.
26. Sengul YS, Ozalevli S, Oztura I, Itil O, Baklan B. The effect of exercise on obstructive sleep apnea: a randomized and controlled trial. Sleep Breath. 2011;15(1):49–56.
27. Arbillaga-Etxarri A, Torrent-Pallicer J, Gimeno-Santos E, Barberan-Garcia A, Delgado A, Balcells E, et al. Validation of walking trails for the urban training™ of chronic obstructive pulmonary disease patients. PloS One. 2016;11(1):e0146705.

Chapter 21
Continuous Positive Airway Pressure, Bilevel, and Supplemental Oxygen: All in One Case!

Liliane P. S. Mendes and Flávia B. Nerbass

Introduction

In this chapter we report a case of a patient who started treatment with continuous positive airway pressure (CPAP) for severe sleep-disordered breathing (SDB). Over 1 year she presented outstanding results in adherence, improvement of the symptoms, and of the obstructive events. However, during an hospitalization, it was necessary to change PAP therapy mode, which required many other adjustments. After hospital discharge, the sleep physiotherapists, along with the multi professional team, faced some challenges, including changes in PAP device, therapy mode, interface, and overnight oxygen titration, which later allowed assertiveness and effectiveness of therapy.

L. P. S. Mendes (✉)
Physiotherapy Department, Federal University of Minas Gerais,
Belo Horizonte, MG, Brazil

F. B. Nerbass
Sleep Laboratory, Pulmonary Division, University of Sao Paulo School of Medicine,
Sao Paulo, SP, Brazil

C. Frange (ed.), *Clinical Cases in Sleep Physical Therapy*,
https://doi.org/10.1007/978-3-031-38340-3_21

Patient Information

F.L.C., woman, 89-year-old, obese (BMI 31.4 kg/m^2), hypertensive, had a previous acute myocardial infarction, complained of snoring, witnessed respiratory pauses, nocturia (once a night), tiredness, and daytime sleepiness (napped twice a day). Her body position in bed was exclusively supine.

Diagnostic Assessment

Her sleep home apnea testing (HSAT) was performed by type III portable monitoring. The results showed an apnea-hypopnea index (AHI) of 118 ev/h, predominantly obstructive, with time of $SpO_2 < 90\% = 476.5$ min, being 180.5 min <80%, with a minimum $SpO_2 = 45\%$ (Table 21.1 and Fig. 21.1).

Table 21.1 Respiratory-related events data from the sleep home apnea testing

	Index (events/ hour)	Total events (number)	Minimum duration (seconds)	Maximum duration (seconds)	Body position events Supine *versus* lateral
Central apneas	0.8	7	11.1	12.5	7
Obstructive apneas	114.2	942	19.1	130	942
Mixed apneas	2.1	17	13.8	18.5	17
Hypopneas	1.2	10	24.3	61	10
Total	118.3	976	19	130	
Time in position (min)					495
Apnea-hypopnea index (ev/h)					118.3

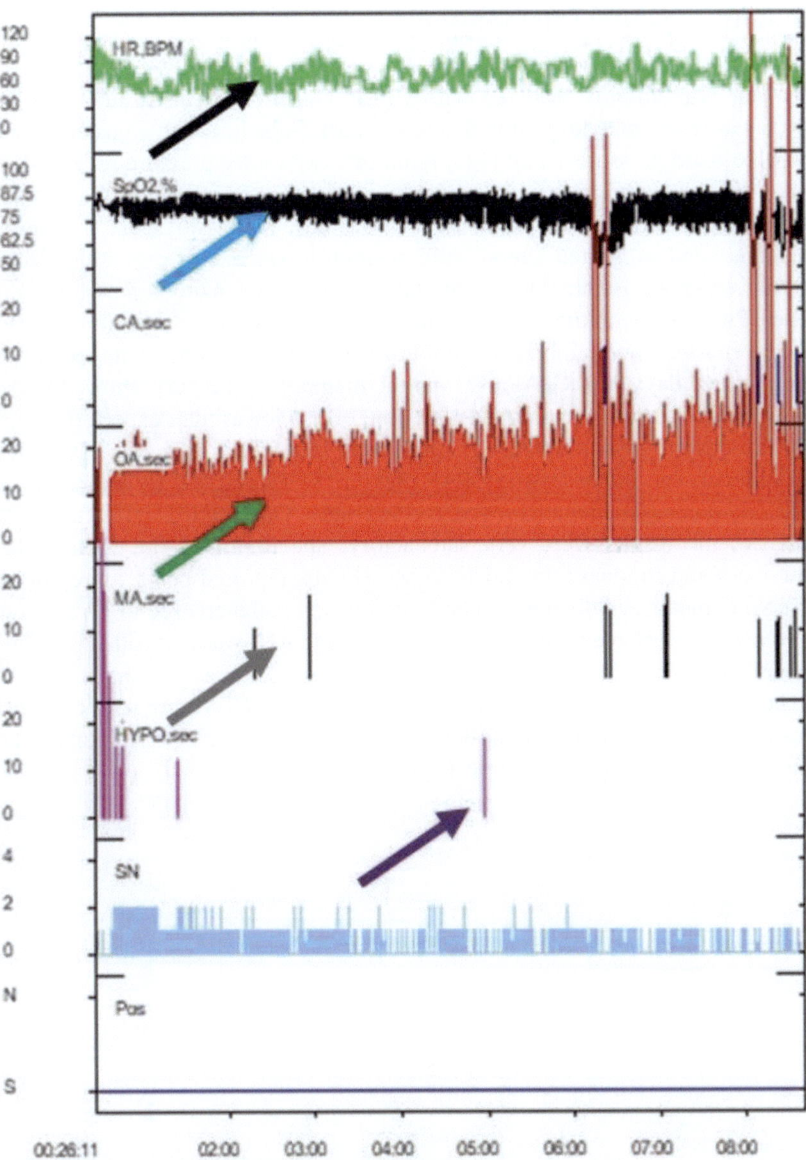

Fig. 21.1 Graph from the HSAT. Black arrow indicates heart hate; blue arrow indicates SpO_2; green arrow indicates obstructive events (red scratches); gray arrow indicates mixed events (black scratches); purple arrow indicates hypopneas (pink scratches); snoring in light blue scratches and supine body position in blue solid line. (Reprinted with permission from F.L.C.)

Physiotherapeutic Intervention

This case was initially resolved with CPAP. On our first visit, automatic PAP device was tested and adapted with a nasal mask (tube up). The adjusted parameters were fixed pressure 10 cmH$_2$O, ramp off, expiratory pressure relief off, and humidity 5. In this initial test, the patient presented a good tolerance. We instructed both family and patient on the correct mask placement, CPAP use during total sleep time, and suggested lateral body position to sleep. However, side sleeping position was not possible due to complaints of low back pain, and mobility difficulties. Phone calls on the first and third days of therapy were performed, and the patient reported good adherence without additional complaints. Our second visit took place 15 days after CPAP use, and the memory card reports showed high air leakage (107.4 L/min), and an average time of use lower than expected (3 h and 32 min), despite a significant AHI reduction (16.2 ev/h). Thus, we associated a chin retainer, and increased the CPAP pressure to 12 cmH$_2$O. By telephone call, the family reported better adherence, and tolerance. On the third visit (after another 15 days), the results were very satisfactory. She improved the complaints of drowsiness and tiredness, the nocturia ceased, she reported being more attentive and communicative. Adherence to pressure therapy had increased to 7 h and 7 min on average, air leakage reduced to 34.8 L/min, and AHI was controlled to 0.7 ev/h (Fig. 21.2).

The detailed graphs below were extracted from the CPAP memory card 1 day before our last visit. Figure 21.3 demonstrates the absence of respiratory events, even in the presence of a high air leakage (Fig. 21.3).

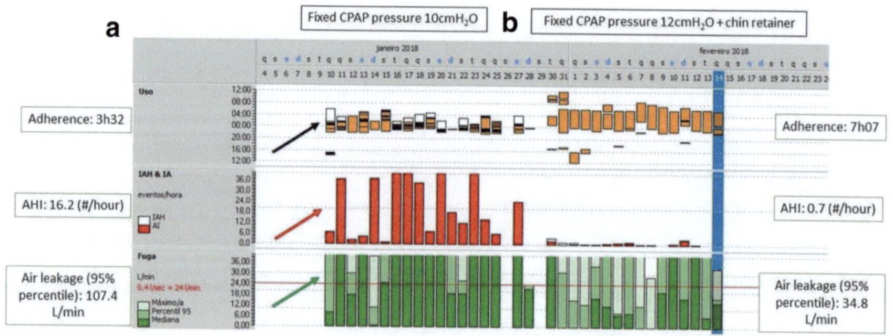

Fig. 21.2 (**a**) Summary graphs from the PAP device, showing the first visit period (15 days), when CPAP therapy was started (fixed pressure of 10 cmH$_2$O). The green arrow indicates that due to high air leakage (dark green bars—107.4 L/min), the patient had poor adherence to treatment (orange bars—3 h 32 min—black arrow), although the mean AHI reduced from 118 to 16.2 events/h (red arrow). (**b**) Data from the second visit period, after associating the chin retainer and increasing the pressure to 12 cmH$_2$O. There was better leakage control, an increase in adherence (7 h 07 min), AHI control (0.7 ev/h), and air leakage reduction (34.8 L/min). (Reprinted with permission from F.L.C.)

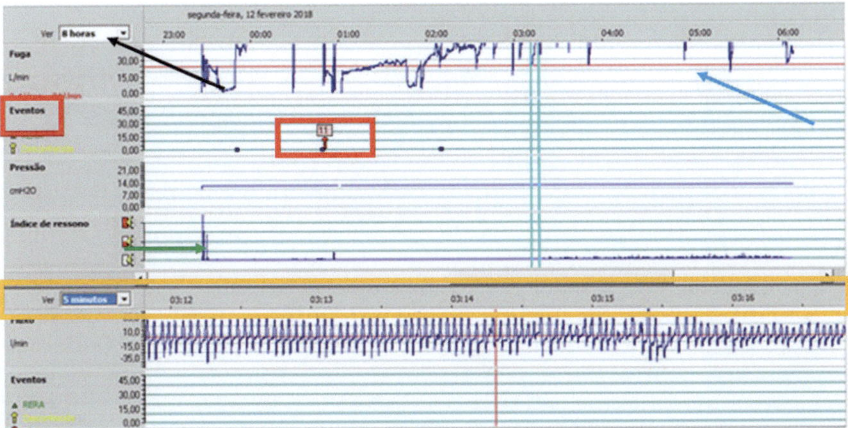

Fig. 21.3 Respiratory flow curve analysis showing the whole night use of PAP device. Black arrow indicates the time of sleeping period, from 23 h to 6 h. Blue arrow indicates air leakage and above the red line indicates high air leakage (>24 L/min). The red boxes show the apnea/hypopnea events. The blue line bellow indicates the CPAP pressure, and the green arrow indicates snoring. The green parallel vertical lines show the zoom interval plotted at the inner 5 min (yellow box). At the bottom, we see the respiratory flow waves in the first line and the apnea events in the second line. We observed that, even with high air leakage, the flow waves were preserved and without residual apnea events, proving that the treatment was adequate. (Reprinted with permission from F.L.C.)

Follow-Up and Outcomes

Follow-up were performed every 3 months during the first year, indicating low AHI and good adherence. However, after that period, the patient was hospitalized because of a hemorrhagic shock (right anterior thoracic hematoma), and pneumonia. She got respiratory failure, and presented drops in O_2 saturation (SpO_2). Bilevel positive pressure therapy was immediately started. In addition, the hospital's clinical team changed her mask to an oronasal route, and associated oxygen at 2.0 L/min to keep her $SpO_2 > 90\%$.

After hospital discharge, the family contacted us because, despite proper use of Bilevel (Inspiratory Positive Airway Pressure (IPAP): 18 cmH$_2$O, Expiratory Positive Airway Pressure (EPAP) 10 cmH$_2$O, + O_2 2 L/min), patient's $SpO_2 = 84\%$, even when she was awake. That way, for 2 consecutive nights, we performed an overnight nocturnal oximetry (attaching to the Bilevel an oximetry module). On the first day, she presented several respiratory events, leading to a drop in SpO_2. The average AHI was 9.6 ev/h, and the highest AHI was 27 ev/h (Fig. 21.4). The mean and minimum SpO_2 reached 85 and 61%, respectively.

With this results, we changed the oronasal route to a nasal, and maintained the same Bilevel pressures and oxygen supply. The goal was to observe the impact of the oronasal route on the obstructive events, considering that previously, the patient had controlled AHI using CPAP 12 cmH$_2$O by nasal mask. Table 21.2 presents the comparative results of 2 nights with the oronasal route, and 2 extra nights with a

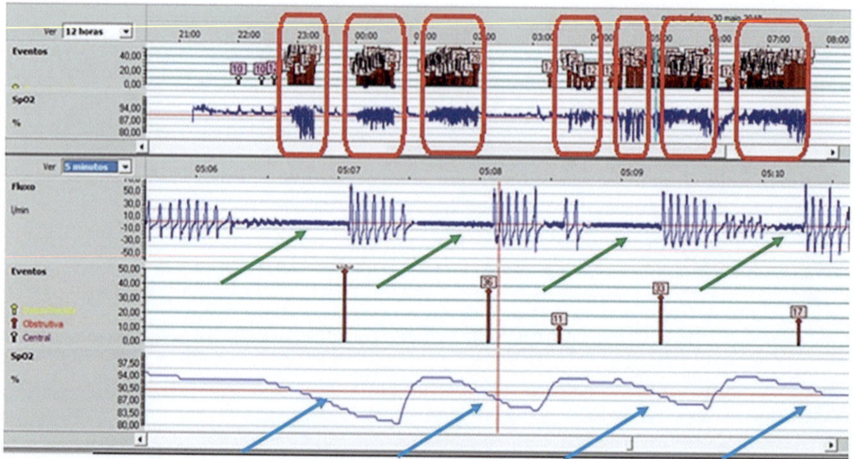

Fig. 21.4 Detailed data from the Bilevel card. At the top are 12 h of sleep. The first line shows apnea events (red boxes), associated with periods of desaturation (second line). Below are the respiratory airflow waves, clearly showing obstructive apnea events (green arrows) followed by synchronous saturation drops (blue arrows). (Reprinted with permission from F.L.C.)

Table 21.2 Comparison between different nights using different interfaces

	Mask route	IPAP/ EPAP	O_2 (L/ min)	AHI (ev/h)	Min SpO_2 (%)	Median SpO_2 (%)	Time SpO_2 < 90%	Time SpO_2 < 80%
Night 1	Oronasal	18/11	2.5	9.6	71	91	00:46:47	00:00:00
Night 2	Oronasal	18/11	2.5	27.5	69	92	01:27:07	00:05:19
Night 3	Nasal	18/11	2.5	1.6	81	86	09:14:58	00:00:00
Night 4	Nasal	18/11	2.5	1.6	78	87	07:36:29	00:00:13

nasal route. All these evaluations were performed without modifications in the Bilevel or oxygen supply parameters.

The results showed that nasal route better controlled AHI (<5 ev/h) and kept the minimum saturation higher than the oronasal route; however, it allowed lower median saturation, and also increased time saturation <90%.

Analyzing the detailed data of the memory card using the nasal route, we observed that the saturation spent most of the time <90% line, although AHI had spent <5 ev/h. However, instead of desaturations being related to obstructive events (as observed with the oronasal mask), desaturations were related to increased time of air leakage with the nasal mask (red boxes). When the air leakage was controlled, the saturation remained at 90%, as shown in Fig. 21.5.

Under the oronasal route, the patient had much more obstructive events followed by hypoxia/reoxygenation. Under nasal route, the desaturations were due to air

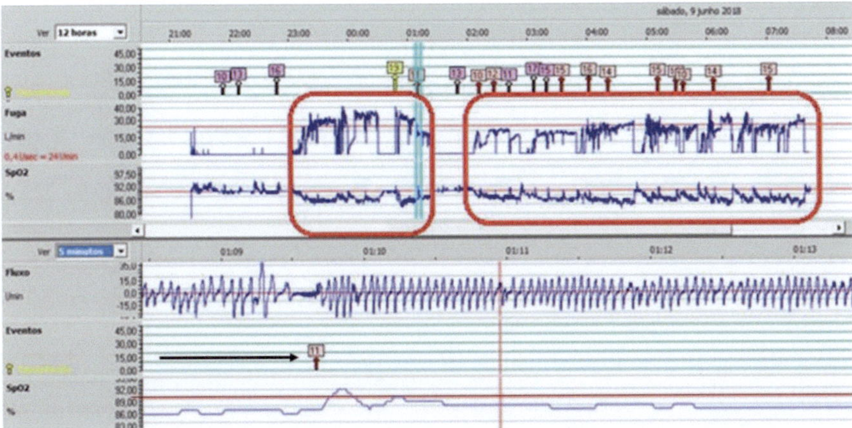

Fig. 21.5 The first line shows the apnea events (on top = obstructive: red sticks, central: black sticks, and unknown: yellow sticks). Signalized by red boxes we can observe that there are periods of increased leakage (second line) associated with simultaneous drops in saturation (third line). Below (5 min of sleep), we can see the respiratory airflow waves, showing only one obstructive event (red stick), followed by a drop in saturation and, even without more events, the saturation remaining <90% (red horizontal line). (Reprinted with permission from F.L.C.)

leakage, despite the patient wearing a chin retainer in both conditions. As the patient spent most of the night in the supine position, it is difficult to control the opening of the mouth, even with a very well-adjusted mask and chin retainer. In this case, the multidisciplinary team decided to maintain the same Bilevel pressures and nasal mask, as arterial blood gas analysis showed adequate partial pressure of carbon dioxide ($PaCO_2$) and pH levels ($PaCO_2$: 45.3/pH: 7.41).

Then, we started an overnight oxygen titration using nocturnal oximetry to guarantee SpO_2 at least 90%. We started with 2 L/min and increased the amount of O_2 offered by 0.5 L/min until we reached the best oxygenation results, which was achieved when under 4.5 L/min, as shown in Fig. 21.6. Even in a high air leaking, the saturation remained >90% all night without obstructive events. Median saturation was 95%, and time of saturation <90% and <80% was 29 and 17 s, respectively.

Discussion

The CPAP device is the gold standard treatment for patients with moderate-to-severe OSA, and the pressure can be delivered through nasal, nasal pillows, oronasal, and oral masks. The oronasal masks were initially described for patients with respiratory failure and high ventilatory demand. Subsequently, they were tested for sleep apnea treatment in those who did not tolerate the nasal route, with good results for AHI correction [1, 2]. However, later studies showed that oronasal masks were

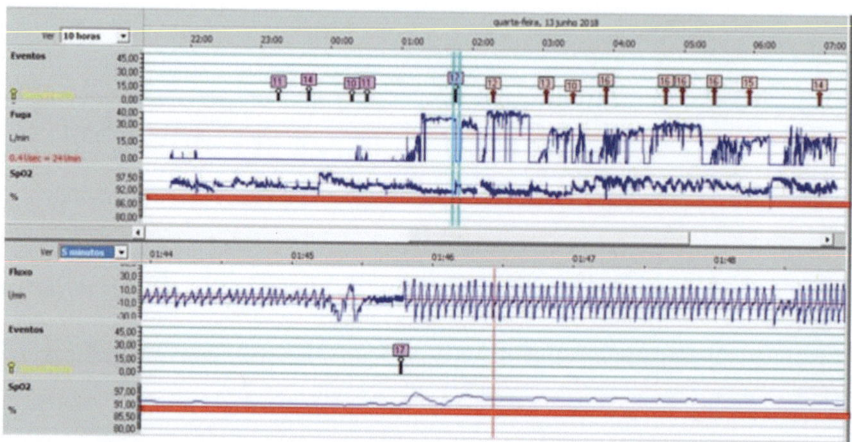

Fig. 21.6 The first line shows the apnea events (on top = obstructive: red sticks, central: black sticks, and unknown: yellow sticks). The second line shows air leakage, and the third one is the O_2 saturation. The horizontal thicker red lines represent the limit of saturation at 90%. Below, we can see the respiratory airflow waves, showing only one central event (black arrow). In the upper and lower image parts, we observe that under 4.5 L/min of oxygen, the patient remained with saturation above 90% all night long. (Reprinted with permission from F.L.C.)

associated with greater patient intolerance, higher leakage, and the need for higher pressure levels, causing lower adherence to treatment [3–5]. The most worrying effect of the oronasal route is the tongue's posterior displacement against the oropharyngeal wall, causing its narrowing and, consequently, more obstruction [4–8]. In this case report, when the nasal mask was changed for the oronasal one (during hospitalization), the patient developed OSA events, despite using Bilevel therapy under higher pressures, as compared to previous period using CPAP. When the air route (oronasal to nasal) was switched again, there was a correction in the AHI and in the intermittent hypoxia caused by those obstructive events (even maintaining the same pressures in the equipment). Recently, The American Thoracic Society published a document recommending the nasal route as the first-line interface to treat SDB [9].

Furthermore, overnight nocturnal oximetry results assessed by detailed data from the Bilevel card (airflow respiratory waves) allowed us to observe that with the nasal mask, the eventual drops in saturation and the sustained saturation time <90% were linked to air leakage (through the mouth). Considering that the oxygen connection is placed at the equipment's air outlet, when under high air leakage, reductions in oxygenation are expected. The patient used a nasal mask and a chin retainer. However, as she slept exclusively in the supine position, the complete closed mouth wase be a challenge, considering her reduced muscle tone.

Considering the positive results, the multidisciplinary team decided to maintain the nasal mask with the chin retainer and adjusted the amount of oxygen offered to 4.5 L/min for good saturation.

In conclusion, the evaluation and follow-up of the sleep physiotherapist was essential to initially ensure adaptation do CPAP, perform adjustments, and optimize adherence. Subsequently, our approach allowed us to recognize that the oronasal route was causing harm to the patient (due to the significant increase in obstructive events, and intermittent hypoxia). Even without modifying parameters in the Bilevel and the amount of O_2 offered, changing the route to the nasal one was able to correct the AHI. Nocturnal oximetry allowed us to observe that lower saturation was related to increased air leakage. Therefore, we emphasize here the importance of a careful and detailed evaluation and patient follow-up, increasing the chances of proper treatment and good adherence to the therapy.

References

1. Sanders MH, Kern NB, Stiller RA, Strollo PJ, Martin TJ, Atwood CW. CPAP therapy via oronasal mask for obstructive sleep apnea. Chest. 1994;106(3):774–9.
2. Prosise GL, Berry RB. Oral-nasal continuous positive airway pressure as a treatment for obstructive sleep apnea. Chest. 1994;106(1):180–6.
3. Teo M, Amis T, Lee S, Falland K, Lambert S, Wheatley J. Equivalence of nasal and oronasal masks during initial CPAP titration for obstructive sleep apnea syndrome. Sleep. 2011;34(7):951–5.
4. Ebben MR, Milrad S, Dyke JP, Phillips CD, Krieger AC. Comparison of the upper airway dynamics of oronasal and nasal masks with positive airway pressure treatment using cine magnetic resonance imaging. Sleep Breath. 2015;20:79.
5. Borel JC, Tamisier R, Dias-Domingos S, Sapene M, Martin F, Stach B, et al. Type of mask may impact on continuous positive airway pressure adherence in apneic patients. PLoS One. 2013;8(5):e64382.
6. Andrade RG, Piccin VS, Nascimento JA, Viana FM, Genta PR, Lorenzi-Filho G. Impact of the type of mask on the effectiveness of and adherence to continuous positive airway pressure treatment for obstructive sleep apnea. J Bras Pneumol. 2014;40(6):658–68.
7. Andrade RG, Madeiro F, Genta PR, Lorenzi-Filho G. Oronasal mask may compromise the efficacy of continuous positive airway pressure on OSA treatment: is there evidence for avoiding the oronasal route? Curr Opin Pulm Med. 2016;22(6):555–62.
8. Schorr F, Genta PR, Gregório MG, Danzi-Soares NJ, Lorenzi-Filho G. Continuous positive airway pressure delivered by oronasal mask may not be effective for obstructive sleep apnoea. Eur Respir J. 2012;40(2):503–5.
9. Genta PR, Kaminska M, Edwards BA, Ebben MR, Krieger AC, Tamisier R, et al. The importance of mask selection on continuous positive airway pressure outcomes for obstructive sleep apnea. An official American Thoracic Society workshop report. Ann Am Thorac Soc. 2020;17(10):1177–85.

Chapter 22
Aligning the Center of Gravity After Stroke: Treatment for Obstructive Sleep Apnea?

Cristina Frange and Sandra Souza de Queiroz

Introduction

In patients with motor dysfunction after stroke (e.g., hemiparesis) the focus of rehabilitation is based on strength training, coordination, and development of skills for functions for activities of daily living (motor control) [1–3], that are frequently measured by the Functional Independence Measure (MIF) [4].

Global postural reeducation (GPR) has been focused on some investigations regarding neurological patients [5, 6]. This method proposes a decrease in muscle tone, and gradual stretching of entire muscle group simultaneously, in an integrated idea of the muscular system formed by muscle chains [7–10], improving mechanics and consequently respiratory and motor function.

Sleep-disordered breathing (i.e., obstructive sleep apnea, OSA) has an alarming prevalence after stroke, as high as 72% [11]. Therefore, treatment of sleep issues is crucial for neurorehabilitation [12–16]. We treated a patient with GPR focusing on posture, center of gravity alignment, respiratory muscle strength, and stretching, for better diaphragm incursion, obstructive sleep apnea, and functional independence.

C. Frange
Neurology and Neurosurgery Department, Federal University of São Paulo (UNIFESP), São Paulo, SP, Brazil

S. S. de Queiroz (✉)
Brazilian Sleep Association, São Paulo, SP, Brazil

C. Frange (ed.), *Clinical Cases in Sleep Physical Therapy*, https://doi.org/10.1007/978-3-031-38340-3_22

Patient Information

M. A. F., a 59-year-old woman, eutrophic (body mass index [BMI] 24.9 kg/m^2) came from the Inpatient Unit of Neurology of Hospital São Paulo, Neurology and Neurosurgery Department of Federal University of São Paulo (UNIFESP). She was attended after 2 months of an ischemic stroke. The stroke event happened in March of 2019. She had left carotid endarterectomy surgery to reduce the risk of another stroke event. She started physical therapy (PT) based on bed mobility training at hospital. The patient presented hypertension, hypercholesterolemia, and diabetes, with regular medication and visits to physicians. Until the stroke event she was sedentary.

Clinical Findings

She presented with incomplete right hemiparesis, with crural predominance. She was able to walk by herself with no assistive devices for walking, and to speak appropriately.

Diagnostic Assessment

The scoring of neurological deficit at clinical admission according to the National Institutes of Health Stroke Scale(NIHSS) [17] was 6 (moderate/severe stroke); no cognitive impairment >18, according to Montreal Cognitive Assessment (MoCA) [18]. The patient underwent measurements pre- and post-20 PT sessions for respiratory muscle strength (manovacuometry) [19], posture and center of gravity alignment (bio photogrammetry) [20, 21], functional independence (functional independence measure) [4, 22], and objective sleep parameters (polysomnography, PSG) [23].

Physiotherapeutic Intervention

The patient received 20 consecutive and individual GPR sessions (60–90 min/week) during the afternoon. The GPR sessions adopted specific postures in dorsal decubitus, aiming to reduce the anterior master neuromuscular coordination chain muscle tone hyperexcitability. The "opening posture" of the hip angle and abducted arms was adopted. In this posture, the retracted muscles related to the central lesion were

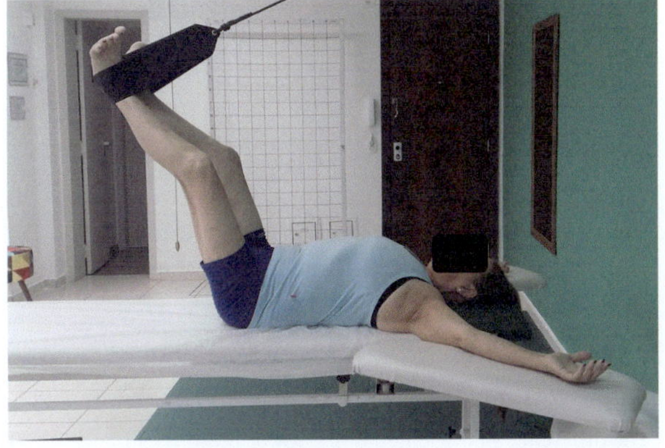

Fig. 22.1 "Opening posture," to reduce muscle tone hyperexcitability of the anterior neuromuscular chain

placed in traction [10]. With the use of cushions, rolls, and elastic bands, the patient stayed in the posture for about 20 min in each session, being corrected where compensation appeared, and whenever the body tried to compensate for that posture. All the time the patient was required to maintain her breath in voluntary control, slowly and deepening, mobilizing the rib cage, activating the diaphragm muscle, and relaxing the accessory muscles of breathing (Fig. 22.1).

Follow-Up and Outcomes

Posture

Lower weight distribution in the affected limb in hemiparetic individuals often generates postural asymmetry and muscle imbalance. Some patients assume a larger base of support to increase their stability. Table 22.1 shows the postural parameters from pre- and post-GPR sessions, extracted from SAPo software (bio photogrammetry).

These measurements showed an objective improvement of the posture (central alignment) of the patient in anterior, posterior, and side views (Fig. 22.2). She reported feeling better, having better balance (although we did not measure it). The intervention improved her posture, reduced shoulder asymmetry (anterior and posterior view), and improved dorsal kyphosis by better vertebral alignment (lateral view). The patient maintained her weight during this intervention time. At the first session, she complained of pain and unpleasant sensation in the neck region of the endarterectomy (fascia adherence?), and with the sessions this pain disappeared completely by the 20th session, although we did not measure it).

Table 22.1 Postural parameters before and after GPR sessions acquired by biophotogammtery

Anterior view	Reference	Pre-GPR	Post-GPR
Head			
Horizontal head alignment	0°	175.2° r	10.1° l
Trunk			
Horizontal acromion alignment	0°	174.9° r	5.4° l
Horizontal alignment of the anterior superior iliac spine	0°	178.0° r	3.1° l
The angle between the two acromion and the two anterior superior iliac spines	0°	3.1° r	2.3° r
Lower limbs			
Left frontal angle	-	1.9° l	7.7° l
Right frontal angle	-	0.2° r	4.0° r
The difference in the length of the lower limbs (right/left)	0 cm	0.3 cm	0 cm
Horizontal alignment of tibial tuberosities	0°	173.5° l	6.1° l
Q angle—right	15°	6.7° r	5.2° r
Q angle—left	15°	4.3° r	6.1° r
Posterior view			
Trunk			
Horizontal asymmetry of the scapula concerning T3 vertebra	0°	1.9° l	8.7° l
Lower limbs			
Hindfoot angle right	–	20.4° r	6.7° r
Hindfoot angle left	–	17.3° r	19.1° r
Right view			
Head			
Horizontal head alignment (C7 vertebra)	–	140.3° l	35.6° r
Vertical head alignment (acromion)	0°	178.3° l	4° r
Trunk			
Vertical trunk alignment	–	175.3° r	1.7° l
Hip angle (trunk and thigh)	–	14.4° l	19.4° l
Vertical body alignment	–	178.6° l	6.1° r
Horizontal alignment of the pelvis	–	160.6° r	9.6° l
Lower limbs			
Knee angle	–	8.2° l	11.7° l
Ankle angle	–	91.6° l	84° r
Left view			
Horizontal head alignment (C7 vertebra)	–	145.7° l	54.1° l
Vertical head alignment (acromion)	0°	171.3° r	5.8° r
Trunk			
Vertical trunk alignment	–	175.0° r	12.1° l
Hip angle (trunk and thigh)	–	11.7° l	20.8° l
Vertical body alignment	–	179.2° l	3.1° l
Horizontal alignment of the pelvis	–	168.5° r	7.6° l
Lower limbs			
Knee angle	–	3° l	11.6° l
Ankle angle	–	93.8° l	92.9° r

Measures expressed angles, except where noted (cm): centimeters. Reference angles and measures are from SAPo software

r: to the right side, l: to the left side

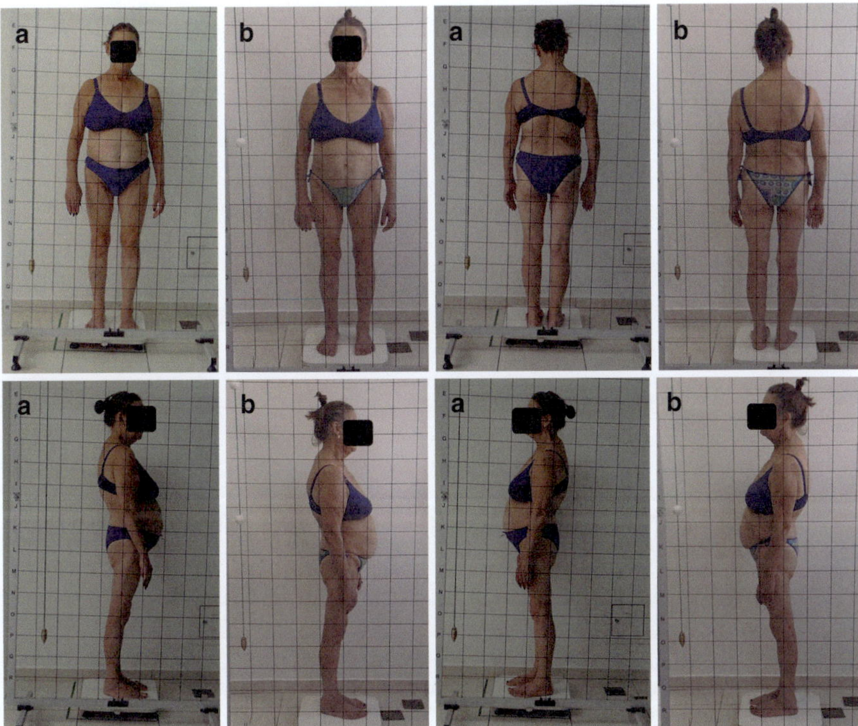

Fig. 22.2 Anterior, posterior, right, and left views pre-GPR (**a**), and post-GPR (**b**) interventions

Center of Gravity

The center of gravity (COG) was anteriorized and left-sided at baseline and after treatment it changed to almost in line and posteriorized. The asymmetry in the frontal plane decreased from 19.3° to the left, to 2.4° to the right; asymmetry in the sagittal plane decreased from 44.3° anteriorly, to 27° posteriorly (Fig. 22.3), indicating an important change of posture and a different load of the muscles to maintain orthostatism after stroke. The position of the COG relative to the mean position of the malleoli (frontal plane) decreased from 0.6 cm to 0, both left; and the position of the COG relative to the mean position of the malleoli (lateral plane) decreased from 0.6 cm to 0.1 cm, both left. Taken together, these measures showed a more aligned posture and imbalance.

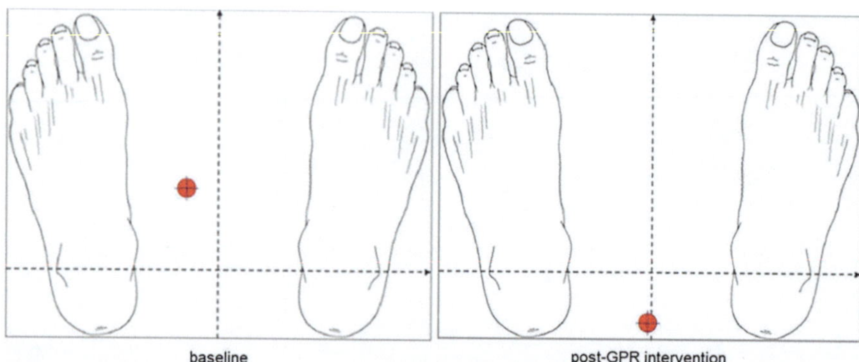

Fig. 22.3 Change in center of gravity (red) at pre- and post-GPR intervention, extracted from SAPo software

Table 22.2 Evaluation of maximum inspiratory and expiratory pressures in the baseline, after treatment, and 1-month follow-up

Maximum inspiratory pressure (cmH$_2$O)			Maximum expiratory pressure (cmH$_2$O)		
Pre-GPR	Post-GPR	1 month follow-up	Pre-GPR	Post-GPR	1 month follow-up
56.7	76.7	60.7	43.3	60.7	70.7

Normal values for the age of the patient are maximum inspiratory pressure 77 ± 26 cmH$_2$O, and maximum expiratory pressure 145 ± 40 cmH$_2$O. Values are expressed in absolute numbers

Respiratory Muscle Strength

We measured respiratory muscle strength via manovacuometry at baseline, after the 20th session and also after 1 month of follow-up after treatment has ended. At baseline, the patient presented respiratory muscle weakness (maximum inspiratory pressure values between 40 and 75 cmH$_2$O [24]); after intervention respiratory muscle strength increased, also indicating better diaphragmatic incursion. However, at 1 month of follow-up respiratory muscle strength decreased (Table 22.2), indicating a dose-dependent response of GPR. We are unaware of data regarding GPR for respiratory muscle strength in patients after stroke.

Table 22.3 Scores of functional independence measure at pre and post-GPR evaluations

	Pre-GPR	Post-GPR
Functional independence measure (total)	102	125
Domain—motor function (total)	75	91
Self-care	38	42
Sphincter control	12	14
Mobility	15	21
Locomotion	10	14
Domain—cognitive function (total)	27	34
Communication	13	14
Social cognition	14	20

Functional Independence and Motor Impairment

Table 22.3 presents the patient's functional independence assessment scores, indicating a slightly improvement in independence of daily life activities

The functional independence measure (FIM) total score varies from 18 to 126, the higher the score, the better is the functionality and independence on activities of daily living. This scale contains 18 items, grouped into 6 dimensions: self-care, locomotion, transference, communication, sphincter control and social cognition and into two subscales: motor subscale will be a value between 13 and 91; cognition subscale will be a value between 5 and 35 [25].

Sleep Pattern

The objective sleep pattern, measured by polysomnographic examination, is summarized in Table 22.4. The main outcome, apnea-hypopnea index (AHI), one of the measures of OSA, changed its classification from severe to moderate, comparing pre- and post-GPR sessions. Interestingly, the obstructive index increased, and the hypopnea index, the desaturation time, and snoring decreased after PT sessions. But contrary to our expectations, other variables of the PGS showed a worsening after PT sessions: sleep efficiency, NREM N3 and REM sleep stage decreased, and REM sleep latency, wake after sleep onset, stages NRENM N1 and N2 increased, indicating a disturbed sleep.

Table 22.4 Objective sleep pattern before and after GPR sessions

	TST (min)	SE (%)	SL (min)	REM SL (min)	WASO (min)	N1 (%)	N2 (%)	N3 (%)	REM (%)	Snore (%)	AHI (n°/h)	OI (n°/h)	HI (n°/h)	CI (n°/h)	SpO_2<90% (min)
Pre-	436.5	89.8	5.3	147.5	28.5	20.3	44.6	10.5	24.6	54.6	16.8	1.4	15.4	0	5.4
Post-	428.0	78.0	1.0	242.0	119.7	24.3	60.9	1.8	13.1	18.6	12.8	10.9	1.8	0	0.1

TST total sleep time: variable within person, *SE* sleep efficiency, the ratio of total sleep time to the total amount of time spent in bed in percentage (>85% of TST), *SL* sleep latency, the length of time in minutes it takes to transits from wake to sleep (<30 min), *REM SL* REM sleep stage latency, the length of time in minutes it takes to first stage of REM sleep (70–120 min), *WASO* wake after sleep onset, the amount of time in minutes spent awake after sleep has been initiated (sleep fragmentation—up to 30 min), *N1* NREM stage N1 sleep (up to 5% of TST), *N2* NREM stage N2 sleep (45–55% of TST), *N3* NREM stage N3 sleep (slow wave sleep or delta sleep—up to 23% of TST), *REM* sleep stage (20–25% of TST), *AHI* apnea-hypopnea index, indicates the mean number of obstructive apneas and hypopneas per hour of sleep (<5/h, normal; ≥5 and <15, mild; ≥15 and <30, moderate; and ≥30, severe); *SpO_2<90%* % of TST spent <90% of oxygen saturation [26]

Discussion

The GPR method is widely used to treat musculoskeletal asymmetries. This condition is common in stroke patients. The 20 GPR sessions were able to show improvement in postural alignment, which can contribute to an improvement in quality of life, especially in terms of functional independence as can be observed in our patient.

Postural imbalance after stroke makes the patient vulnerable to the risk of falls, which makes them more likely to adopt a sedentary lifestyle—which can lead to several other health problems regarding inactivity [27].

The gain in muscular strength of the inspiratory muscles, evidenced by the increase in the maximum inspiratory pressure, leads us to consider that the breathing exercises of the GPR sessions were able to promote an increase in the resistance and in the incursion of the diaphragm muscle. This resulted in an improvement in patency of the upper airways, with consequent improvement in airflow fluidity, also during sleep, and thus promoting a decrease in the AHI [28]. In addition, caudal tracheal traction may have happened due to a better incursion of the trachea and diaphragm [29], gained with the PT sessions.

One question that came to our mind was: did the patient improve because of GPR or because of time? There is a hypothetical model of functional recovery postulating that activities and function after a stroke reach a maximum peak between 3 and 6 months after the event, that is, in the subacute phase [30], phase of this patient. However, the degree of recovery and the phase are still uncertain, not only depending very much on the injury itself but also depending on the environment, rehabilitation, and mainly on the rehabilitation intensity and frequency to which the patient is destined [31, 32].

In this case report, the GPR method was able to improve postural alignment and thus OSA classification based on AHI, and functional Independence. Sleep must be investigated in patients after stroke, and treated using PT approaches [33, 34]. Rehabilitation processes and reintegration of the patient to functional, personal activities, and social participation must be reestablished as soon as possible—and sleep is imperative to rehabilitate.

References

1. Winstein CJ, et al. Guidelines for adult stroke rehabilitation and recovery: a guideline for healthcare professionals From the American Heart Association/American Stroke Association. Stroke. 2016;47(6):e98–e169.
2. Duncan PW, et al. Management of adult stroke rehabilitation care: a clinical practice guideline. Stroke. 2005;36(9):e100–43.
3. National Institute for Health and Care Excellence. Stroke rehabilitation in adults. In: Clinical guideline. London: National Institute for Health and Care Excellence; 2013. p. 39.
4. Riberto M, et al. Validação da versão brasileira da medida de independência funcional. Acta Fisiatr. 2004;11(2):72–6.

5. Todri J, Lena O, Martinez Gil JL. An experimental pilot study of global postural reeducation concerning the cognitive approach of patients with Alzheimer's disease. Am J Alzheimers Dis Other Dement. 2020;35:1533317519867824.

6. Todri J, Todri A, Lena O. Why not a global postural reeducation as an alternative therapy applied to Alzheimer's patients in nursing homes? A pioneer randomized controlled trial. Dement Geriatr Cogn Disord. 2019;48(3-4):172–9.

7. Souchard PE. Global postural re-education. Available from https://abrir.link/eUkLo.

8. Moreno MA, et al. Effect of a muscle stretching program using the global postural reeducation method on respiratory muscle strength and thoracoabdominal mobility of sedentary young males. J Bras Pneumol. 2007;33(6):679–86.

9. Mandanmohan, et al. Effect of yoga training on handgrip, respiratory pressures and pulmonary function. Indian J Physiol Pharmacol. 2003;47(4):387–92.

10. Souchard PE. Reeducação postural global: método do campo fechado. 4th ed. São Paulo: Ícone; 2001.

11. Johnson KG, Johnson DC. Frequency of sleep apnea in stroke and TIA patients: a meta-analysis. J Clin Sleep Med. 2010;6(2):131–7.

12. Backhaus W, et al. Can daytime napping assist the process of skills acquisition after stroke? Front Neurol. 2018;9:1002.

13. Siengsukon C, Boyd LA. Sleep enhances off-line spatial and temporal motor learning after stroke. Neurorehabil Neural Repair. 2009;23(4):327–35.

14. Siengsukon CF, Boyd LA. Sleep to learn after stroke: implicit and explicit off-line motor learning. Neurosci Lett. 2009;451(1):1–5.

15. Al-Dughmi M, et al. Executive function is associated with off-line motor learning in people with chronic stroke. J Neurol Phys Ther. 2017;41(2):101–6.

16. Lubart AA et al. Action observation of motor skills followed by immediate sleep enhances the motor rehabilitation of older adults with stroke. J Geriatr Phys Ther. 2017. https://doi.org/10.1519/JPT.0000000000000136.

17. Cincura C, et al. Validation of the National Institutes of Health stroke scale, modified Rankin scale and Barthel index in Brazil: the role of cultural adaptation and structured interviewing. Cerebrovasc Dis. 2009;27(2):119–22.

18. Freitas S, et al. Montreal cognitive assessment (MoCA): normative study for the Portuguese population. J Clin Exp Neuropsychol. 2011;33(9):989–96.

19. Neder JA, et al. Reference values for lung function tests. II. Maximal respiratory pressures and voluntary ventilation. Braz J Med Biol Res. 1999;32(6):719–27.

20. Ferreira EA, et al. Quantitative assessment of postural alignment in young adults based on photographs of anterior, posterior, and lateral views. J Manip Physiol Ther. 2011;34(6):371–80.

21. Souza JA, et al. Biophotogrammetry: reliability of measurements obtained with a posture assessment software (SAPO). Rev Bras Cineantropom Desempenho Hum. 2011;13:299–305.

22. Maki T, et al. Estudo de confiabilidade da aplicação da escala de Fugl-Meyer no Brasil. Braz J Phys Ther. 2006;10:2.

23. Berry RB, et al. Rules for scoring respiratory events in sleep: update of the 2007 AASM Manual for the Scoring of Sleep and Associated Events. Deliberations of the Sleep Apnea Definitions Task Force of the American Academy of Sleep Medicine. J Clin Sleep Med. 2012;8(5):597–619.

24. Souza R. Pressões respiratórias estáticas máximas. J Pneumol. 2002;28:155.

25. Linacre JM, et al. The structure and stability of the functional independence measure. Arch Phys Med Rehabil. 1994;75(2):127–32.

26. Berry RB, Abreu AR, et al. The AASM manual for the scoring of sleep and associated events: rules, terminology and technical specifications. Darien: AASM; 2020.

27. Schmid AA, et al. Balance is associated with quality of life in chronic stroke. Top Stroke Rehabil. 2013;20(4):340–6.

28. Giebelhaus V, et al. Physical exercise as an adjunct therapy in sleep apnea-an open trial. Sleep Breath. 2000;4(4):173–6.

29. Tong J, et al. Respiratory-related displacement of the trachea in obstructive sleep apnea. J Appl Physiol. 2019;127(5):1307–16.
30. Langhorne P, Bernhardt J, Kwakkel G. Stroke rehabilitation. Lancet. 2011;377(9778):1693–702.
31. Scrivener K. Don't underestimate the power of one arm: living independently after stroke. J Physiother. 2016;62(4):234.
32. Scrivener K, Sherrington C, Schurr K. Exercise dose and mobility outcome in a comprehensive stroke unit: description and prediction from a prospective cohort study. J Rehabil Med. 2012;44(10):824–9.
33. Fulk G. Is sleep the next frontier in movement science? J Neurol Phys Ther. 2022;46(3):187–8.
34. Frange C, et al. Practice recommendations for the role of physiotherapy in the management of sleep disorders: the 2022 Brazilian Sleep Association Guidelines. Sleep Sci. 2022;15(4):515–73.

Chapter 23
No Residual Apnea-Hypopnea Index and the Epiglottis Prolapse: The Need for an Interprofessional Collaboration

Camila F. Leite ⓘ and Juliana A. Lino ⓘ

Introduction

Information guided by simple parameters and analyzed separately can lead professionals to false perceptions that their patients' cases are resolved and that the best therapeutic option is being offered to them. This clinical case reveals that the use of the apnea-hypopnea index (AHI) as the only parameter for analyzing therapeutic effectiveness can lead to failures in the management of the case. Detailed information collected from careful anamnesis and adequate physical examination allow the physiotherapist, in some cases, to adjust conducts. In others, they allow the formulation of some hypotheses that will be elucidated and properly conducted in interprofessional follow-up. In any professional approach scenario, it is imperative that the patient be at the center of therapy [1]. Their complaints, difficulties, and limitations need to be understood, as well as their treatment goals to maximize outcomes and, from then on, therapeutic goals should be outlined to improve its functioning. Excellence in sleep treatment is often dependent on the integration of knowledge obtained through an inter or transdisciplinary approach. In the case presented here, the patient has a diagnosis obstructive sleep apnea (OSA), treated with continuous positive airway pressure (CPAP). In clinical follow-up, considerable complaints were noted after the initial process of adaptation to positive airway pressure (PAP) therapy, such as *"I clearly feel as if my throat is closing"* or *"I get suffocated and I*

C. F. Leite (✉)
Physical Therapy Department, Federal University of Ceara, Fortaleza, CE, Brazil

J. A. Lino
Federal University of Ceara, Fortaleza, CE, Brazil

© The Author(s), under exclusive license to Springer Nature Switzerland AG 2023

C. Frange (ed.), *Clinical Cases in Sleep Physical Therapy*,
https://doi.org/10.1007/978-3-031-38340-3_23

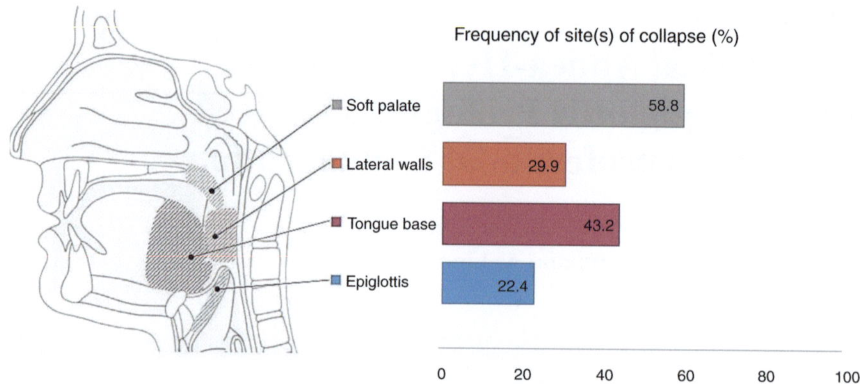

Fig. 23.1 Overall frequency of site(s) of collapse during natural sleep endoscopy. Values are presented as mean percentage of patients with upper airway collapse at each level. Reprinted with permission from [5]

realize the time when the closure is undone." In the PAP reports, patients had obstructive events adequately controlled (AHI within normal range) with PAP treatment, showing good adherence to pressure therapy. After patient evaluation and qualified listening to her complaints, hypotheses were considered, and it was concluded that the case also needed to be followed up by an otorhinolaryngologist with training in sleep, since the patient's airway needed to be investigated. In situations where CPAP therapy is not tolerated, a thorough clinical history and examination are necessary to obtain potential therapeutic targets [2]. The use of Drug-Induced Sleep Endoscopy (DISE) combined with CPAP may serve as a first step in understanding why some patients fail to adapt to CPAP treatment. This approach can help identify patterns of airway collapse (Fig. 23.1), which may require different pressures from those the patient is using, or even identify anatomical factors that can be corrected in surgical processes [3], for example. In addition to the DISE, other ways of evaluating the airways that would help elucidate this case would be the drug-induced sleep computed tomography (DI-SCT cephalometry). Alternatively, the epiglottic collapse can be identified from the airflow signal measured during a sleep study [4].

Patient Information

This was a 44-year-old female patient, body mass index (BMI) = 27 kg/m^2, who sought care from a sleep doctor, presenting as main complaints fragmented sleep due to snoring, worse in the supine position, in addition to excessive daytime sleepiness (Epworth Sleep Scale (ESS) = 16). As comorbidities, the patient had asthma, allergic rhinitis, and systemic arterial hypertension. She was using medication to treat bronchial asthma (beclomethasone dipropionate, salbutamol, fluticasone furoate), losartan, and hydrochlorothiazide for blood pressure control. There were no cases of sleep disorder in her family history. There was no previous treatment performed by the patient aiming to improve sleep quality. Regarding sleep habits, the patient claimed to have a regular bedtime, going to bed at 23 h and falling asleep at 23:15. She usually woke up at 4:40 and stayed in bed until 5:30. She referred to wake up during the night 2–3 times; the reason for waking up was her own snoring. She mentioned not feeling that sleep was repaired when waking up. She napped throughout the day for 20 min on most days of the week.

Concerning sleep hygiene education, she denied watching TV in bed, lying in bed sleepless, or reading in bed. She did not consume alcohol or tobacco, as well as denying the practice of physical activity and the habit of eating large meals at night. However, she reported consuming caffeine after 18 h on most days of the week. She considered her sleeping environment adequate. Regarding snoring, she reported an audible intensity throughout the house.

Clinical Findings

In the initial assessment, the patient was in good general condition, communicative and with an adequate cognitive level. The measurement of the cervical circumference was 37 cm.

As complementary exams, chest tomography revealed discrete bronchiectasis with signs of mucoid impaction in the middle lobe of the right lung, with the rest of the lung parenchyma without significant alterations. Virtual pleural spaces, normal cardiac area, thoracic aorta, and pulmonary artery trunk with normal calibers were also observed. Spirometry showed normal values in relation to the predicted value. Transthoracic echocardiography showed normal findings. Nasofibroscopy revealed an elongated palate, with Muller retropalatal 4/4+ circumferential/retrolingual 2/4+ anteroposterior. Friedman tong position [6] grade was III.

Timeline

The patient started the follow-up of the sleep disorder in a tertiary public hospital. Screening and initial assessment were performed by a sleep physician. After performing type I polysomnography, the patient was diagnosed with moderate OSA (AHI = 25.8 ev/h), the use of CPAP was indicated, and she was referred to physical therapy assessment and for CPAP adaptation (Fig. 23.2). CPAP eliminates snoring, awakenings, and nocturia [1] in addition to improving sleep architecture, which has a positive impact on the waking period, with an improvement in daytime somnolence.

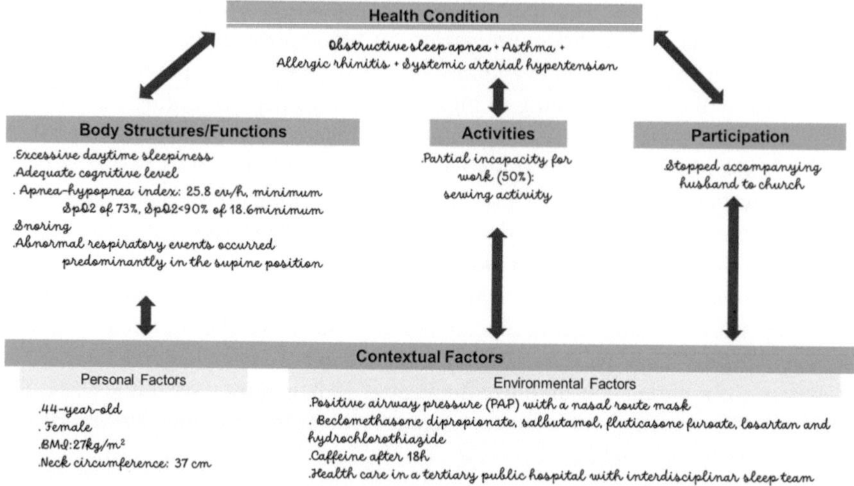

Fig. 23.2 Information collected in the patient's physiotherapeutic assessment, grouped according to the International Classification of Functioning, Disability, and Health (ICF)—model of functioning and disability. Image courtesy from the authors

Diagnostic Assessment

Type 1 polysomnography showed a sleep efficiency of 93.5%, with a total sleep time of 428 min, reduced sleep latency (4.4 min), rapid eye movement (REM) sleep latency of 80.5 min. Concerning sleep phases, 7.2% of the sleep time occurred in non-rapid eye movement (NREM) N1 sleep stage, 47.1% in NREM N2 sleep stage, 22% in NREM N3 sleep stage and 23.7% in REM sleep stage. The AHI was 25.8 ev/h, with minimum saturation of peripheral oxygen (SpO_2) of 73%; basal SpO_2 of 95%, and mean SpO_2 of 94%, and time spent with $SpO_2 < 90\%$ of 18.6 min. The awakening rate was 25.2 ev/h. Snoring and abnormal respiratory events occurred predominantly in the supine position.

Physiotherapeutic Intervention

Acceptance of the PAP with a nasal route interface occurred immediately. According to the transtheoretical model of behavioral change [7, 8], the patient was perceived to be in the preparation stage, already committed to the action to be instituted. The patient initially received an orientation session [9], including education intervention.

Types of Therapeutic Intervention

Since the beginning of the treatment, the patient presented with adequate frequency of CPAP related to the day of use and daily time of use. Initially, the device was set in automatic mode (APAP), with (pressure range from 4 to 12 cm H_2O) with automatic ramp. The device did not have a heated humidifier and did not allow obtaining data for telemonitoring.

After a week using CPAP, the patient returned to the office with no complaints related to the use of the equipment. She reported sleeping better and showing reduced daytime sleepiness (ESS = 6). Data are satisfactory in terms of time and frequency, and apnea events are satisfactorily controlled. Here, it was decided to adjust the mode to CPAP, with fixed pressure at 12 cmH_2O, based on the P95 obtained from the CPAP equipment report.

Changes in Therapeutic Intervention

After 2 weeks, the patient returned to the office complaining of air leakage through the mouth and oral dryness. She maintained a good adherence to CPAP. We used a chin strap to control leaks, and the therapeutic pressure was reduced to 11 cmH_2O.

One month after this episode, the patient returned to the outpatient clinic complaining of a claustrophobic feeling when using the chin strap. Furthermore, she maintained the complaint of oral dryness, and exhibited symptoms of daytime sleepiness. The data from the device revealed adequate time using CPAP (more than 5 h/day), without significant leaks, and controlled AHI (1.3 ev/h), with the occurrence of snoring on some nights. To increase comfort, the use of a humidifier was indicated, and the chin strap was suspended.

In the subsequent follow-up, the patient maintained high leaks in the nasal mask and AHI control. On that occasion, the pressure was reduced to 10 cmH_2O, to improve patient comfort since higher pressures lead to more patient discomfort and side effects [1]. In this consultation, the complaint presented by the patient was a feeling of suffocation when using CPAP, as something that caused asphyxiation, which was reversed after a few seconds. Faced with these complaints, sleep ergonomics orientations were reinforced, asking the patient to adopt strategies for sleeping in the lateral decubitus position.

Follow-Up and Outcomes

During the clinical follow-up of the patient using CPAP, adequate adherence was observed, with control of respiratory events, with high unintentional leakage, despite attempts to change the mask (different models of nasal route) and use of a chin strap. The initial complaint of excessive daytime sleepiness, which had been controlled at the beginning of PAP therapy, was again present. It was evident that the patient needed to be evaluated by another professional to confirm hypotheses that were raised in the dialog with the patient during physical therapy reassessment, mainly related to the complaint of asphyxia/suffocation evidenced during the use of CPAP.

Discussion

The feeling of suffocation reported by the patient using PAP signaled the need for investigation. This asphyxia is uncomfortable and may even represent a cause of non-tolerance to CPAP. One hypothesis raised was that the patient could have epiglottis collapse. The data suggests that the prevalence of epiglottis collapse occurs in 12% of cases of snoring, and sound originating from it has a higher pitch than palatal snoring [10]. In situations of epiglottis prolapse, PAP pushes the epiglottis posteriorly, creating a complete seal in the throat. The anatomical shape of the epiglottis is contradictory to the airflow generated by CPAP, so it acts as a CPAP barrier [11]. This barrier is not relieved with higher PAP pressures (as would occur, for example, if the structures that would perform this blockade were the soft palate or tongue) and, in contrast, higher pressures lead to even more unpleasant sensations in cases of collapse of the epiglottis [12, 13]. Decreasing the CPAP pressures also does not usually work in these cases, since there is a need of enough pressure to open the airway. As alternatives, mandibular advancement device (oral device), hyoid suspension, or partial epiglottectomy are possible solutions to epiglottic obstruction. Six different surgical techniques were described, considered safe, and effective, including partial epiglottectomy, epiglottis stiffening operation, glosso-epiglottopexy, supraglottoplasty, transoral robotic surgery, maxillomandibular advancement, and hypoglossal nerve stimulation. The selection of the appropriate surgical technique should be part of an individualized, patient-specific therapeutic approach [14]. The surgical management of epiglottic collapse can improve OSA severity or even cure OSA, but can also improve CPAP compliance [14].

The interdisciplinary approach made it possible to direct a new therapeutic approach to the patient. The performance of DISE confirmed the presence of epiglottic collapse, and after the diagnosis, behavioral measures were reinforced, such as weight reduction, recommendations to avoid dorsal decubitus when sleeping, having in mind that these measures were not specifically directed to the epiglottis.

The patient was referred to the sleep dentist for the evaluation of the use of the oral device [15]. Notably, this resource can confer benefits to the patient, but it also does not address the epiglottis directly. The incorporation of these feature is still under evaluation.

If behavioral strategies and the use of an oral device do not obtain a beneficial response, the surgical option must be evaluated. We rarely see patients with OSA having isolated epiglottis collapse, which explains why we currently don't have enough evidence to support any treatment that might specifically address this problem.

For each strategy applied to the clinical case, the importance of clinical follow-up by a different sleep professional is observed. Here, a sleep physician, a physiotherapist, a dentist, and a otolaryngology surgeon were integrated [1]. If the surgical option will be chosen, the postoperative period might include treatment with myofunctional therapy, adding the speech therapist [16] to the team. At the beginning of this patient's treatment, the professional assistance received through a physician and a physiotherapist was multidisciplinary. Here, the different disciplines acted in a juxtaposed and non-integrative manner, with professionals working as independent specialists. The professionals' objective for this clinical case was common, but it did not advance due to their own disciplinary limitations.

Faced with the complaint presented by the patient, the physiotherapeutic action could no longer progress since it was on the margins of its own fields of activity. At this point, in a meeting with the other specialists, the case was discussed interdisciplinarily, and a new level of conversation/discourse was established after the integration of different knowledge.

There is no need to involve multiple professionals in cases of simple management. However, it is imperative that each professional knows the principles, concepts, and field of action of the colleague from another faculty so that difficult situations can be properly handled, and that the appropriate professional to integrate the case or conduct specific investigations is incorporated into the team. Specifically in sleep, there is a lack of evidence on the health team's approach, although empirically, greater patient engagement and, consequently, better results from the therapy instituted are noticeable [17]. Given the multidimensionality of sleep disorders, this integration of knowledge seems to make sense. In addition to this aspect, the case presented here highlights that qualified listening in the patient follow-up process is fundamental. The information collected from the patient guides the therapeutic adjustment. Any professional needs to listen to his patient and associate the responses of independent variables in all situations. If the patient's initial sleep complaint persists, even if the patient has the best AHI, he or she cannot be considered adequately treated. Considering this context, associating many variables with the exam findings, and always having the idea that OSA is a prevalent disease, which influences social relations and quality of life with major health impact [16], this needs to be investigated in the clinical follow-up of patients.

What is strongly encouraged from this chapter is that sleep physiotherapists consider patient-centered practice as an essential attribute in their professional practice [18].

The way the therapy is instituted will have a very significant impact on the patient's engagement with the treatment [19]. The professional scope is limited and keeping patients getting the best of their specific actions may not be enough. Finally, there are cases where CPAP may not be a good choice for patients with epiglottic collapse since the anatomical shape of the epiglottis is contradictory to the airflow generated by CPAP.

References

1. Steiner WA, et al. Use of the ICF model as a clinical problem-solving tool in physical therapy and rehabilitation medicine. Phys Ther. 2002;82(11):1098–107.
2. Virk JS, Kotecha B. When continuous positive airway pressure (CPAP) fails. J Thorac Dis. 2016;8(10):E1112–21.
3. Torre C, et al. Impact of continuous positive airway pressure in patients with obstructive sleep apnea during drug-induced sleep endoscopy. Clin Otolaryngol. 2017;42(6):1218–23.
4. Azarbarzin A, et al. Predicting epiglottic collapse in patients with obstructive sleep apnoea. Eur Respir J. 2017;50(3):1700345.
5. Van den Bossche K, et al. Natural sleep endoscopy in obstructive sleep apnea: a systematic review. Sleep Med Rev. 2021;60:101534.
6. Yu JL, Rosen I. Utility of the modified Mallampati grade and Friedman tongue position in the assessment of obstructive sleep apnea. J Clin Sleep Med. 2020;16(2):303–8.
7. DiClemente CC, Prochaska JO. Self-change and therapy change of smoking behavior: a comparison of processes of change in cessation and maintenance. Addict Behav. 1982;7(2):133–42.
8. Velicer WF, et al. An empirical typology of subjects within stage of change. Addict Behav. 1995;20(3):299–320.
9. Silva RS, et al. An orientation session improves objective sleep quality and mask acceptance during positive airway pressure titration. Sleep Breath. 2008;12(1):85–9.
10. Torre C, et al. Epiglottis collapse in adult obstructive sleep apnea: a systematic review. Laryngoscope. 2016;126(2):515–23.
11. Jeong SH, et al. Partial epiglottectomy improves residual apnea-hypopnea index in patients with epiglottis collapse. J Clin Sleep Med. 2020;16(9):1607–10.
12. Sung CM, Kim HC, Yang HC. The clinical characteristics of patients with an isolate epiglottic collapse. Auris Nasus Larynx. 2020;47(3):450–7.
13. Genta PR, et al. Airflow shape is associated with the pharyngeal structure causing OSA. Chest. 2017;152(3):537–46.
14. Vallianou K, Chaidas K. Surgical treatment options for epiglottic collapse in adult obstructive sleep apnoea: a systematic review. Life. 2022;12(11):1845.
15. Giles TL, et al. Continuous positive airways pressure for obstructive sleep apnoea in adults. Cochrane Database Syst Rev. 2006;3:CD001106.
16. Li HY, et al. How to manage continuous positive airway pressure (CPAP) failure-hybrid surgery and integrated treatment. Auris Nasus Larynx. 2020;47(3):335–42.
17. Frange C, et al. Practice recommendations for the role of physiotherapy in the management of sleep disorders: the 2022 Brazilian Sleep Association Guidelines. Sleep Sci. 2022;15(4):515–73.
18. Darrah J, et al. Role of conceptual models in a physical therapy curriculum: application of an integrated model of theory, research, and clinical practice. Physiother Theory Pract. 2006;22(5):239–50.
19. Baker SM, et al. Patient participation in physical therapy goal setting. Phys Ther. 2001;81(5):1118–26.

Part VIII
Clinical Cases: Central Sleep Apnea

Chapter 24
Central Sleep Apnea: Less is More

Juliana A. Lino ⓘ and Camila F. Leite ⓘ

Introduction

Although central sleep apnea (CSA) is less frequent than obstructive sleep apnea (OSA) in the general population, it is common in specific subpopulations, including patients with cardiovascular and neurological diseases and those with chronic use of opioids. Treating patients with CSA remains a challenge since different pathophysiological mechanisms resulting from central respiratory instability and reduction in the ventilatory drive are involved in the development of CSA [1, 2].

In clinical practice, continuous positive airway pressure (CPAP) has been the first choice in the treatment of the main subtypes of CSA and can be used combined with other therapies [3]. However, the management of CPAP parameters must be performed individually, by a qualified professional, considering not only isolated parameters, such as time and frequency CPAP use, apnea and hypopnea index (AHI), and unintentional airflow leakage, but the set of information collected from the anamnesis added to the sleep study's findings and the complaints presented by the patient, considering their disabilities and individual needs.

In this chapter, the clinical case to be discussed refers to a patient using CPAP for the treatment of severe sleep-disordered breathing (SDB), with high therapeutic pressures and periodic breathing pattern, presenting important complaints of discomfort with the therapy. In this case, careful evaluation of the patient and periodic clinical follow-up was essential to ensure therapeutic efficacy and treatment tolerance.

J. A. Lino (✉)
Federal University of Ceara, Fortaleza, CE, Brazil

C. F. Leite
Physical Therapy Department, Federal University of Ceara, Fortaleza, CE, Brazil

221

C. Frange (ed.), *Clinical Cases in Sleep Physical Therapy*,
https://doi.org/10.1007/978-3-031-38340-3_24

Patient Information

This is a male patient, 90-year-old, widowed, independent in activities of daily living, good cognition, and using CPAP. He was referred by a cardiologist and accompanied by his children, who reported as main complaints residual daytime sleepiness, especially in the morning, the presence of sporadic snoring, and discomfort with the mask and chin strap used. The patient had been using CPAP for some years, without follow-up with a sleep physiotherapist. As morbidities, he presented systemic arterial hypertension, cardiac arrhythmia, previous transient ischemic attack, aortic aneurysm, and had already undergone coronary artery bypass graft surgery 20 years ago. He used medication to control his blood pressure and heart function.

Regarding sleep habits, the patient slept in a bed, in a comfortable room, with a caregiver. According to family members, he had regular sleep and wake times. He usually went to bed at 20:30 and started sleeping around 21:30, after putting on the CPAP; he woke up and got out of bed at 07:00. During the night, he woke up 2–3 times to go to the bathroom. Despite not reporting periods of sleep during the day, his children reported daytime sleepiness, especially in the morning. He did not consume alcohol or tobacco, or caffeinated drinks. He performed motor physiotherapy 3 times a week and speech therapy 2 times a week. The patient lived with his daughter and had a dedicated and present family. He was very fond of reading and doing crosswords during the day.

Clinical Findings

During the initial evaluation, the patient presented a body mass index (BMI) = 29.4 kg/m^2, neck circumference = 44 cm, and Friedman tong position [4] was grade II. Blood pressure = 140 × 80 mmHg, heart rate = 78 bpm, and peripheral oxyhemoglobin saturation (SpO_2) = 96% in ambient air. On inspection, there were no important anatomical changes, such as retrognathia or micrognathia. Edema was observed in both legs.

Timeline

After performing a respiratory polygraphy test (type 3 polysomnographic sleep study), the patient was diagnosed with severe SDB (AHI = 57 ev/h) and was referred to a private service for treatment with CPAP. After a few years of positive airway pressure (PAP) treatment, without sleep physiotherapist follow-up, during a new medical appointment, he reported daytime sleepiness, nighttime snoring, oral dryness, and discomfort with the mask and chin strap. Then he was referred to sleep physiotherapist, already using CPAP, for evaluation and clinical follow-up.

Diagnostic Assessment

The respiratory polygraphy showed 432 respiratory events, being 346 OSA, 04 CSA, 15 mixed apneas, and 67 hypopneas during sleep, making up an AHI = 57 ev/h. There was moderate SpO_2 associated with respiratory events (mean SpO_2 during sleep = 94%, and minimum SpO_2 = 78%), being 57 min (12%) of the recorded time with SpO_2 < 90%. Heart rate (HR) remained within normal limits, with a minimum HR = 66 bpm and maximum HR = 81 bpm.

According to the type 3 sleep study, the patient was diagnosed with severe SDB, considering the AHI classification: <4.9 ev/h = normal AHI; between 5 to 14.9 ev/h = mild AHI; between 15 and 29 ev/h = moderate AHI, and ≥ 30 ev/h = severe AHI. There was a predominance of OSA, with central and mixed respiratory events. The sleep study report showed a period of Cheyne-Stokes breathing (CSB).

Despite its portability, one of the limitations of respiratory polygraphy is that it only comprises the recording of airflow, respiratory effort, and oximetry. Some devices allow recording of body position and snoring. In addition, the absence of electroencephalogram recording prevents the identification of sleep stages and arousals, compromising the marking of arousal events related to respiratory effort-related arousals (RERA) and hypopneas validated by arousal [5]. The American Academy Sleep Medicine (AASM) classifies central hypopnea by the absence of the following criteria: snoring, paradoxical thoracic-abdominal patterns, and flattening of respiratory flow during the event [6]. However, the AASM doesn't make recommendations for central or obstructive hypopneas to be marked. This can also be a limiting factor that can compromise the diagnostic test interpretation.

He scored 18 on the Epworth Sleepiness Scale (ESS), suggesting the presence of excessive daytime sleepiness [7].

Physiotherapeutic Intervention

During the first consultation, the patient and his family received information about his diagnosis, with an explanation of respiratory polygraphy findings, the possible systemic consequences of sleep apnea, and the importance of adequate treatment in improving his quality of life. He was also guided on healthy sleep habits and the importance of a proper sleep routine.

The patient was already undergoing treatment with CPAP with oronasal interface and chin strap. Therefore, after talking to him about his complaints and clarifying all doubts, the CPAP data was evaluated. The parameters were set to automatic CPAP (APAP), with pressure range from 14 to 19 cmH_2O, pressure at the 95th percentile (P95) = 19 cmH_2O, ramp time = 20min, expiratory relief = 1 cmH_2O only during ramp time, and humidification = 4. Despite complaints presented by the patient, data from CPAP device revealed adequate time using CPAP, with an average use of 6 h 32 min, a 96% adherence rate (% days of use ≥4 h), without unintentional airflow leakage. However, he presented residual AHI (14 ev/h), with a record of 14.9% of CSB. The respiratory flow waveform analysis showed an increasing-decreasing breathing pattern, alternating hyperventilation and central apnea and hypopnea events, in addition to RERA events (Fig. 24.1a).

The initial approach was to change the oronasal to a nasal mask, and it was suggested to stop using the chin strap, to assess the breathing pattern and unintentional airflow leakage during sleep. The APAP was set with lower pressure range from 5 to 10 cmH$_2$O and the ramp time and expiratory relief were turned off. Humidification was increased from 4 to 6.

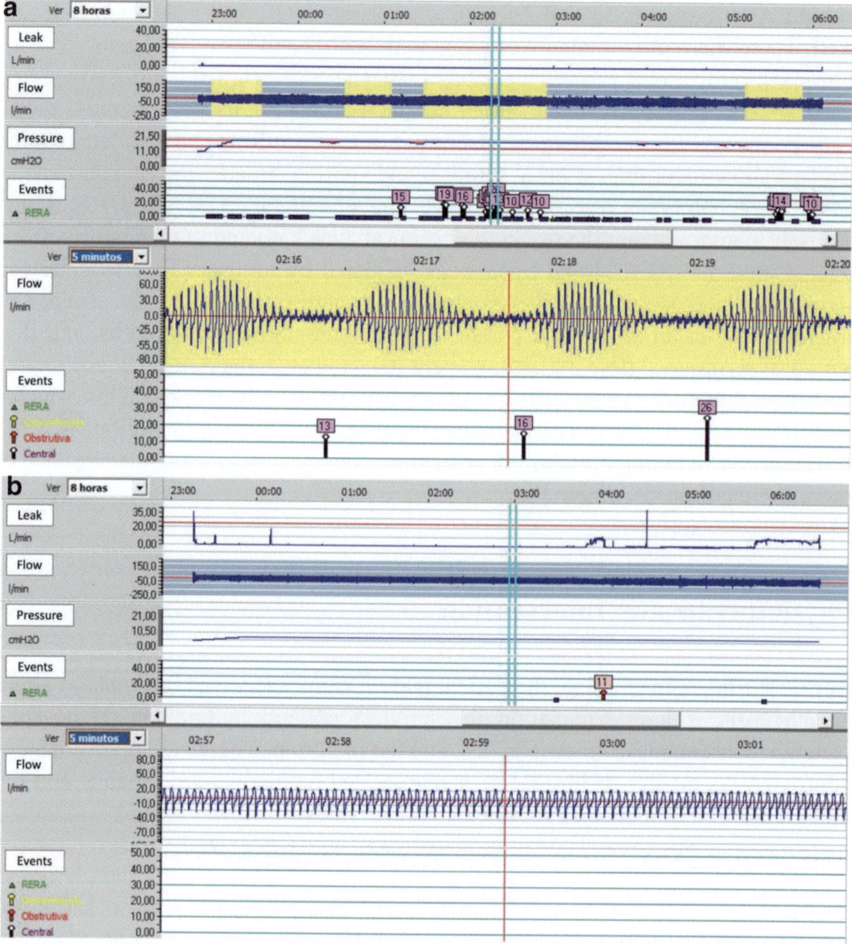

Fig. 24.1 Sample of 5-min respiratory waveform, extracted from positive pressure equipment. (**a**) shows an increasing-decreasing breathing pattern, indicative of respiratory instability, with the patient using APAP, expiratory relief, oronasal mask and chin strap; (**b**) shows a normalized breathing pattern during sleep, after fixed CPAP pressure and nasal mask. Image courtesy of the authors

The clinical follow-up to evaluate changes in mask and therapeutic pressure would initially occur once a week and that, after acceptation and therapeutic efficacy, the clinical follow-up would occur with a longer interval between appointments.

Changes in Therapeutic Intervention

After a week, the patient returned to the office for a new clinical evaluation, reporting greater comfort with the nasal mask, without the chin strap. He also reported having slept better and that he was no longer experiencing oral dryness. The patient maintained good adherence (average time of use of 6h48min), with a median unintentional airflow leakage = 1.2 L/min, AHI = 11.2 ev/h, with a predominance of hypopneas and 17.2% of CSB. The CPAP was set at fixed pressure at 7 cmH_2O, based on the P95 obtained from the CPAP equipment report, with a 40-min ramp time. Elevation of the head of the bed by 15 cm (equivalent to 45°) was also recommended to reduce the rostral displacement of liquid during the night to the chest region, preventing the appearance of central events.

In the following week, the patient reported better acceptance and comfort with the PAP, with no relevant complaints related to the interface or oral dryness. The daughter informed he was in a better mood during the day, with reduced daytime sleepiness, being able to read books and crossword puzzles, as he enjoyed. She also no longer heard the snoring-like noise while using CPAP. He maintained a good adherence to CPAP, with an increase in the average time of use to 7 h 32 min, low unintentional airflow leakage (4.8 L/min) with a significant reduction in AHI to 1.7 ev/h, without CSB recording. The respiratory flow waveform showed a regular breathing pattern, without inspiratory flow restriction and periodic breathing pattern on most nights.

Thus, the patient was instructed to continue using fixed CPAP at 7 cmH_2O, 40-min ramp time, and humidification = 6. Orientations on the importance of healthy sleep habits and positioning in bed were reinforced. He was informed about clinical follow-up through remote monitoring and periodic face-to-face consultations.

Follow-Up and Outcomes

After replacing the interface to a nasal model, without a chin strap, and fixed CPAP pressure, the patient presented better acceptance to the treatment, with good adherence to PAP, control of respiratory events, and minimal unintentional airflow leakage (Fig. 24.1b). He reported greater comfort with the nasal mask, with lower therapeutic pressure, and without complaining of oral dryness. He reports sleeping better, getting up only once during the night to go to the bathroom, and showed reduced daytime sleepiness (ESS = 8). He can do his readings and crossword puzzles, with a better quality of life with his family.

Discussion

In patients with SDB, conducting treatment based only on isolated variables can compromise therapeutic efficacy and lead to false interpretations regarding the resolution of the problem.

In the clinical case discussed, despite good adherence to CPAP, the patient presented a high residual AHI, with periodic breathing pattern, and relevant clinical complaints. A careful initial assessment reveals this patient already had significant cardiovascular morbidities, in addition to presence of central respiratory events observed in the respiratory polygraphy, which may lead to a greater propensity for ventilatory instability during treatment with PAP. In this case, the patient used APAP, with high therapeutic pressures and exhalation relief adjustment during the ramp time. The AASM recommends the use of fixed or automatic CPAP for ongoing treatment of OSA in adults but emphasizes that this recommendation was based on studies that excluded patients with morbidities, including those with CSA [8]. Therefore, in clinical practice, the use of fixed CPAP is recommended, since pressure variation can contribute to the appearance of arousals and the perpetuation of central events in patients with ventilatory instability and low arousal threshold, which can lead to sleep fragmentation and daytime sleepiness, one of the main complaints presented by the patient. The lowest possible therapeutic pressure that is effective in suppressing obstructive events and reducing the respiratory control instability should be used. Ventilatory stimuli such as automatic ramping, exhalation relief, and responsive pressure relief should be avoided in these patients [1, 9].

Although it has been discussed the use of APAP, especially with high pressures, can contribute to ventilatory instability and the appearance of central events, it is important to emphasize that high therapeutic pressures should be avoided, whenever possible, in any other condition, since they can increase the unintentional airflow leakage and cause discomfort for the patient.

In the clinical case presented, one of the main complaints of the patient was associated with discomfort with his oronasal interface. Despite the low unintentional airflow leakage, possibly due to the association with the use of a chin strap, the patient reported considerable discomfort. Several studies recommend the use of a nasal mask as the first choice in the treatment of SDB and demonstrate that oronasal masks require higher levels of therapeutic pressure, increase unintentional airflow leakage, and residual respiratory events due to posterior displacement of the tongue and soft palate and less adherence to treatment [10, 11]. In the analysis of the respiratory flow waveform, periods of inspiratory flow limitation were observed. Additionally, the increased inspiratory flow resistance can trigger an increase in the patient's inspiratory effort, with consequent arousals, hyperventilation, and central events.

In addition to pressure adjustment, therapeutic alternatives may be necessary for the treatment of CSA. In the clinical case discussed, the patient, who already had leg edema during the clinical evaluation, was instructed to raise the head of the bed to avoid the rostral displacement of liquid to the chest region and the appearance of central events. This simple non-pharmacological and non-invasive intervention can reduce the rostral displacement of fluids to the lungs, contributing to a reduction in central, mainly concentrated at the end of the night [12].

In this context, optimization of therapeutic pressure with fixed CPAP, prolonged ramp time, off-exhalation relief, adequate humidification, nasal interface, and positional therapy was effective in controlling respiratory events and reducing periodic breathing periods. The patient reported greater comfort and tolerance to the treatment, reduced daytime sleepiness, fewer nighttime arousals, and better functioning and quality of life in their daily activities. So, it was not just a single adjustment that made the difference, but a set of actions, centered on the patient, that resulted in therapeutic efficacy and improvement of the patient's symptoms.

In this clinical case, there was total control of AHI values (<5 ev/h). However, when it comes to CSA, normalizing the AHI is not the main goal, since the management of this disorder requires greater parsimony on the part of the sleep professional and a higher AHI can be tolerated once the primary cause of CSA is resolved, and symptoms are under control. In the Canadian Continuous Positive Airway Pressure for Patients with Central Sleep Apnea and Heart Failure (CANPAP) post hoc analysis, there was early suppression of CSA by CPAP, with an AHI <15 events/h being associated with an improvement in left ventricular ejection fraction and survival of the patient with heart failure [13].

The basis of treatment for CSA is the optimization of the underlying cause. Considering the etiological heterogeneity of patients with CSA, the combination of therapies with an interdisciplinary approach, such as optimization of pharmacological therapy, positional therapy, and PAP treatment, can control residual respiratory events and improve the patient's quality of life. Despite this, the treatment of CSA remains a challenge for sleep professionals. Therefore, knowledge of the pathophysiology involved in this SDB, which is associated with careful clinical assessment, correct interpretation of sleep studies, and patient follow-up, is essential for adequate management of CSA. In addition, it is important to consider each patient's individual needs and disabilities and their expectations regarding treatment.

References

1. Frange C, et al. Practice recommendations for the role of physiotherapy in the management of sleep disorders: the 2022 Brazilian Sleep Association Guidelines. Sleep Sci. 2022;15(4):515–73.
2. Nerbass FB, Mendes LPDS. Apneia Central do Sono: Mecanismos e Intervenção. in PROFISIO C8V2. 2022.
3. Aurora RN, et al. The treatment of central sleep apnea syndromes in adults: practice parameters with an evidence-based literature review and meta-analyses. Sleep. 2012;35(1):17–40.
4. Yu JL, Rosen I. Utility of the modified Mallampati grade and Friedman tongue position in the assessment of obstructive sleep apnea. J Clin Sleep Med. 2020;16(2):303–8.
5. Mortari DM, Lino JA, Santos SB. Estratégias atuais de avaliação da apneia obstrutiva do sono. In: PROFISIO Programa de Atualização em Fisioterapia Cardiovascular e Respiratória: Ciclo 8. Porto Alegre: Artmed Panamericana; 2021. p. 85–127.

6. Berry RB, et al. Rules for scoring respiratory events in sleep: update of the 2007 AASM Manual for the Scoring of Sleep and Associated Events. Deliberations of the Sleep Apnea Definitions Task Force of the American Academy of Sleep Medicine. J Clin Sleep Med. 2012;8(5):597–619.
7. Bertolazi AN, et al. Portuguese-language version of the Epworth sleepiness scale: validation for use in Brazil. J Bras Pneumol. 2009;35(9):877–83.
8. Patil SP, et al. Treatment of adult obstructive sleep apnea with positive airway pressure: an American Academy of Sleep Medicine Clinical Practice Guideline. J Clin Sleep Med. 2019;15(2):335–43.
9. Lino JA, Piccin VS. Central sleep apnea: physiotherapeutic approach. In: Nature S, editor. Sleep medicine and physical therapy. A comprehensive guide for practitioners. Cham: Springer; 2022.
10. Andrade RG, et al. Impact of the type of mask on the effectiveness of and adherence to continuous positive airway pressure treatment for obstructive sleep apnea. J Bras Pneumol. 2014;40(6):658–68.
11. Genta PR, et al. The importance of mask selection on continuous positive airway pressure outcomes for obstructive sleep apnea. An Official American Thoracic Society Workshop Report. Ann Am Thorac Soc. 2020;17(10):1177–85.
12. White LH, Bradley TD. Role of nocturnal rostral fluid shift in the pathogenesis of obstructive and central sleep apnoea. J Physiol. 2013;591(5):1179–93.
13. Arzt M, et al. Suppression of central sleep apnea by continuous positive airway pressure and transplant-free survival in heart failure: a post hoc analysis of the Canadian Continuous Positive Airway Pressure for Patients with Central Sleep Apnea and Heart Failure Trial (CANPAP). Circulation. 2007;115(25):3173–80.

Chapter 25
The Positioning Approach is Not Only a Marketing Strategy

Vivien S. Piccin ⓘ, Maria José Perrelli ⓘ, and Rafaela G. S. de Andrade ⓘ

Introduction

Since the beginning of CPAP (continuous positive airway pressure) use in the 1980s, by Dr. Colin Sullivan [1], until the mid-2000s, sleep-disordered breathing treatment primarily focused on obstructive sleep apnea (OSA). Central respiratory events, including complex apnea (known today as treatment-emergent central apnea) were targeted for servo-ventilator treatment. Little was known about the sleep physiology and pathophysiology. Phenotypic characteristics and overlap with other pathologies were timidly explored. Mixed apneas were treated as obstructive events since knowledge and access to respiratory flow curves during sleep were basically limited to clinical research (algorithms of the positive pressure devices were difficult to access, their limitations for the interpretation of respiratory events during sleep were not known) [2]. Over the years, studies onto respiratory disturbances during sleep have deepened. The precision medicine concept in sleep area has begun and nowadays; it is necessary to have a broad knowledge of both pathophysiological processes and individual characteristics for effective and assertive treatment of respiratory disorders by using positive pressure.

Treatment-emergent central sleep apnea (TECSA) is characterized by the appearance of central sleep apnea/hypopnea (CSA) while undergoing treatment for OSA was initially observed in some patients who primarily had OSA after the significant resolution of the obstructive events by treatment with a positive airway pressure (PAP) device. Although it is more commonly reported during the initiation of PAP

V. S. Piccin (✉) · R. G. S. de Andrade
Sleep Medicine, Pulmonary Division, Heart Institute, Faculdade de Medicina da Universidade Federal de São Paulo (InCor-FMUSP), São Paulo, SP, Brazil

M. J. Perrelli
Brazilian College of Systemic Studies (CBES), Curitiba, PR, Brazil
e-mail: mariajose@respcare.com.br

C. Frange (ed.), *Clinical Cases in Sleep Physical Therapy*,
https://doi.org/10.1007/978-3-031-38340-3_25

therapy, it is currently known that the TECSA could occur after various treatment modalities for OSA, including the use of a mandibular advancement device (MAD), maxillomandibular advancement surgery, sinus or nasal surgery, and also myofunctional therapy [3, 4]. The prevalence of TECSA vary widely among different studies ranging from 0.56 to 20.3% and it is considered a non-hypercapnia-induced central sleep-disordered breathing [3, 5].

Potential pathophysiological mechanisms for TECSA include low arousal threshold, ventilatory control instability (expressed by high loop gain in patients with OSA and the presence of upper airway narrowing during central apneas and hypopneas), prolonged circulation time, and activation of lung stretch receptors [3, 6, 7]. The central respiratory events seen in TECSA may be transient and resolve spontaneously through strict adherence to the assigned therapy, but in some patients, they persist even with regular therapy maintenance [3, 5].

There is controversy about the optimal method for treating TECSA. With regard to PAP treatment, studies have shown that CSA events naturally disappear after few months with the maintenance of CPAP. Bilevel PAP (Bilevel) with or without a back-up respiratory rate can be an effective alternative for treating TECSA in patients who do not respond to CPAP. And Adaptive Servo-Ventilation (ASV) could be a treatment option for patients whose TECSA does not improve after use of CPAP or Bilevel. Medications could be selected to improve ventilatory control stability or elevate the arousal threshold for TECSA patients, which may be a supplement to PAP therapy, but there are no large sample clinical trials to confirm the effectiveness and safety of such therapeutic options. More evidence is needed before recommending oxygen therapy or carbon dioxide (CO_2) supplementation as viable treatments options for TECSA [3, 7, 8].

Specifically in relation to pressure therapy, the development of TECSA may affect the effectiveness of OSA treatment and patient compliance [3]. Inadequate ventilation strategies can, in turn, trigger central respiratory events, if the emergence of these events is associated with ventilatory control instability or a high arousal threshold. Thus, it is extremely necessary to identify TECSA, as well as to conduct a detailed analysis of the facts for an adequate resolution of the problem.

Patient Information

A.C.G., a 59-year-old man, was referred to the PAP therapy adaptation program, complaining of non-restful sleep, nightmares, snoring, and hypersomnia. Diagnostic polysomnography (PSG) presented an apnea-hypopnea index (AHI) of 32.0 respiratory events/hour and titration study suggested a CPAP pressure of 13 cmH$_2$O. The patient started pressure therapy with an Auto-PAP at 5.6–13 cmH$_2$O. During a follow-up visit at 2 weeks with an average of hours of CPAP use of 5:14 h and residual AHI of 3.3/h, the patient still complained of non-restorative sleep and daytime sleepiness. At the respiratory flow curve analysis, we observed central sleep apneas typical of TECSA events.

Diagnostic Assessment

Basal Polysomnographic Examination

The total recording time was 494.9 min. Stage N1 latency was 9.5 min (normal <30 min), and rapid eye movement (REM) sleep latency (REMSL) was 137.0 min (normal = 70–120 min). The total sleep time (TST) was 389.5 min (78.7% sleep efficiency (SE); normal >85%) and the percentages of sleep stages in relation to TST were N1: 12.3%; N2: 49.0%; N3: 18.2% REM sleep: 20.4%. Wake time after sleep onset (WASO) was 95.9 min. 223 registered micro-awakenings (duration <15 s), with an index of 34.4/h (normal <10/h). Two-hundred eight breathing pauses were recorded during sleep, divided into 62 apneas (4 obstructive, 38 mixed, 20 central) and 146 hypopneas. These breaks lasted between 10.0 and 59.0 s (average duration = 18.0 s), with an average oxygen saturation (SaO_2) of 95% and a minimum of 85%. The SaO_2 remained below 90% during 0.4% of total sleep time. The index of apnea-hypopnea was 32.0/h (normal <5/h). Moderate-to-high snoring intensity was recorded. Mean heart rate was 55.2 bpm (sinus rhythm). There were 69 periodic movements of the lower limbs, with 2 events associated with awakening. The index of periodic limb movements (PLMi) was 10.6/h (normal <15/h). The sleep laboratory evaluation showed: (1) Marked increase in AHI (32.0/h), with respiratory pauses associated with oxyhemoglobin desaturation (minimum SaO_2 of 85%) and/ or micro-awakenings; (2) Constant, moderate-high intensity snoring on the night of assessment; (3) Normal movement index (10.6/h); (4) Sleep architecture with: (a) reduced SE (78.7%), (b) increased WASO (95.9 min), (c) normal NREM sleep latency (9.5 min), (d) increased REMSL (137.0 min), (e) percentage of N3 normal (18.2%), (f) increased N1 percentage (12.3%), (g) percentage of normal REM sleep stage (20.4%); (5) Increased micro-awakening rate (34.4/h).

Polysomnography for CPAP Titration

A new PSG was conducted to regulate CPAP pressute. The total registration time was 401.2 min. Stage N1 latency was 4.5 min (normal <30 min), and REM sleep was 55.0 min (normal = 70–120 min). The TST was 329.5 min (82.1% efficiency; normal >85%) and the percentages of sleep stages in relation to total sleep time were N1: 4.1%; N2: 49.0%; N3: 26.4%; REM sleep: 20.5%. The WASO was 67.2 min. One-hundred sixty-three micro-awakenings were recorded (duration <15 s), with an index of 24.9/h (normal <10/h). A nasal mask (size XL) (Fig. 25.1a) was used until 2:25h when it was changed to another model of nasal mask from other brand (size L) (Fig. 25.1b), with manual pressure adjustment. With CPAP pressure set at 13 cmH$_2$O, the patient did not snore, and no significant oxyhemoglobin desaturation was observed (minimum SaO_2 = 88%). In the total night (assessment of all pressure levels), 66 respiratory pauses were recorded during sleep, divided into 17

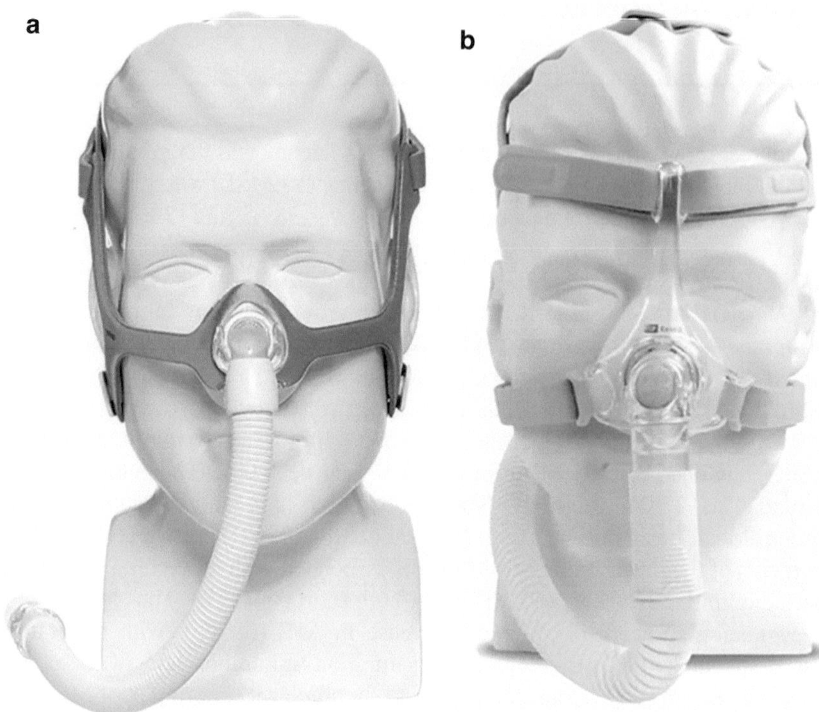

Fig. 25.1 (**a, b**) Different nasal route masks from different brands. The main difference between these two models of nasal masks is the forehead support. Original figure. Image courtesy of Dr. Vivien Schmeling Piccin

apneas (2 obstructive, 0 mixed, 15 central) and 49 hypopneas. These pauses lasted between 10.0 and 26.5 s (average duration = 18.1 s), with mean SaO_2 of 94% and minimum of 88%. SaO_2 remained below 90% during 0.3% of TST. The AHI was 12.0/h (normal <5/h). Mean heart rate was 54.8 bpm (sinus rhythm). There were observed 116 periodic lower limbs movements, with 20 events associated with awakening. The total rate of periodic was 17.7/h (normal <15/h). The evaluation showed: (1) Considering, in each therapeutic adjustment evaluated, the sleep time, the presence of REM sleep and supine position, better control of breathing events occurred with CPAP at a pressure of 13 cmH_2O; (2) With CPAP at a pressure of 13 cmH_2O: normal AHI (4/h), associated with no relevant oxyhemoglobin desaturation and/or micro-arousals (snoring abolished); (3) Slight increase in PLMi (17.7/h); (4) Increased micro-awakening rate (24.9/h).

Computed Tomography of the Face and Paranasal Sinuses

The face computed tomography (CT), prescribed by the otorhinolaryngologist, was performed without contrast (Fig. 25.2) and revealed nasal septum inclined to the left in the anterior cartilaginous portion and deviated to the right in the other portions, with a bone spur to the left that remodels the inferior nasal turbinate on this side.

- Asymmetrical ethmoid fovea, lower on the right
- Pneumatization of the vertical lamella of the right middle concha
- Bilateral wide ethmoid bulla
- Prominence of the mucous component of the turbinates and nasal cavities
- Slight thickening of the mucous lining of all paranasal cavities, with probable small retention cyst/polyp in the left maxillary sinus
- Discreet amount of secretion with bullae in right posterior ethmoid cell
- There is no liquid level
- Infundibulum, frontal and sphenoethmoidal recesses patent
- Rhinopharynx of regular contours
- Elongated soft palate
- Tongue with increased dimensions and verticalization of its longitudinal axis
- Topical hyoid bone
- And prominent palatine and lingual tonsils, with reduced pharyngeal air column caliber (these findings can be found in individuals who snore or have OSA).

Additional findings: Hypoattenuating material fills some mastoid cells and coats the right tympanic cavity. The anteroposterior diameter of the left eyeball is increased.

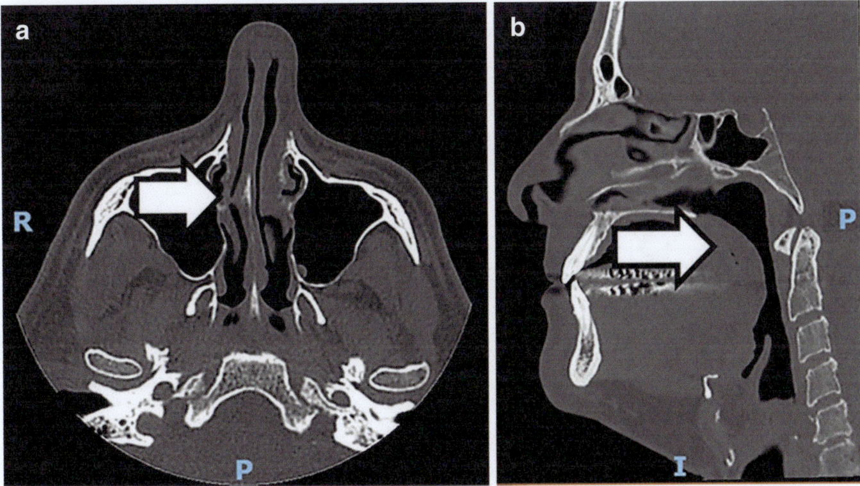

Fig. 25.2 Computed tomography of sinuses and face showing (white arrows): (**a**) Nasal septum inclined to the left in the anterior cartilaginous portion and deviated to the right in the other portions and (**b**) Elongated soft palate with reduced pharyngeal air column caliber. *R* right, *P* posterior, *I* inferior. Reprinted with permission from A.C.G

Clinical Findings

The patient reported that he usually goes to sleep at 22:00 and wakes up at 5:30. He reported fragmented sleep, snoring, nightmares, and daytime sleepiness. He also reported previous hernia treatment in the lumbar spine and pituitary adenoma. The patient was in treatment with pantoprazole, rosuvastatin and cabergoline. Previously underwent surgery to lumbar hernia correction and arthroscopy in the right knee. He reported moderate alcohol consumption (4 times a week) and moderate physical activity. He never smoked. The physical examination presented weight of 94 kg, height of 178 cm, BMI of 29.7 kg/m^2, modified Mallampatti score III, SaO$_2$ of 97%, HR of 65 bpm, and Epworth scale of 10.

Timeline

The timeline show the historical and current information of this case report is depicted in Fig. 25.3.

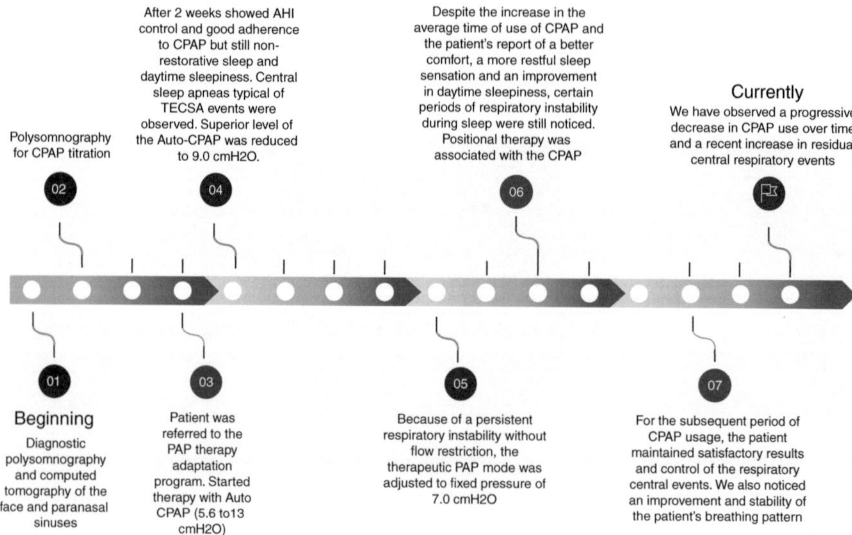

Fig. 25.3 Timeline panel showing the historical and current information from this case report. *CPAP* continuous positive airway pressure, *PAP* positive airway pressure, *AHI* apnea hypopnea index, *TECSA* treatment-emergent central sleep apnea

Physiotherapeutic Intervention

As previously described, the patient started pressure therapy with an Auto-PAP between 5.6 and 13 cmH_2O. In a follow-up visit after 2 weeks, he still complained of non-restorative sleep and the same daytime sleepiness. Moreover, at respiratory flow curve analysis, we observed central sleep apneas typical of TECSA events (Fig. 25.4).

Considering the respiratory instability observed at the beginning of the Auto-CPAP treatment, the superior level of the Auto-CPAP was reduced to 9.0 cmH_2O. We observed a persistent respiratory instability, but without inspiratory flow restriction. On the other hand, we observed a slight increase in the number of residual central respiratory events and patient reported still a little daytime sleepiness. So, aiming a breathing pattern improvement and patient comfort, and considering the existence of a probable instability of the respiratory center (increased by excessive pressure support), the therapeutic mode was adjusted to a fixed pressure of 7.0 cmH_2O.

Despite patient comfort and improvement in sleepiness symptoms, respiratory instability during sleep was still noticed (distributed at specific night periods). We raised the hypothesis of the upper airway collapse related to sleep positioning (due to palatal prolapse, because CT showed an elongated soft palate). Moreover, we

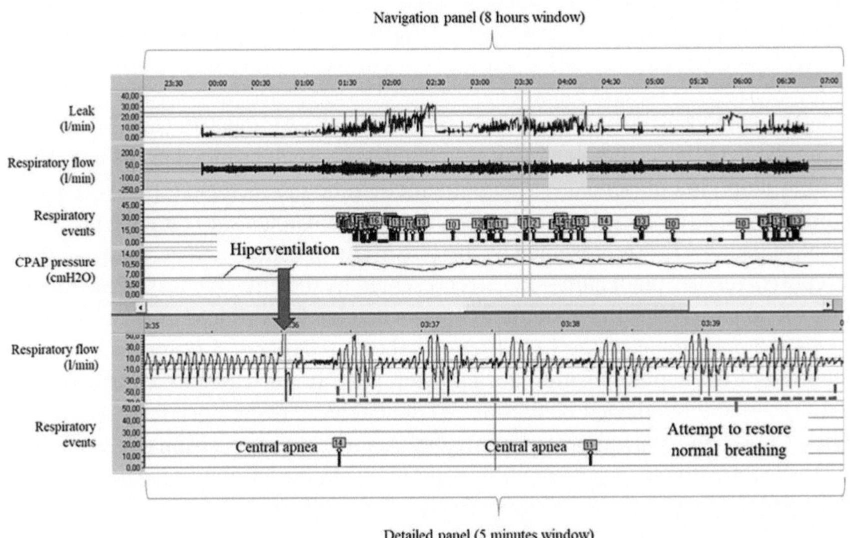

Fig. 25.4 Screen of a graphical data presentation, extracted from positive pressure equipment. The arrow shows a physiological sigh event, with a considerable increase in respiratory flow (hyperventilation). Next, we observe that the inspiratory flow curve diminishes, in response to the carbon dioxide level decrease caused by the increase in respiratory amplitude, as observed in the previous respiratory cycle. In a 5-min window, we observed the maintenance of a subsequent respiratory instability, including two central apnea events triggering detected by the equipment algorithm. Reprinted with permission from A.C.G

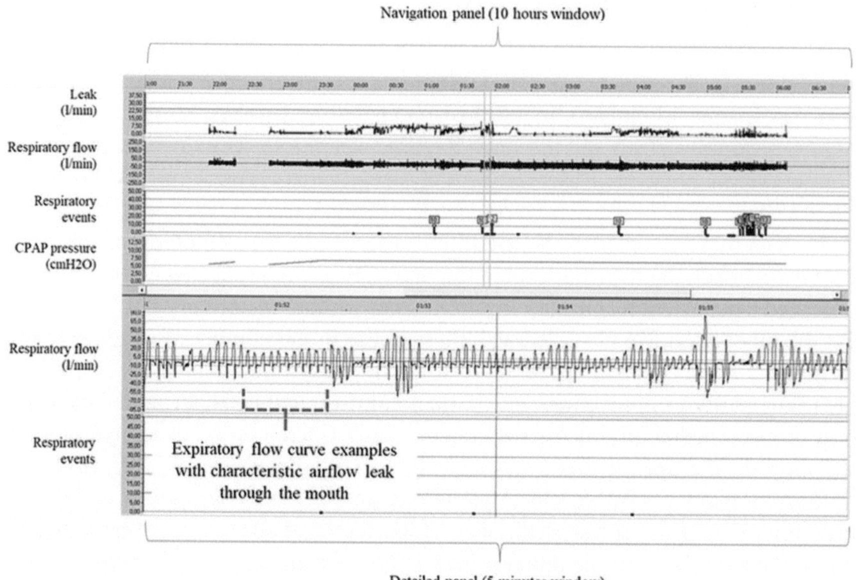

Fig. 25.5 Oral leakage can also occur due to prolapse of the soft palate during expiration, causing obstruction of the nasopharynx and air leakage through the mouth. This specific type of mouth leak can be detected by analyzing the airflow shape obtained on CPAP data card. Reprinted with permission from A.C.G

found a characteristic expiratory flow curve at the CPAP data (Fig. 25.5), corroborating the hypothesis of palatal prolapse [9, 10]. These data added to the hypothesis of high loop gain presented by the patient could be the factors responsible for the ventilatory disorder, resulting in the emergent central apneas. In fact, the product of "control gain—CG" (represented by the sensitivity of central and peripheral chemoreceptors) versus "plain gain—PG" (represented by the effectiveness of the lungs to alter blood gases, plus the increase in factors that lead to collapse of the UA), determines the magnitude of the LG. There might be a dynamic LG increase with the adoption of the supine position during sleep [11]. In our case, we considered that adding a positional device could infer to the decrease respiratory response magnitude to a probable palatal prolapse (maybe, due to a supine position). As an adjunct to the PAP treatment, a positional therapy was introduced with a positioning vest, maintaining the therapeutic pressure fixed at 7.0 cmH$_2$O.

Follow-Up and Outcomes

Without pressure adjustments, just adding the positional therapy along CPAP use, a good therapeutic result was observed and for the subsequent period of CPAP usage, the patient maintained satisfactory results and control of the respiratory central events (Table 25.1). We also observed an improvement and stability of the patient's breathing pattern, as seen in Fig. 25.6.

During the patient follow-up, we performed a small increment in the therapeutic pressure, to correct inspiratory flow curve limitation during sleep. Unfortunately, we have observed a progressive decrease in CPAP use over time and a recent increase in residual central respiratory events (Table 25.1).

Table 25.1 Main results of the initial period of CPAP usage and subsequent follow-up

	Two-week period of initial CPAP use	Subsequent period of CPAP use	Subsequent period of CPAP use	Subsequent period of CPAP use	Subsequent period of CPAP use
Usage days/total days (percentile of more than 4 h of usage per night)	15/15 (100%)	2/2 (100%)	7/77 (84%)	142/386 (60%)	176/300 (54%)
Mask	Nasal	Nasal	Nasal	Nasal	Nasal
Pressure (cmH$_2$O)	5.6–13.0	5.6–9.0	7.0	7.0	7.2
95th percentile pressure (cmH$_2$O)	11.2	8.9	7.0	7.0	7.2
Median pressure—cmH$_2$O	9.4	8.0	7.0	7.0	7.2
Average usage (total days) (h)	6:46	6:50	7:13	4:00	3:34
Median usage (days used) (h)	6:42	6:50	6:11	6:30	6:11
Expiratory relief	Off	Off	Off	Off	Off
95th percentile leaks (L/min)	13.2	14.4	6.6	6.0	7.5
Median leaks (L/min)	3.6	4.2	2.4	0.0	0.6
Events per hour (residual AHI)	8.5	8.8	9.4	4.8	6.3
Central apnea index	4.0	4.4	3.7	1.4	3.1
Obstructive apnea index	0.6	0.6	0.8	0.3	0.4
Obstructive hypopnea index	3.8	3.8	4.8	3.0	2.7
Unknown apnea index	0.0	0.0	0.0	0.0	0.0

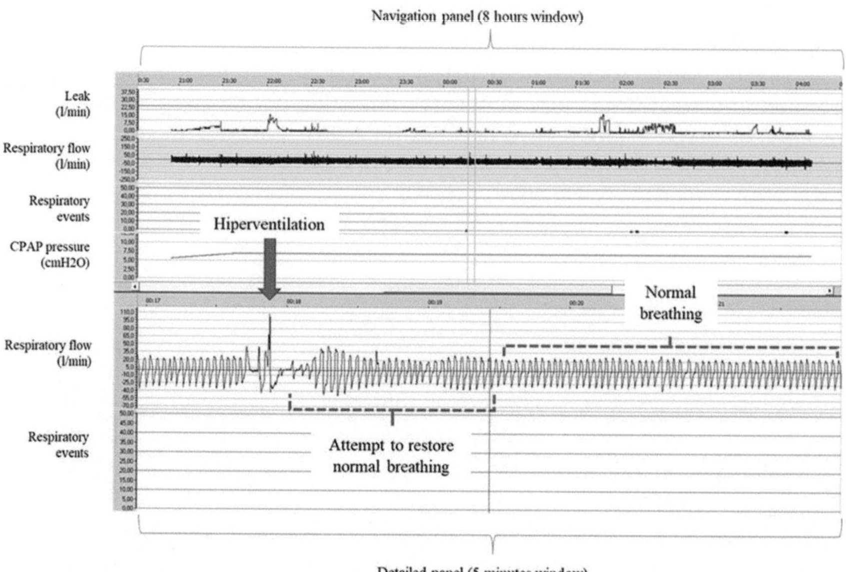

Fig. 25.6 Screen of a graphical data presentation, extracted from positive pressure equipment. The arrow shows a physiological sigh event, with a considerable increase in respiratory flow (hyperventilation). Next, we observe that the inspiratory flow curve diminishes, in response to the carbon dioxide level decrease caused by the increase in respiratory amplitude, as observed in the previous respiratory cycle. In a 5-min window, we observed a faster recover of the normal respiratory flow curve, in relation of what was observed at initial period of CPAP use, as showed before in Fig. 25.4. Reprinted with permission from A.C.G

Discussion

It is important to observe that central apnea rarely occurs as a single event; instead, it occurs in cycles of apneas or hypopneas, alternating with hyperpnea, a reflection of the negative feedback closed-loop cycle that characterizes ventilatory control (often described by using the concept of "loop gain") [6]. In our case report, it seems that TECSA was a loop gain event mainly caused by two factors: (a) chemoreflex sensitivity (controller gain) reflecting the response of the ventilatory system to changing pressure of end tidal carbon dioxide (the controller); and (b) the upper airway anatomy causing the inspiratory flow restriction on the supine position by palatal prolapse [11, 12].

TESCA treatment remains a gray area, and caution is recommended when a therapeutic approach is extrapolated from other forms of central apnea. Increased pressure or Auto-CPAP for patients with respiratory instability may not be a good therapeutic alternative [13], as it may trigger more central respiratory events, the association of positional therapy to control palatal prolapse, and, consequently, maintain upper airway permeability during sleep seems reasonable. In fact, the literature shows that in 61.5% of patients with primary CSA, positioning during sleep is the main causal factor of central respiratory events [14] and the positional therapy could improve CSA optimizing the treatment of associated comorbid conditions [15].

In this case report, positional therapy associated with CPAP improved TECSA, but still with residual CSA events. The literature shows that about a third of patients with TECSA may continue to exhibit persistence of CSA on reevaluation, and the pathophysiological mechanisms for that remain unknown [3, 5]. But, in our case, one plausible explanation for the residual central apneas observed could be that the CO_2 reservoir and the apnea threshold for the patient are labile as a direct consequence of the intermittent PAP usage and CPAP use decrease over time (as presented on Table 25.1). This view is supported by experiments that have demonstrated that the magnitude of reduction in $PaCO_2$ below eupneic $PaCO_2$ and the transient increase in alveolar ventilation required to attain the apneic threshold is not a constant value. This variability in the apneic threshold by the non-regular CPAP use could lead to persistence of central apneas on PAP therapy depending on the degree of patient adaptation of chemoreceptors to the fluctuating CO_2 reservoir and the apneic threshold [5]. Another justification for central respiratory events is that, over time, the patient no longer uses positional therapy associated with CPAP.

In fact CPAP compliance is still a challenge and has been reported to range from 40 to 84% [16]. Adherence to long-term positional therapy was hampered by patient-reported discomfort, and the reliability of adherence information is also hampered by the subjective assessment of the data. One study evaluated tennis ball technique and found that long-term adherence was less than 10%. Another group studied patients wearing a supine sleeping position preventive vest and found adherence lower than 30%, in an average period of 24 months of use of positional therapy [17].

In our case, the patient reported that traveled often for work and the equipment size was an impediment to take it on his travels. He was currently considering the possibility of purchasing a mini-CPAP to make it easier to carry on when traveling. The patient also reported that he is no longer using positional therapy .

Take-Away Messages

1. TECSA is a complex process that can combine central respiratory instability as well as unfavorable upper airway structure and function.
2. It requires a careful assessment of the patient, including, in addition to polysomnographic examinations, information of the upper airway anatomy.
3. Treatment includes identifying the underlying causes and treating any precipitating factors.
4. The use of combined therapies can be a simple and cost-effective solution for treatment-emerging central apnea management.
5. Therapy compliance is still a challenge.

Patient Perspective

"Around 2015, I started to suffer with tiredness and drowsiness during the day. My endocrinologist, in mid-2019, referred me to a sleep doctor. It was found that there were several apneas during my night's sleep, and this was the cause of my daily discomfort. I was then referred to a sleep physiotherapist to start the CPAP therapy. With the frequent use of the equipment, I have had very regular periods of sleep, with a much lower number of respiratory events that occurred in the period when I did not use the device. The consequence of this continuous CPAP use is that I no longer suffer from tiredness and drowsiness during the day."

References

1. Sullivan CE, Issa FG, Berthon-Jones M, Eves L. Reversal of obstructive sleep apnoea by continuous positive airway pressure applied through the nares. Lancet. 1981;1(8225):862–5.
2. Issa FG, Sullivan CE. Reversal of central sleep apnea using nasal CPAP. Chest. 1986;90(2):165–71. https://doi.org/10.1378/chest.90.2.165.
3. Zhang J, Wang L, Guo HJ, Wang Y, Cao J, Chen BY. Treatment-emergent central sleep apnea: a unique sleep-disordered breathing. Chin Med J. 2020;133(22):2721–30. https://doi.org/10.1097/CM9.0000000000001125.
4. American Academy of Sleep Medicine, editor. The International Classification of Sleep Disorders (ICSD-3). 3rd ed. Darien: American Academy of Sleep Medicine; 2014.
5. Nigam G, Riaz M, Chang ET, Camacho M. Natural history of treatment-emergent central sleep apnea on positive airway pressure: a systematic review. Ann Thorac Med. 2018;13(2):86–91. https://doi.org/10.4103/atm.ATM_321_17.
6. Zeineddine S, Badr MS. Treatment-emergent central apnea. Chest. 2021;159(6):2449–57. https://doi.org/10.1016/j.chest.2021.01.036.
7. Stanchina M, Robinson K, Corrao W, Donat W, Sands S, Malhotra A. Clinical use of loop gain measures to determine continuous positive airway pressure efficacy in patients with complex sleep apnea. A pilot study. Ann Am Thorac Soc. 2015;12(9):1351–7. https://doi.org/10.1513/AnnalsATS.201410-469BC.
8. Kuźniar TJ, Morgenthaler TI. Treatment of complex sleep apnea syndrome. Chest. 2012;142(4):1049–57. https://doi.org/10.1378/chest.11-3223.
9. Genta PR, Kaminska M, Edwards BA, Ebben MR, Krieger AC, Tamisier R, et al. The importance of mask selection on continuous positive airway pressure outcomes for obstructive sleep apnea. An official American Thoracic Society workshop report. Ann Am Thorac Soc. 2020;17(10):1177–85. https://doi.org/10.1513/AnnalsATS.202007-864ST.
10. Genta PR, Sands SA, Butler JP, Loring SH, Katz ES, Demko BG, et al. Airflow shape is associated with the pharyngeal structure causing OSA. Chest. 2017;152(3):537–46. https://doi.org/10.1016/j.chest.2017.06.017.
11. Joosten SA, Landry SA, Sands SA, Terrill PI, Mann D, Andara C, et al. Dynamic loop gain increases upon adopting the supine body position during sleep in patients with obstructive sleep apnoea. Respirology. 2017;22(8):1662–9. https://doi.org/10.1111/resp.13108.
12. Joosten SA, O'Driscoll DM, Berger PJ, Hamilton GS. Supine position related obstructive sleep apnea in adults: pathogenesis and treatment. Sleep Med Rev. 2014;18(1):7–17. https://doi.org/10.1016/j.smrv.2013.01.005.

13. Nigam G, Riaz M, Pathak C, Malaiya N, Shelgikar AV. Use of auto-titrating positive airway pressure devices for sleep-disordered breathing: the good, the bad and the ugly. J Pulm Respir Med. 2016;6:1000336.
14. Oktay Arslan B, Ucar Hosgor ZZ, Ekinci S, Cetinkol I. Evaluation of the impact of body position on primary central sleep apnea syndrome. Arch Bronconeumol. 2021;57(6):393–8. https://doi.org/10.1016/j.arbr.2020.03.030.
15. Benoist LBL, Vonk PE, de Vries N, Janssen HCJP, Verbraecken J. New-generation positional therapy in patients with positional central sleep apnea. Eur Arch Otorhinolaryngol. 2019;276(9):2611–9. https://doi.org/10.1007/s00405-019-05545-y.
16. Russell T. Enhancing adherence to positive airway pressure therapy for sleep disordered breathing. Semin Respir Crit Care Med. 2014;35(5):604–12. https://doi.org/10.1055/s-0034-1390070.
17. van Maanen JP, de Vries N. Long-term effectiveness and compliance of positional therapy with the sleep position trainer in the treatment of positional obstructive sleep apnea syndrome. Sleep. 2014;37(7):1209–15. https://doi.org/10.5665/sleep.3840.

Chapter 26
Central Apnea and Neurological Impairment: An Individual Management with Something More…

Rafaela G. S. de Andrade ⓘ, Maria José Perrelli ⓘ, and Vivien S. Piccin ⓘ

Introduction

The association of sleep-related breathing disorders (SBD) and stroke is bidirectional. SBD is a risk factor for stroke and patients with acute stroke and post-stroke have SBD [1]. In turn, strokes disrupt multiple respiratory functions (Table 26.1), depending on the site and extent of the neurological injury. Disorders of respiratory mechanics, pattern, and control result from lesions affecting respiratory control centers and/or respiratory muscles. The prevalence of SBD varies widely (3–72%) on patients with stroke [2].

Supra or infratentorial bilateral lesions have been associated with Cheyne-Stokes breathing (CSB), while unilateral infratentorial strokes have been linked with central hyperventilation, irregular (ataxic or Biot's) breathing, apneustic breathing, and sleep apnea disordered breathing [3, 4]. CSB and central sleep apnea (CSA) are common after stroke. CSB is regarded as a characteristic sequel of an extensive cerebrovascular accident and regularly found immediately after the stroke, while it declines markedly 3 and 6 months into recovery [4–6] and it is characterized by a hyperventilation, hypoventilation, in a crescendo-decrescendo fashion, followed by an apnea. This breathing pattern reflects the instability of the ventilatory control system [7] with a cycle length of at least 40 s [7] On the other hand, CSA in briefer cycle and can be related to unstable breathing caused by high loop gain or to a decreased output from the central neurons (Fig. 26.1).

R. G. S. de Andrade (✉) · V. S. Piccin (✉)
Sleep Medicine, Pulmonary Division, Heart Institute, Faculdade de Medicina da Universidade de São Paulo (InCor-FMUSP), Sao Paulo, SP, Brazil

M. J. Perrelli
Brazilian College of Systemic Studies (CBES), Curitiba, PR, Brazil

C. Frange (ed.), *Clinical Cases in Sleep Physical Therapy*,
https://doi.org/10.1007/978-3-031-38340-3_26

Table 26.1 Respiratory complications of neurological impairment

(a) Impaired chest wall mechanics and diaphragm function
(b) Abnormal breathing patterns
Cheyne-Stokes respiration (CSB)
Central apnea syndrome (CSA)
Central neurogenic hyperventilation
Apneustic breathing
Ataxic breathing
Hypoventilation or apnea sleep-disordered breathing
Others

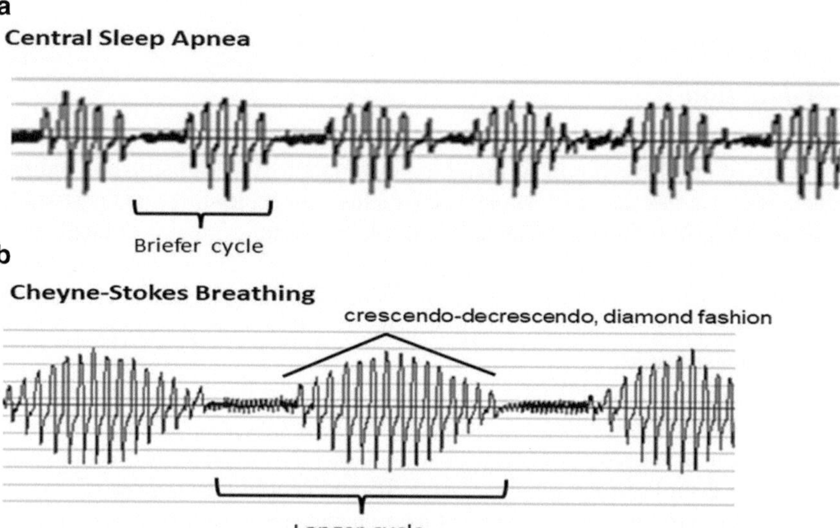

Fig. 26.1 A schematic illustration from airway flow curve shape of CSA in (**a**) and CSB in (**b**)

In addition, delays due to hemoglobin binding, prolonged circulation time, and increase in ventilatory drive may play a role in this physiopathology. All these may predispose hyperventilation and subsequent lowering of PCO_2 below the apneic threshold [8, 9]. Primary CSA has a different pattern with the apnea often terminated abruptly by a normal breath [1]. Both CSB and CSA have been associated with congestive heart failure and have been observed after history of stroke [1]. Next, we describe a clinical scenario where CSA was found, discussing the management approach in detail and timeline events (Fig. 26.2).

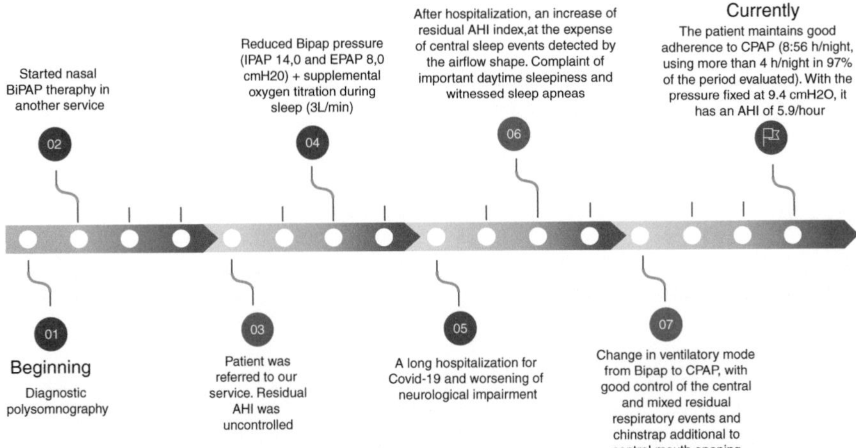

Fig. 26.2 Timeline panel showing the historical and current information from this case report. *CPAP* continuous positive airway pressure, *Bilevel PAP* (positive airway pressure); *IPAP* inspiratory positive airway pressure), *EPAP* expiratory positive airway pressure), *AHI* apnea hypopnea index

Patient Information

L.D.R., an 88-year-old man, married, affected by diabetes, hypertension, dyslipidemia, vascular impairment, depression, and pulmonary emphysema had a recent infection by coronavirus disease 2019 (COVID-19) (May 2022) with a long time of hospitalization. Patient reported four previous ischemic strokes and complaint of somnolence in the morning and during the day with interference in patient's activities. Additionally, the patient's wife has observed a respiratory effort during sleep, even with Bilevel (a device that works with two distinct levels of positive airway pressure known as IPAP/inspiratory airway pressure and EPAP/expiratory airways pressure). He reported waking up frequently during the night to urinate and having nightmares.

Clinical Findings

The patient reported that he usually goes to sleep at 11:00 pm and wakes up at 6:00 am. Patient underwent treatment with pioglitazone hydrochloride, chlorthalidone, ramipril, atenolol, acetylsalicylic acid, aluminum glycinate, magnesium carbonate, apixaban, paroxetine hydrochloride, rosuvastatin, quetiapine, and vortioxetine. Previously, he underwent surgery to tonsillectomy a long time ago. The patient reported alcohol consumption sometimes and light physical activity 3 times/week.

He smoked an average of 3 packs/days and quitted at least 40 years. The physical examination presented weight of 87 kg, height of 180 cm, body mass index (BMI) of 26.9 kg/m^2, modified Mallampati score IV, oxygen saturation (SaO2) of 92%, heart rate (HR) of 78 bpm, during attendance.

Timeline

Diagnostic Assessment

Diagnostic Polysomnography

Stage N1 latency was 14.3 min (normal < 30 min), and rapid eye movement (REM) sleep was 114.5 min (normal = 70–120 min). The total sleep time was 413.5 min (76.6% efficiency; normal >85%) and the percentages of sleep stages in relation to total sleep time were: N1: 2.4%; N2: 48.0%; N3: 16.3% REM sleep: 33.3%. Wake time after sleep onset was 111.9 min. There were 458 registered micro-awakenings (duration<15 s), with an index of 66.5/h (normal <10/h). Four-hundred forty-nine breathing pauses were recorded during sleep, with an apnea hypopnea index (AHI) of 65.2 ev/h. The average SaO_2 was 88.8%. The oxyhemoglobin saturation remained below 90% during 61.1% of sleep time. The mean heart rate was 80.4 bpm. The sleep laboratory evaluation showed: (a) Marked increase in apnea-hypopnea index (65.2 ev/h), with respiratory pauses associated with oxyhemoglobin desaturation (minimum SaO_2 of 66%); (b) Fragmented sleep with an increase in micro-awakenings rate, increased wake time after sleep onset (11.9 min); (c) Reduced sleep efficiency (76.6%); (d) Increased REM percentage (33.3%). Patient diagnosed with severe obstructive sleep apnea (AHI 65.2 e/h)—central apnea index was 1 e/h, patient had more events from hypopnea than apnea as illustrated in Fig. 26.3 and poor sleep saturation.

Computed Tomography

Computed tomography of the skull was performed during hospitalization by COVID-19 (Fig. 26.2, step 5). Clinical context: vascular dementia, prolonged hospitalization by COVID-19 with various infectious complications and delirium. Diagnostic impression: enlargement of intracranial routes of cerebrospinal fluid circulation, without hypertensive signs, related to reduction brain volumetric. Confluent hypodensities of the bi-hemispheric periventricular white matter, usually related

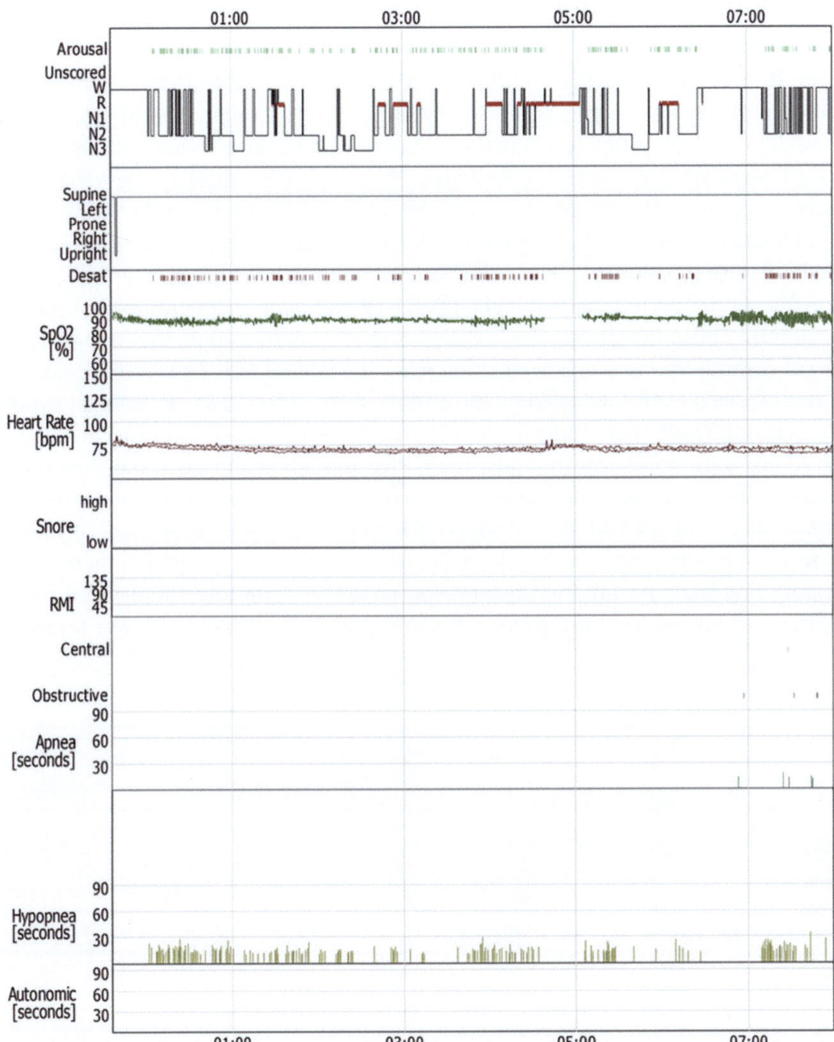

Fig. 26.3 Patient hypnogram from polysomnographic examination showing sleep fragmentation, desaturations and hypopneas events during all polysomnographic examination. Reprinted with permission from L.D.R

gliosis and/or myelin thinning. Areas of medial occipital and anterior temporal gliosis/encephalomalacia on the right. Nucleocapsular ischemic gaps in the radiated crowns and cerebellar hemispheres. Vertebral and intracranial carotid atheromatosis.

Physiotherapeutic Intervention

Nasal Bilevel therapy (IPAP 15.0/EPAP 7.0 cmH$_2$O) started in another service with decrease in respiratory events, residual AHI 12.9 e/h. Compliance of Bilevel was around 11 h/night. After few months, patient came to our service with an uncontrolled respiratory residual events index even with PAP therapy. We decided to decrease de nasal Bilevel pressure to IPAP 14.0 and EPAP 8.0 cmH$_2$O. We added supplemental oxygen (3 L/min) during sleep since the patient presented poor oxygenation during majority of sleep time according to polysomnography.

After a brief period, patient had COVID-19 and increased neurological impairment during hospitalization. The first nights after hospitalization, the Bilevel detection of respiratory events showed an increase in residual AHI index, at the expense of central sleep events detected by the airflow shape (Fig. 26.4), with apnea hypopnea index of 52 e/h (Fig. 26.5). Then, with the patient at home, three physical therapist visits were necessary to adjust the CPAP therapy to improve the therapeutic results. We changed the ventilation mode to obtain an optimal control of the respiratory events, using a CPAP device adjusted in 9.4 cmH$_2$O + supplemental oxygen in 3 L/min + chinstrap, to mouth leakage control. Additionally, positional therapy was proposed by the physiotherapist; however, patient did not tolerate elevated lateral (right or left) decubitus during sleep due to vascular impairment of lower limbs.

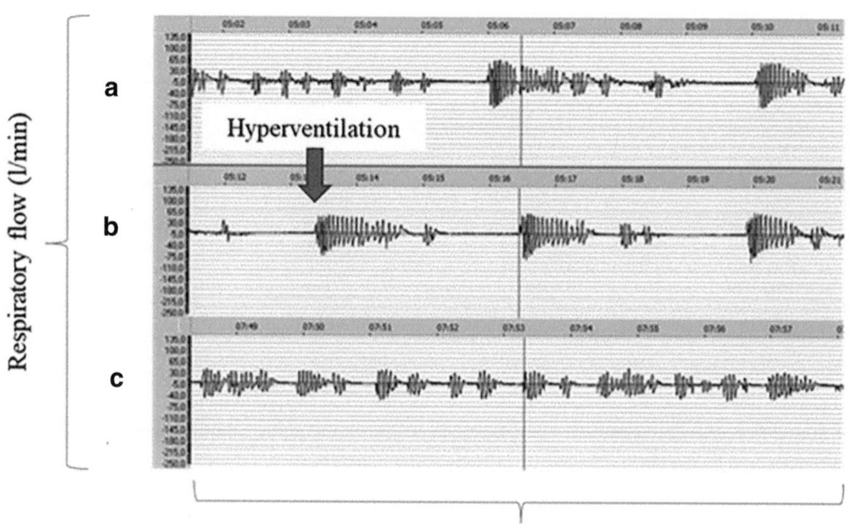

Fig. 26.4 Respiratory airflow curve (l/min) with a periodic pattern. Central apneas can be observed in (**a**) and (**c**). In (**b**) we can see mixed apneas with an abrupt opening of the upper airway causing hyperventilation

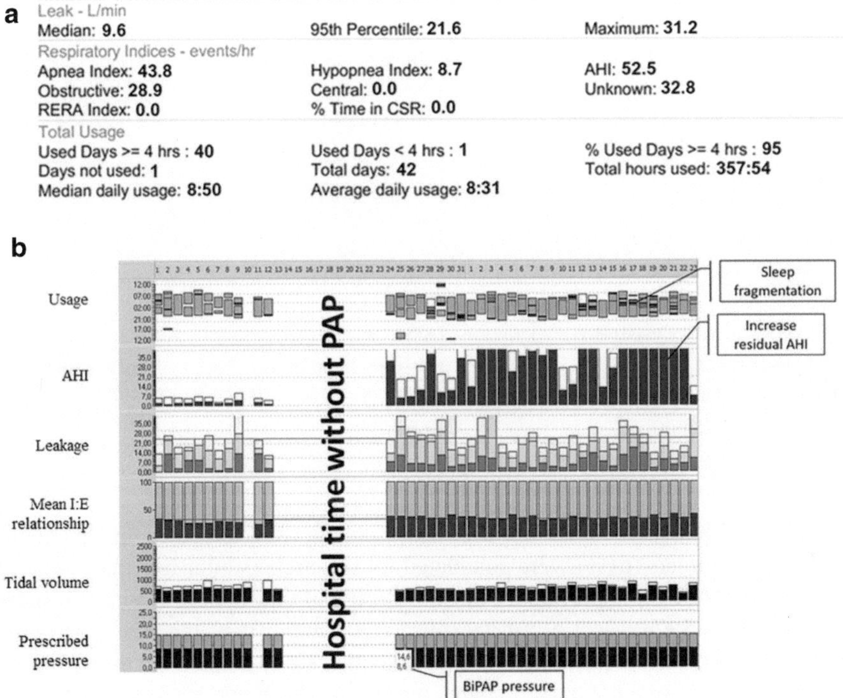

Fig. 26.5 Bilevel statistics (**a**) and summary report (**b**). In (**b**) from top to bottom: Compliance (usage) with therapy interruptions in black, residual AHI, leakage, inspiratory expiratory relationship, tidal volume and Bilevel pressure (inspiratory pressure in black and expiratory pressure in gray). After hospital time and a new stroke history, we can see a clearly increase of the respiratory events

Follow-Up and Outcomes

After intervention (CPAP pressure of 9.4 cmH$_2$0 + supplemental oxygen of 3L/min + chinstrap), we obtained a residual AHI of 5.9 ev/h, a compliance of 8.56 h/night, the 95th percentile of leakage was 11.6L/min, and SpO$_2$ of 94% during sleep, recorded by high resolution pulse oximetry (Table 26.2).

Discussion

An early study [9] reported that CSB was present in as many as 26% of 161 patients in the first 48–72 h after admission to the stroke unit, presumably within the first 5 days post-stroke [10]. On the same line, a meta-analysis of 86 studies showed the

Table 26.2 Statistics report about compliance data, device configuration, lea and residual apnea-hypopnea index

	Bilevel evaluation after hospital discharge	30 days period of initial CPAP use
Usage days/total days (percentile of more than 4 hours of usage per night)	40/42 (95%)	29/30 (97%)
Mask	Nasal	Nasal
Pressure (cmH$_2$O)	IPAP 14.6/EPAP 8.6	9.4
95th percentile pressure (cmH$_2$O)	–	9.4
Median pressure (cmH$_2$O)	–	9.4
Average usage (total days) (h)	8:31	8:56
Median usage (days used) (h)	8:50	8:54
Expiratory relief	1—only ramp time	1—only ramp time
95th percentile leaks (L/min)	21.6	11.6
Median leaks (L/min)	9.6	3.5
Events per hour (residual AHI)	52.5	5.9

prevalence CSA after stroke or transient ischemic attack (TIA). In this meta-analysis, 54 studies (61%) were conducted for researchers after less than 1-month post-stroke. The overall prevalence of CSA ($\geq$50% of total apneas scored as central) with an AHI >5 e/h was 12%; it was observed a major prevalence of obstructive events in these patients [11]. In accordance, another study pointed out that CSA was uncommon in a large cohort of patients with recent ischemic stroke event [12]. In conclusion, CSB-CSA appears to occur during the acute stage of less than 5 days post-stroke with a clinically significant prevalence. CSB-CSA tends to decline in prevalence and severity as the post-stroke period evolves and may become negligible later. With all these concepts in mind, we will discuss this case report.

This interplay between hypocapnia and central apneic threshold is an important factor in determining periodic breathing and central apneas [13]. The implications for treatment are important because, sometimes the ventilatory mode can concur to ventilatory instability. Clinicians may be tempted to use auto CPAP initially in the absence of conventional PAP [1]. Patients with CSB-CSA fare poorly with auto CPAP and this device should not be applied to patients with CSB-CSA [14]. On the other hand, Bilevel, in this case, can converge with a hyperventilation and changes in PaCO$_2$ culminating with central events and instability of the ventilatory control system perpetuating more central and mixed events with an abrupt opening of the upper airway.

SDB treatment must be personally and individualized, considering the history, medication, and comorbidities of each patient. Knowledge about sleep physiology and pathophysiology of sleep breathing disorders will be the foundation of the patient treatment conduction.

Take-Home Messages

1. Sleep-related breathing disorders and stroke are bidirectional, SBD can be a risk factor for stroke, and patients with acute stroke and post-stroke can present SBD.
2. Periodic breathing is a quite common manifestation in patients after stroke.
3. Patients with CSB-CSA fare poorly with PAP modes that destabilize the ventilatory center (as auto-CPAP and expiratory relief technology).

Treatment must be personally and individualized, considering the history, medication, and comorbidities of each patient.

Patient Perspective

Patient says he is sleeping much better, without having so many apneas and awakenings. However, he reports that he wakes up approximately three times in the middle of the night to eat. The patient's wife reports that her husband is experiencing less daytime sleepiness.

References

1. Culebras A. Central sleep apnea may be central to acute stroke. Sleep Med. 2021;77:302–3. https://doi.org/10.1016/j.sleep.2020.10.006.
2. Johnson KG, Johnson DC. Frequency of sleep apnea in stroke and TIA patients: a meta-analysis. J Clin Sleep Med. 2010;6(2):131–7.
3. Bassetti C, Aldrich MS, Quint D. Sleep-disordered breathing in patients with acute supra- and infratentorial strokes. A prospective study of 39 patients. Stroke. 1997;28(9):1765–72. https://doi.org/10.1161/01.str.28.9.1765.
4. Nachtmann A, Siebler M, Rose G, Sitzer M, Steinmetz H. Cheyne-Stokes respiration in ischemic stroke. Neurology. 1995;45(4):820–1. https://doi.org/10.1212/wnl.45.4.820.
5. Brack T, Randerath W, Bloch KE. Cheyne-Stokes respiration in patients with heart failure: prevalence, causes, consequences and treatments. Respiration. 2012;83(2):165–76. https://doi.org/10.1159/000331457.
6. Lipford MC, Park JG, Ramar K. Sleep-disordered breathing and stroke: therapeutic approaches. Curr Neurol Neurosci Rep. 2014;14(2):431. https://doi.org/10.1007/s11910-013-0431-7.
7. Bassetti CL. Sleep and stroke. In: Kryger MH, Dement WC, editors. Priciples and practice of sleep medicine. St Louis: Elsevier; 2011. p. 993–1015.
8. Randerath W, Verbraecken J, Andreas S, Arzt M, Bloch KE, Brack T, et al. Definition, discrimination, diagnosis and treatment of central breathing disturbances during sleep. Eur Respir J. 2017;49(1):1600959. https://doi.org/10.1183/13993003.00959-2016.
9. Malhotra A, Owens RL. What is central sleep apnea? Respir Care. 2010;55(9):1168–78.
10. Parra O, Arboix A, Bechich S, García-Eroles L, Montserrat JM, López JA, et al. Time course of sleep-related breathing disorders in first-ever stroke or transient ischemic attack. Am J Respir Crit Care Med. 2000;161(2):375–80. https://doi.org/10.1164/ajrccm.161.2.9903139.

11. Seiler A, Camilo M, Korostovtseva L, Haynes AG, Brill AK, Horvath T, et al. Prevalence of sleep-disordered breathing after stroke and TIA: a meta-analysis. Neurology. 2019;92(7):e648–54. https://doi.org/10.1212/WNL.0000000000006904.
12. Schütz SG, Lisabeth LD, Hsu CW, Kim S, Chervin RD, Brown DL. Central sleep apnea is uncommon after stroke. Sleep Med. 2021;77:304–6. https://doi.org/10.1016/j.sleep.2020.08.025.
13. Eckert DJ, Malhotra A, Jordan AS. Mechanisms of apnea. Prog Cardiovasc Dis. 2009;51(4):313–23. https://doi.org/10.1016/j.pcad.2008.02.003.
14. Morgenthaler TI, Aurora RN, Brown T, Zak R, Alessi C, Boehlecke B, et al. Practice parameters for the use of autotitrating continuous positive airway pressure devices for titrating pressures and treating adult patients with obstructive sleep apnea syndrome: an update for 2007. An American Academy of Sleep Medicine report. Sleep. 2008;31(1):141–7. https://doi.org/10.1093/sleep/31.1.141.

Chapter 27
Crescendo–Decrescendo: The Heart Manifests Itself

Maria José Perrelli ⓘ, Rafaela G. S. de Andrade ⓘ, and Vivien S. Piccin ⓘ

Introduction

Central sleep apnea (CSA) commonly occurs in patients with heart failure, especially in a pattern of Cheyne-Stokes Breathing (CSB), a well-described phenomenon in the current literature. CSB shows an increasing–decreasing respiratory pattern (known as a diamond-patterned respiratory flow) influenced by ventilatory drive instability and nocturnal rostral fluid shift, and affects about 20–40% of patients with left ventricular systolic dysfunction. Cardiac resynchronization and reduction in cardiac post load tends to improve CSA in patients with cardiovascular dysfunction [1].

Diagnosis of CSA with CSB requires the criteria of primary CSA ($\geq$5 central apneas and/or central hypopneas per hour of sleep, with a total number of these central events being >50% of total respiratory events in the apnea–hypopnea index [AHI]) with three or more consecutive central apneas or hypopneas separated by a *crescendo–decrescendo* respiratory pattern with a cycle length of $\geq$40 s [2]. Nevertheless, there is a great underreporting of central hypopnea in sleep exams since respiratory effort is not measured directly via electromyogram or esophageal pressure during polysomnography (PSG) [1]. Heart failure is the leading cause of CSA–CSB and common symptoms are excessive daytime sleepiness, insomnia, nocturnal dyspnea, and frequent awakenings. This respiratory pattern may also occur during wakefulness and some studies suggest a worse prognosis of the disease [3].

The main treatment for CSA in patients with cardiovascular dysfunction is drug optimization. The literature shows that the continuous positive airway pressure

M. J. Perrelli (✉)
Brazilian College of Systemic Studies (CBES), Curitiba, PR, Brazil

R. G. S. de Andrade · V. S. Piccin
Sleep Medicine, Pulmonary Division, Heart Institute (InCor-FMUSP), Faculdade de Medicina da Universidade de São Paulo, Sao Paulo, SP, Brazil

C. Frange (ed.), *Clinical Cases in Sleep Physical Therapy*,
https://doi.org/10.1007/978-3-031-38340-3_27

(CPAP) therapy targeted to normalize the apnea–hypopnea index (AHI) is indicated for the treatment of CSA in these patients [4]. Despite the fact that there is no evidence in the literature that CPAP decreases the mortality rate [5], the post-hoc analysis of the Canadian Continuous Positive Airway Pressure (CANPAP), study suggests that early suppression of CSA by CPAP to an AHI below 15/h may improve both left ventricular ejection fraction (LVEF) and heart transplant-free survival [1, 4]. Here, we describe a clinical scenario where CSA was found in a patient with heart failure and atrial fibrillation, discussing the physiotherapeutic approach.

Patient Information

C.M.P., an 82-year-old man, presented with atrial flutter and fibrillation, sustained atrial tachycardia and supraventricular tachycardia, LVEF 61%, mild edema in lower limbs, sedentarism, complaint of daytime fatigue, dyspnea on mild efforts, non-restorative sleep, daytime sleepiness, recent memory deficit, nocturia, oral mucosa dryness, and moderate snoring, and was diagnosed with moderate sleep apnea. Patient was referred for CPAP adaptation program by his physician due to a baseline PSG presenting AHI = 23/h with predominance of unclassified hypopneas.

Diagnostic Assessment

Diagnostic Polysomnography

The PSG examination was performed in a Sleep Laboratory following the criteria of the International Classification Sleep Disorders [2]. The patient had a sleep latency of 23 min, rapid eye movement (REM) sleep latency of 95 min, sleep efficiency of 64.9%, and wake after sleep onset (WASO) of 151 min. The sleep stages distribution was: N1 = 10.6%, N2 = 63.8%, N3 = 9.6%, and REM = 16%. Awakening index was 13.6/h, lasting between 3 and 15 s. Apnea–hypopnea index (AHI) was 23 ev/h (Fig. 27.1), being 8.2/h for apneas and 14.9/h for hypopneas. In supine position, AHI was 21 ev/h; considering only lateral decubitus and prone position, the AIH was 24 ev/h. The number of respiratory events was 124 (80 hypopneas, 24 obstructive apneas, 10 central apneas, and 10 mixed apneas). Maximum duration was 43 s. Oxyhemoglobin saturation (SpO_2) in wakefulness before sleep onset was 95%, mean SpO2 during non-REM (NREM) and REM sleep was 95% and 94%, respectively, and minimum SpO_2 was 87%. Patient remained 0.2% of the sleep time with SpO_2 <90%. Mean heart rate during non-NREM sleep and REM sleep was 62 and 65 breaths per minute (BPM), respectively. Periodic movement of the lower limbs index was 16/h, and 0.2% associated with awakenings.

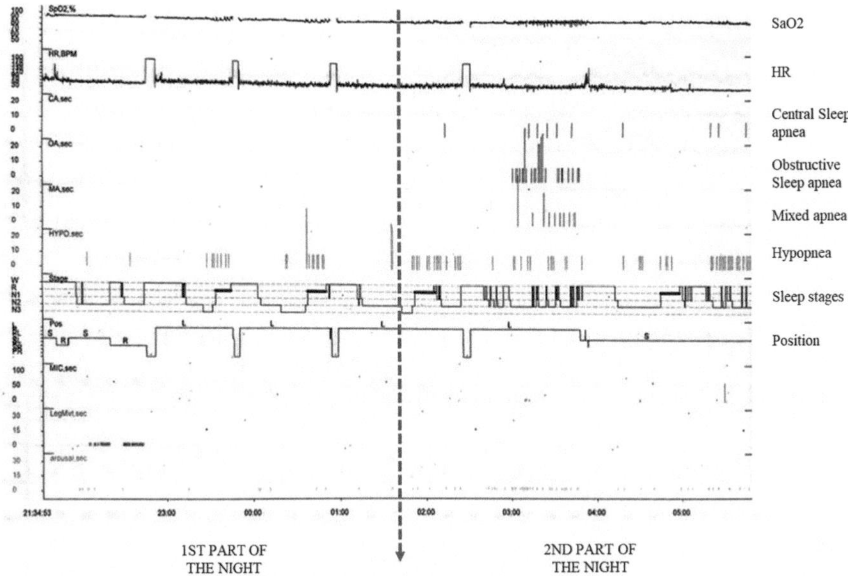

Fig. 27.1 Hypnogram of baseline polysomnography. Observe the increase in respiratory events at the second half of the night. (Reprinted with permission from C.M.P.)

PSG demonstrated reduced sleep efficiency due to frequent periods of wakefulness throughout the night, sleep architecture showing decreased stages NREM N3 and R, sporadic snoring, and moderate sleep apnea. Episodes of heart rhythm alteration were observed.

Echocardiogram

Echocardiogram showed left ventricle with geometric pattern of concentric remodeling, segmental contractility, and normal systolic function. Left atrium was enlarged, with normal right chambers. Mild pulmonary hypertension, mild to moderate mitral reflux, and no thrombus were observed.

Holter 24 Hours

It showed predominant sinus rhythm, paroxysmal atrial flutter, atrial fibrillation, and sustained atrial tachycardia. Periods of isorhythmic dissociation/junctional rhythm, moderate supraventricular ectopy, and tachycardia episodes/non-sustained atrial ectopic rhythm were observed.

Clinical Findings

On the first day of CPAP adherence program, patient was evaluated and presented with body mass index (BMI) of 21 kg/m^2, modified Mallampati score III, and $SpO_2 = 95\%$ at rest. He was regularly treated with medications such as dabigatran, diltiazem, metoprolol, empagliflozin, and rosuvastatin. After CPAP initiation, the patient underwent cardiac ablation for flutter correction.

Timeline

Historical and current information are depicted in Fig. 27.2.

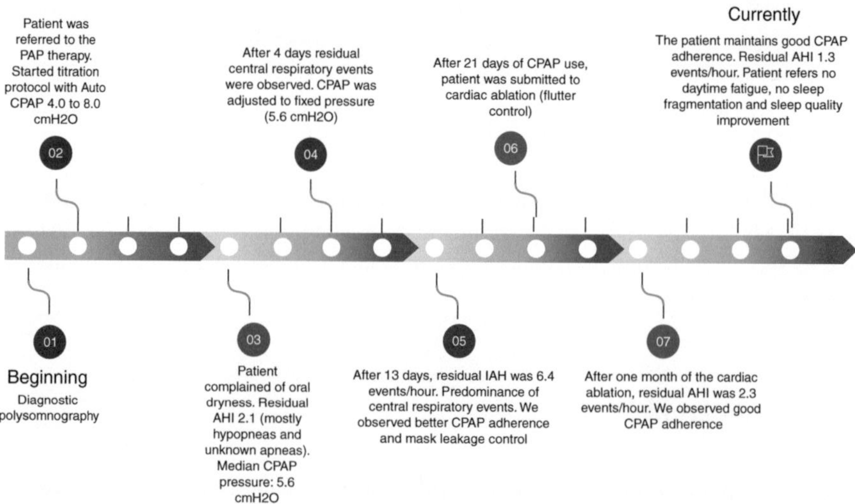

Fig. 27.2 Timeline panel showing the historical and current information from this case report. *AHI* apnea–hypopnea index, *CPAP* continuous positive airway pressure, *PAP* positive airway pressure

Physiotherapeutic Intervention

The CPAP program started with home APAP—automatic continuous positive airway pressure—titration at minimum pressure adjustment of 4.0 cmH$_2$O and maximum of 8.0 cmH$_2$O, with a nasal mask.

At the beginning of the CPAP program, patient complained of mouth dryness. We observed central apnea events in the CPAP reports (and witnessed by patient's wife). Analyzing the respiratory flow curves obtained from the CPAP memory card, we observed periods of CSA (Fig. 27.3). Also, the patient complained of wearing and adjusting the CPAP mask, leading to an excessive air leakage during the CPAP use.

CPAP follow-up occurred weekly, trying to achieve the optimal CPAP pressure adjustment for AHI control (below 5 ev/h) and patient comfort. We changed the CPAP mode to fixed pressure after 5 days due to the presence of CSA in the flow curves. Reassessments were made both remotely and personally (Table 27.1).

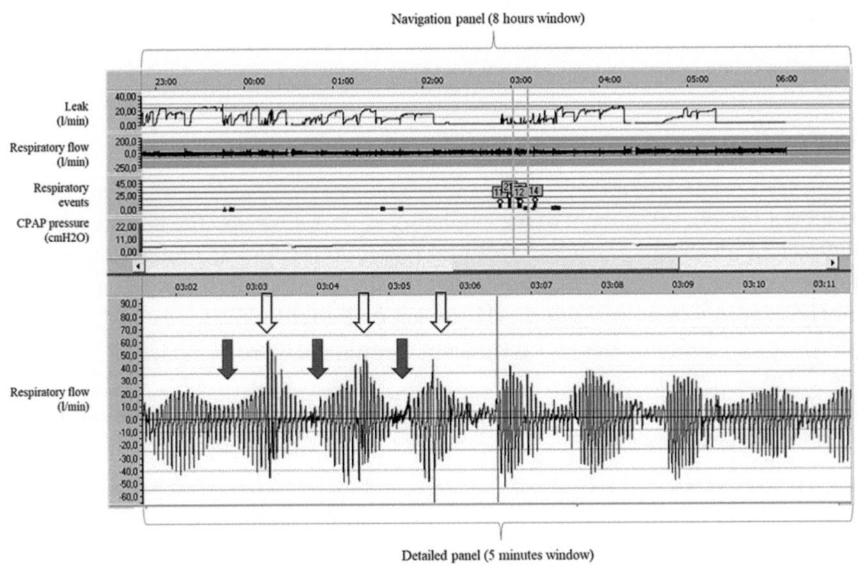

Fig. 27.3 Respiratory flow curve showing ventilatory instability by periodic events of hypoventilation (dark arrow) and hyperventilation (open arrow). (Reprinted with permission from C.M.P.)

Table 27.1 Data obtained during the beginning of the CPAP program

	First day of CPAP usage	Subsequent period of CPAP usage	Subsequent period of CPAP usage
Usage days/total days (percentile of more than 4 h of usage per night)	1/1 (100%)	5/5 (100%)	20/20 (100%)
Mask	Nasal	Nasal	Nasal
Pressure (cmH$_2$O)	4.0–8.0	4.0–6.0	5.6
95th percentile pressure (cmH$_2$O)	7.2	5.8	5.6
Median pressure (cmH$_2$O)	5.3	4.3	5.6
Average usage (total days)—in hours	3:19	6:55	6:41
Median usage (days used)—in hours	3:19	7:36	7:16
Expiratory relief	3; only during ramp	3; only during ramp	3; only during ramp
95th percentile leaks (L/min)	22.8	45.6	49.2
Median leaks (L/min)	7.2	13.2	18.0
Events per hour (residual apnea-hypopnea index AHI)	2.1	6.7	6.4
Humidification	Level 5	Level 5	Level 5

Follow-Up and Outcomes

In a brief period, subsequent of the beginning of the CPAP use, the patient was submitted to a procedure of cardiac ablation (flutter correction) and referred to cardio-respiratory rehabilitation. We maintained the CPAP mode in fixed pressure of 5.6 cmH$_2$O and observed a residual AHI of 1.3 ev/h (Table 27.2). Also, after family guidance and reinforcement for the patient regarding the use of the CPAP mask, the air leak was controlled.

In Fig. 27.4, we compare details of sleep quality and CPAP use pre- and post-cardiac ablation procedure.

Table 27.2 Data of CPAP use after cardiac ablation demonstrating AHI and leakage control, and CPAP adherence

	Period of CPAP usage after cardiac ablation	Subsequent period of CPAP usage after cardiac ablation	Subsequent period of CPAP usage after cardiac ablation
Usage days/total days (percentile of more than 4 h of usage per night)	32/32 (100%)	61/61 (100%)	120/122 (93%)
Mask	Nasal	Nasal	Nasal
Pressure (cmH$_2$O)	5.6	5.6	5.6
Average usage (total days)—in hours	7:33	7:51	7:16
Median usage (days used)—in hours	7:32	8:03	8:02
Expiratory relief	3; only during ramp	Off	Off
95th percentile leaks (L/min)	48.0	42.0	25.2
Median leaks (L/min)	22.8	16.8	4.8
Events per hour (residual AHI)	2.8	1.2	1.1
Humidification	Level 5	Level 5	Level 5

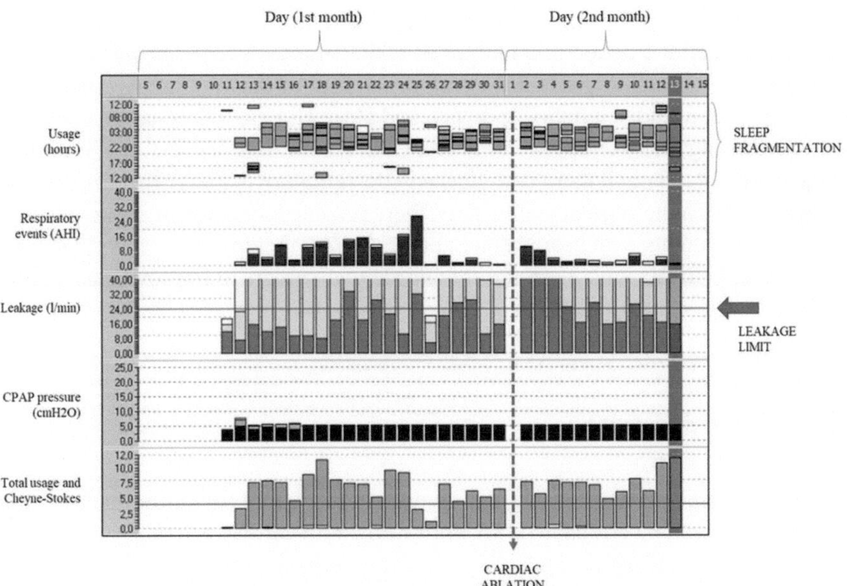

Fig. 27.4 This graph demonstrates sleep fragmentation (probably due to excessive leakage), and residual respiratory events (*AHI* apnea–hypopnea index) with CPAP use (pre- and post-cardiac ablation). (Reprinted with permission from C.M.P.)

Discussion

The primary goals in CSA management are the control of abnormal respiratory events and treatment optimization for comorbid conditions. The American Academy of Sleep Medicine (AASM) recommends CPAP as the initial choice for CSA treatment, but Bilevel Pressure Airway Positive (Bilevel) therapy and adaptive servo-ventilation (ASV) could be considered by physical therapists when the CPAP cannot control residual respiratory events. Apart from PAP devices, therapeutical options include supplemental oxygen, carbon dioxide, and pharmacologic agents. The heterogeneity of disease requires individualized therapies for the proper management of CSA rather than a homogenous treatment approach [4, 6–8].

In a clinical trial the short term CPAP use plus the best supportive care reduced the central AHI because it resulted in little or no difference in cardiovascular mortality and no adverse effects were observed with CPAP [9].

Even though we used the APAP mode for CPAP titration, after 5 days we considered the use of fixed CPAP to prevent ventilatory instability. The literature considers that CPAP treatment in patients with CSA stabilizes lung volumes by reducing the changes in partial pressure of carbon dioxide responsible for the abnormal respiratory rhythm [10, 11]. On the other hand, we consider that in this case the cardiac ablation procedure was essential to stabilize the patient organism, resulting in successful control of CSA-CSB with the CPAP device.

In our case study, the respiratory stabilization at the central nervous system level was achieved after a period of 5 months of PAP therapy, since treatment with CPAP requires some period to gradually promote stability of the ventilatory control system [12]. The multidisciplinary approach and close clinical follow-up by the phsiotherapist during PAP therapy were fundamental for the case success. It is important to mention that although there is evidence in the literature that PAP therapy does not reduce the risk of heart-related mortality, there is some indication of improved quality of life in patients with heart failure and CSA. PAP therapy may be worth considering for individuals with heart failure and sleep disorders to improve their quality of life [13, 14].

Take-Home Message

1. Drugs administration or surgical compensation for heart failure and/or atrial fibrillation can be critical to CSA improvement in cardiac patients.
2. APAP in cardiac patients may worsen central events.
3. The respiratory stability as well as the control of CSA demand a period of adaptation of CPAP. The fixed pressure mode is recommended to limit ventilatory stimulus variations during the sleep.
4. Close monitoring of respiratory events and patient complaints are important for PAP adherence.

Patient Perspective

Nowadays the patient extensively uses CPAP device without complaints. The patient reports sleep and quality of life improvement.

References

1. Roberts EG, Raphelson JR, Orr JE, LaBuzetta JN, Malhotra A. The pathogenesis of central and complex sleep apnea. Curr Neurol Neurosci Rep. 2022;22(7):405–12. https://doi.org/10.1007/s11910-022-01199-2.
2. Berry RB, Brooks R, Gamaldo C, Harding SM, Lloyd RM, Quan SF, et al. AASM scoring manual updates for 2017 (version 2.4). J Clin Sleep Med. 2017;13(5):665–6. https://doi.org/10.5664/jcsm.6576.
3. American Academy of Sleep Medicine, editor. The International classification of sleep disorders (ICSD-3). 3rd ed. Darien: American Academy of Sleep Medicine; 2014.
4. Aurora RN, Chowdhuri S, Ramar K, Bista SR, Casey KR, Lamm CI, et al. The treatment of central sleep apnea syndromes in adults: practice parameters with an evidence-based literature review and meta-analyses. Sleep. 2012;35(1):17–40. https://doi.org/10.5665/sleep.1580.
5. Bradley TD, Logan AG, Kimoff RJ, Sériès F, Morrison D, Ferguson K, et al. Continuous positive airway pressure for central sleep apnea and heart failure. N Engl J Med. 2005;353(19):2025–33. https://doi.org/10.1056/NEJMoa051001.
6. Eckert DJ, Jordan AS, Merchia P, Malhotra A. Central sleep apnea: pathophysiology and treatment. Chest. 2007;131(2):595–607. https://doi.org/10.1378/chest.06.2287.
7. Iftikhar IH, Khayat RN. Central sleep apnea treatment in patients with heart failure with reduced ejection fraction: a network meta-analysis. Sleep Breath. 2022;26(3):1227–35. https://doi.org/10.1007/s11325-021-02512-y.
8. Sadeghi Y, Sedaghat M, Majedi MA, Pakzad B, Ghaderi A, Raeisi A. Comparative evaluation of therapeutic approaches to central sleep apnea. Adv Biomed Res. 2019;8:13. https://doi.org/10.4103/abr.abr_173_18.
9. Pinto ACPN, Rocha A, Pachito DV, Drager LF, Lorenzi-Filho G. Non-invasive positive pressure ventilation for central sleep apnoea in adults. Cochrane Database Syst Rev. 2022;10(10):CD012889 https://doi.org/10.1002/14651858.CD012889.pub2.
10. Arzt M, Floras JS, Logan AG, Kimoff RJ, Series F, Morrison D, et al. Suppression of central sleep apnea by continuous positive airway pressure and transplant-free survival in heart failure: a post hoc analysis of the Canadian Continuous Positive Airway Pressure for Patients with Central Sleep Apnea and Heart Failure Trial (CANPAP). Circulation. 2007;115(25):3173–80. https://doi.org/10.1161/CIRCULATIONAHA.106.683482.
11. Terziyski K, Draganova A. Central sleep apnea with Cheyne-Stokes breathing in heart failure - from research to clinical practice and beyond. Adv Exp Med Biol. 2018;1067:327–51. https://doi.org/10.1007/5584_2018_146.
12. Stanchina M, Robinson K, Corrao W, Donat W, Sands S, Malhotra A. Clinical use of loop gain measures to determine continuous positive airway pressure efficacy in patients with complex sleep apnea. A pilot study. Ann Am Thorac Soc. 2015;12(9):1351–7. https://doi.org/10.1513/AnnalsATS.201410-469BC.
13. Yamamoto S, Yamaga T, Nishie K, Nagata C, Mori R. Positive airway pressure therapy for the treatment of central sleep apnoea associated with heart failure. Cochrane Database Syst Rev. 2019;12(12):CD012803. https://doi.org/10.1002/14651858.CD012803.pub2.
14. Voigt J, Emani S, Gupta S, Germany R, Khayat R. Meta-analysis comparing outcomes of therapies for patients with central sleep apnea and heart failure with reduced ejection fraction. Am J Cardiol. 2020;127:73–83. https://doi.org/10.1016/j.amjcard.2020.04.011.

Part IX
Clinical Cases: Other Sleep-Breathing Disorders

Chapter 28
Non-invasive Ventilation for Stable Hypercapnic Chronic Obstructive Pulmonary Disease

Amanda J. Piper ⓘ

Introduction

Although non-invasive ventilation (NIV) is widely used in patients with chronic obstructive pulmonary disease (COPD) and stable hypercapnia, there remain several questions regarding the phenotype that may be most responsive to treatment, timing of intervention, and mode of therapy that may produce the best outcomes. The current case serves to illustrate a few issues requiring consideration when using nocturnal NIV in patients with stable chronic hypercapnic respiratory failure, including sufficient inspiratory support to reduce nocturnal carbon dioxide (CO_2) and the role of remote monitoring.

Patient Information

A 56-year-old woman, ex-smoker, residing in a regional town was referred to a quaternary center for review and management of her NIV. The patient had been diagnosed with severe COPD some years earlier. She had been on oxygen therapy for around 8 months. More recently she reported increasing exertional breathlessness and was found to be in chronic hypercapnic respiratory failure, with a $PaCO_2$ (partial pressure of carbon dioxide) of 54 mmHg sampled with the patient awake. She was commenced on nocturnal NIV by her local respiratory care team. However, higher levels of inspiratory support were not tolerated and despite extended use of NIV, the awake CO_2 continued to rise to 60 mmHg with bicarbonate 41 mmol/L.

A. J. Piper (✉)
Respiratory Support Service, Department of Respiratory and Sleep Medicine, Royal Prince Alfred Hospital, Camperdown, NSW, Australia

C. Frange (ed.), *Clinical Cases in Sleep Physical Therapy*,
https://doi.org/10.1007/978-3-031-38340-3_28

She resided with her husband, who was very supportive. Her usual medications included Panadol, Aspirin, Ostelin, and Trelegy. She reported two episodes of respiratory arrest in the past when given intravenous (IV) midazolam, and stated she was intolerant of other benzodiazepines.

Clinical Findings

On the afternoon prior to her sleep study, her resting SpO_2 (oxygen saturation measured by pulse oximetry) on 3 L/min was 89%, with normal sinus rhythm and a heart rate of 100 bpm. Her jugular venous pressure was not raised. On auscultation, breath sounds were reduced with an occasional inspiratory wheeze. Her body mass index was 27 kg/m^2.

Timeline

2014	Diagnosed with COPD
2017	Osteoporosis identified
2019	Emergency Department admission with tibia and fibula fracture; respiratory arrest after administration of midazolam
2019	Commenced on aclasta (zoledronic acid) infusion yearly
2020	Increasing complaints of exertional breathlessness; patient becoming increasingly hypoxic; arterial blood gas confirmed chronic stable hypercapnic respiratory failure
2020	Non-invasive ventilation initiated as an outpatient locally

Diagnostic Assessment

Lung function testing performed prior to commencing NIV showed significant obstruction with an FEV_1 of 1.2 L (45% of predicted), and a ratio of forced expiratory volume in one second to forced vital capacity (FEV_1/FVC) of 63%. Total lung capacity was 106% of predicted while residual volume was 187% of predicted, indicating significant air trapping.

A chest X-ray was performed, which showed a mildly enlarged heart with pulmonary venous congestion but no interstitial or pulmonary edema. An echocardiogram showed no evidence of pulmonary hypertension nor any significant valve defects.

Following the initial blood gas showing chronically raised $PaCO_2$, a diagnosis of severe hypercapnic respiratory failure secondary to COPD was confirmed. The patient agreed to a trial of nocturnal NIV.

Physiotherapeutic Intervention

She was commenced on NIV as an outpatient using a spontaneous timed (ST) mode with a backup rate of 16 bpm and a rise time of "3." The inspiratory positive airway pressure (IPAP) was set initially at 10 cmH$_2$O and expiratory positive airway pressure (EPAP) at 6 cmH$_2$O. Over the next 8 weeks numerous attempts were made to increase the IPAP above 11 cmH$_2$O, but the patient was unable to tolerate this, complaining of significant aerophagia and discomfort at each attempt. Overnight oximetry on NIV was arranged by the local care team. This showed ongoing severe nocturnal hypoxemia despite NIV and 4 L/min of supplemental oxygen. Ninety-nine percent of the recording time was spent with SpO$_2$ <85% (Fig. 28.1). Nocturnal carbon dioxide monitoring on NIV could not be performed locally. Although the patient was using NIV therapy for more than 12 h per 24-hour period, the awake PaCO$_2$ remained between 55 and 60 mmHg, with bicarbonate of 35 mmol/L and pH 7.35. She was referred to a quaternary home NIV service.

A Level 1 polysomnogram (PSG) including transcutaneous carbon dioxide (TcCO$_2$) was arranged by the quaternary service to review and further titrate NIV. The goal was to identify any issues contributing to intolerance of higher levels of pressure support. A download from the device showed no unintentional leak with the nasal mask; it was not clear if this would still be the case when higher inspiratory pressures were used. She was trialed with an oronasal mask but did not tolerate this, feeling claustrophobic. A chinstrap was fitted and trialed in case significant mouth leak occurred with her nasal mask during the study. She commenced the sleep study using her usual home NIV settings with the exceptions of the inspiratory time, which was reduced from 1.4 to 1.2 s, and an increase in the rise time from a setting of 3 to 2. Once asleep, pressure support was gradually increased. There was

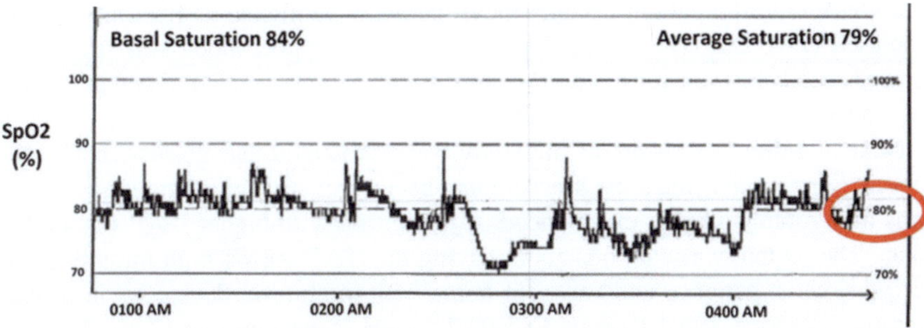

Fig. 28.1 Nocturnal oximetry recording of the patient on NIV and 4 L/min of supplemental oxygen after a few weeks of low-span bilevel therapy. The patient was compliant with therapy but no improvements in daytime PaCO$_2$ occurred. The patient remained extremely hypoxic during sleep. *PaCO$_2$* partial pressure of carbon dioxide, *SpO$_2$* oxygen saturation measured by pulse oximetry

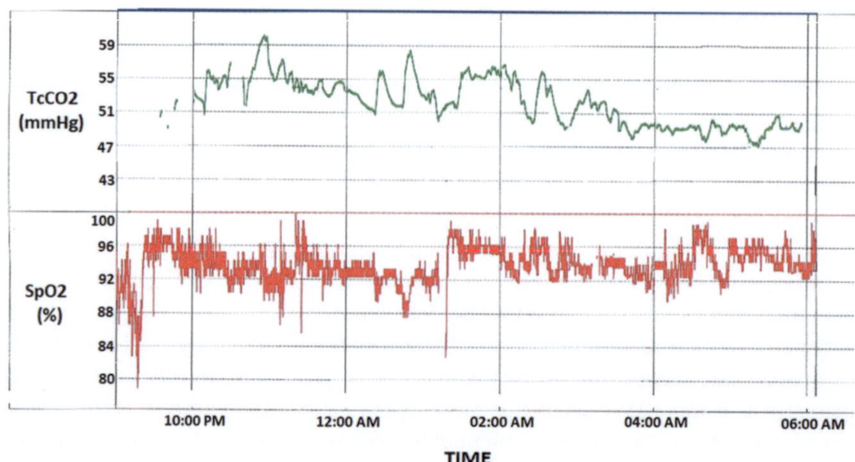

Fig. 28.2 Overnight SpO_2 and $TcCO_2$ monitoring during the polysomnographically guided NIV titration study showing the gradual reduction in $TcCO_2$ as the level of pressure support was increased. SpO_2 oxygen saturation measured by pulse oximetry, $TcCO_2$ transcutaneous carbon dioxide monitoring

no evidence of any patient–ventilator asynchrony or upper airway obstruction during the study. Consequently, expiratory positive airway pressure (EPAP) was reduced to 5 cmH_2O. Consistent with the device download data, tidal volumes remained below 300 mL with pressure support levels of 5–9 cmH_2O, with failure to reduce $TcCO_2$ levels. IPAP was gradually increased to 21 cmH_2O, resulting in tidal volumes of around 500 mL.

There was a gradual reduction in $TcCO_2$ at the higher inspiratory pressures (Fig. 28.2), and the patient became more passively ventilated as pressure support increased (Fig. 28.3). A volume-targeted pressure support mode was trialed but showed no advantage over fixed pressure support. Supplemental oxygen at 2L/min was added to maintain a baseline of 88–92%.

Next morning the results of the study were explained and discussed with the patient. She was surprised the pressure had been taken so high without any symptoms of aerophagia being experienced. A home trial with higher IPAP was undertaken. The patient was cautious about having the IPAP set too high initially given her previous experience and was sent home with the bilevel device set in a fixed pressure ST mode, IPAP 19 cmH_2O, EPAP 5 cmH_2O, backup rate 17 pm, Ti 1.2 s, and rise time 2. Supplemental oxygen at 2 L/min was added.

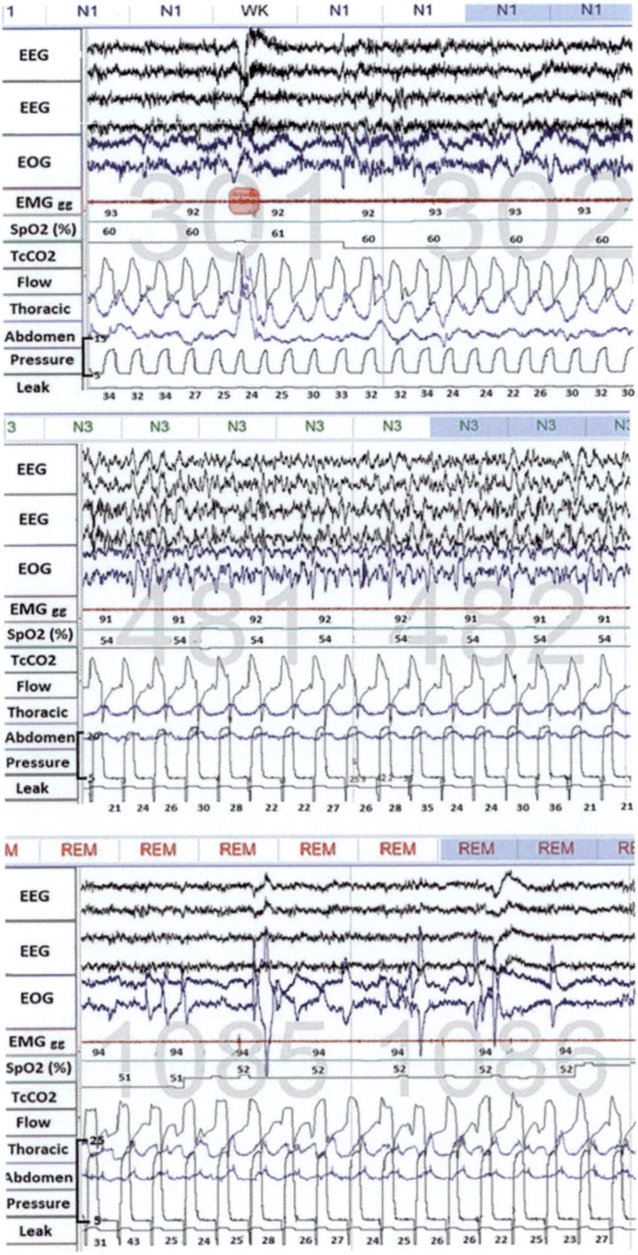

Fig. 28.3 One-minute epochs of Wake, N3, and rapid eye movement (REM) sleep showing the impact of increasing pressure support on lowering TcCO₂. During the transition between wake and sleep, TcCO₂ rose to 60 mmHg with low-span bilevel ventilation. As the pressure support increased, TcCO₂ gradually fell and ventilation became more passive, with an increasing number of breaths being machine triggered. *EEG* electroencephalogram, *EOG* electro-oculogram, *EMGgg* electromyogram genioglossus, *SpO₂* oxygen saturation, *TcCO₂* transcutaneous carbon dioxide

Follow-Up and Outcomes

Progress with therapy was monitored remotely with data on ventilation being sent to and stored on the cloud for regular review, looking at unintentional leak, tidal volumes, and usage. Over the next 2 weeks, IPAP was increased in 1 cmH$_2$O weekly increments to 21 cmH$_2$O, without any adverse impact on the patient in terms of aerophagia or increased mask leak. Even the small increase in IPAP from 19 to 21 cmH$_2$O produced important increases in average tidal volumes (Fig. 28.4). She reported sleeping well on therapy and found she did not need to use the device as much during the day for breathlessness. Her mean usage fell to 7 h and 55 min/ night. A repeat blood gas taken 3 months later showed awake PaCO$_2$ had fallen to 45 mmHg and bicarbonate to 28 mmol/L.

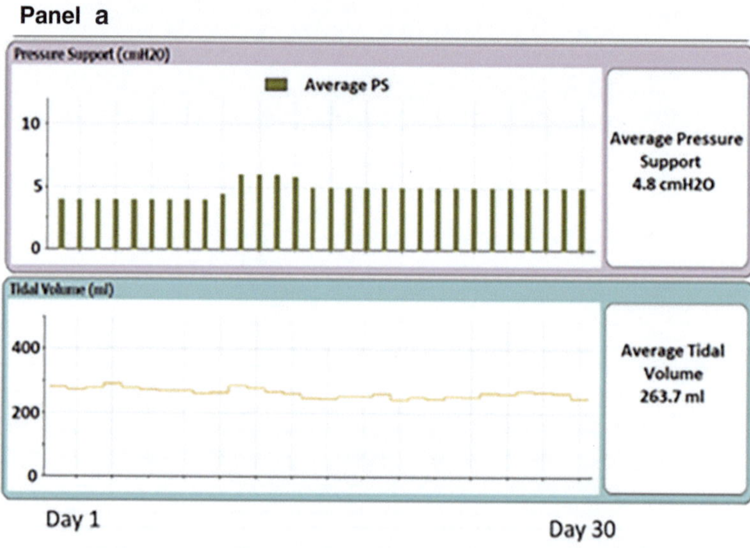

Fig. 28.4 (**a**) Delivery of low-average tidal volumes when low-span bilevel therapy was used initially. (**b**) During the 4 weeks following the PSG-titrated NIV review, average tidal volumes were substantially higher with the increased level of pressure support. The higher-intensity NIV produced more passive ventilatory support, with more breaths machine triggered

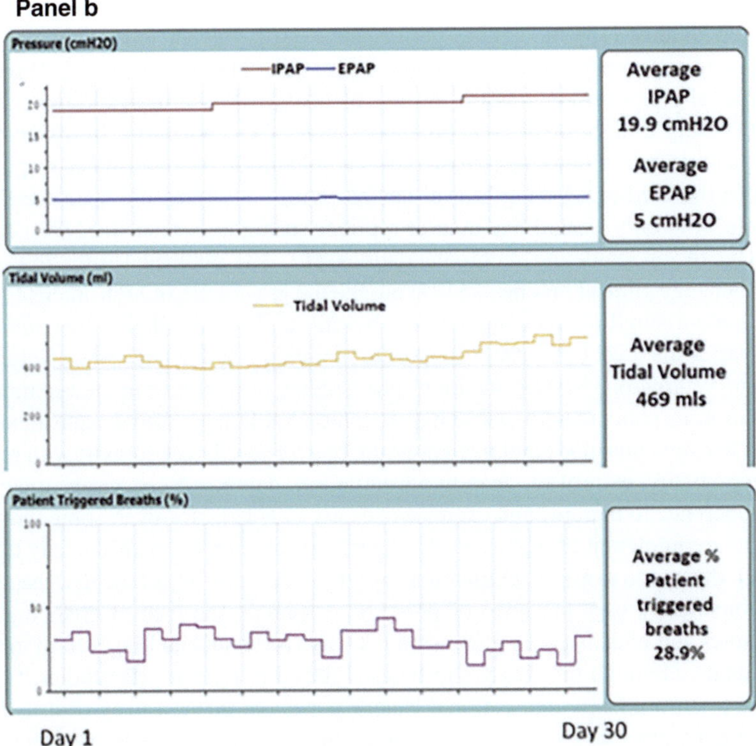

Fig. 28.4 (continued)

Discussion

Chronic obstructive pulmonary disease is a common indication for home non-invasive ventilation (NIV), accounting for more than 30% of prescriptions in many regions [1, 2]. Until recently, uncertainty existed around the clinical benefits of using NIV for the long-term management of stable hypercapnic COPD [3]. This contrasts significantly with the strong evidence underlying the use of NIV for acute hypercapnic exacerbations of COPD [4]. Early studies evaluating home NIV in patients with COPD frequently used modest levels of pressure support (often <10 cmH$_2$0), which may have accounted for the limited clinical benefits found compared to standard oxygen therapy alone [5–7]. More recent studies have used a ventilation strategy of high-intensity NIV (HI-NIV), which focusses on using the highest levels of pressure support tolerated by the patient with the aim of maximizing the reduction in CO$_2$ [8–11]. These studies have demonstrated significantly greater benefits including better health-related quality of life [8, 12–14], reduced hospital admissions [9, 14], exercise tolerance [12], and improved survival [8, 13], although the impact on this latter outcome may be modest [12]. While there were initial concerns patients would be unable to tolerate high inspiratory pressures, it has been subsequently shown that compliance is not compromised, with no adverse effects on sleep quality [15] or cardiac performance [16]. Recent guidelines from the European Respiratory Society [12] and the American Thoracic Society [13] provide conditional recommendations for the use of nocturnal NIV in stable hypercapnic COPD, using a high-intensity approach to target CO_2 reduction. In a web-based survey conducted prior to the release of these guidelines, the majority of responders (44.4%) reported prescribing bilevel devices with a low-pressure span for COPD patients, with only around one-quarter routinely using high-intensity NIV (26.9%) [1]. The recent guideline recommendations [12, 13] published after this study should change clinical practice and encourage the greater use of high-intensity NIV.

Volume-assured pressure support is a hybrid mode of ventilation that automatically varies the level of pressure support to maintain a stable target tidal volume or alveolar ventilation. Several medium-term studies evaluating this newer mode of ventilation in patients with stable hypercapnic COPD have found equivalent outcomes between this mode and fixed pressure bilevel ventilatory support with respect to sleep quality, control of sleep hypoventilation, daytime blood gases, quality of life, adherence to therapy, and exercise capacity [17–19]. However, some individuals who are intolerant of higher levels of pressure support when awake may do better with this mode to assist acclimation to therapy [17, 20]. Theoretically, the ability to automatically vary the level of pressure support in the face of changing lung mechanics and with disease progression may also be beneficial longer term in some individuals, although this has yet to be established in longer-term studies. Care is needed to ensure large unintentional leak or persistent upper airway obstruction is not present when using volume-assured pressure support as these issues can impact the effectiveness of therapy [21].

The interface used for NIV is seen as a key element in the success of therapy [22], influencing both patient comfort and the degree of unintentional leak seen during treatment. A large European study surveying home NIV practices from two decades ago reported the use of nasal masks in around 80% of patients diagnosed with lung disease [2]. In contrast, more recent studies have described oronasal masks being used in 80–90% of patients with COPD [23–25]. However, good-quality data to guide choice are limited. A small randomized crossover trial found both oronasal and nasal masks were capable of delivering effective NIV in patients with COPD, but authors commented that an individual's response to different interfaces was extremely heterogeneous [26]. Patients who are older, who require higher IPAP levels, or who commence home NIV due to persisting hypercapnia after acute respiratory failure are more likely to be prescribed an oronasal mask [23]. A recent meta-analysis of eight randomized controlled trials assessing the efficacy of NIV in patients with obesity hypoventilation syndrome (OHS) and COPD found no difference between the mask types with respect to improvements in awake blood gases or adherence to therapy [24].

In the past, routine clinical practice was to admit patients with COPD for inpatient NIV acclimation and titration, with some studies reporting mean inpatient stays of 5–7 days [8, 27] especially when setting up high-intensity NIV. Given resource constraints in many centers this is not always feasible, resulting in delays in initiating NIV while waiting for an in-patient bed. Such delays have been shown to impact survival in neuromuscular [28] and COPD patients [29]. Consequently, investigators have looked at the feasibility of initiating and titrating NIV in the outpatient [25, 28, 30, 31] or home [27] settings and have reported similar clinical outcomes irrespective of the location of initial trials of NIV. A study of 67 stable hypercapnic COPD patients who were randomized to NIV initiation either as an inpatient or at-home with the use of telemedicine found no difference in gas exchange, health-related quality of life, symptoms, hospitalizations, or therapy compliance at 6 months, with substantially lower costs to initiate therapy in the at-home group [27].

The use of an attended polysomnogram (PSG) to initiate and titrate NIV in patients with COPD is no longer considered necessary to optimize therapy [12, 13]. Rather the goal is to target the normalization of CO_2, or at least reduce it significantly [8, 10, 12, 13]. This can be carried out during daytime sessions, although it may take longer to finalize settings compared to an in-patient approach [27]. In a randomized study of non-COPD patients, Hannan et al. [32] reported patients undergoing PSG-guided titration of NIV had less patient–ventilator asynchrony compared to those undergoing daytime titration only, although this did not translate to better clinical outcomes. However, patients with low initial adherence to NIV significantly improved average daily use after undergoing a PSG-guided titration. In a small observational study of COPD patients experiencing dyspnea after coming off NIV, use of PSG to review and guide NIV settings improved patient comfort and led to a marked reduction in morning breathlessness [33]. Consequently, PSG to titrate NIV settings in patients with COPD may be reserved for those experiencing problems either adapting to therapy or experiencing side effects from it. Rather, daytime titration with the goal of reducing CO_2 to within or close to normal values is recommended [8, 10, 12, 13, 27].

Interest in two-way remote monitoring of patients using home NIV has increased in recent years, with many bilevel devices designed for domiciliary NIV now routinely equipped with in-built modems and software capable of capturing, storing, and analyzing ventilation data. This technology provides the opportunity to set up NIV remotely, either by gradually adjusting settings manually or using auto-adjusting bilevel modes. Either approach reduces the need to admit patients to the hospital for NIV acclimation, with ongoing monitoring of basic ventilation data such as leak, tidal volume, upper airway obstruction, and usage to guide care. Data from a retrospective cohort study demonstrated this approach is not only feasible but also prolongs time to readmission or death within 12 months of commencing NIV compared to a comparator group of patients not using NIV [34]. Once established on home NIV, close outpatient review of patients is necessary to identify and correct ventilation issues that could impact on adherence or effectiveness of therapy, including patient–ventilator asynchronies and leak. However, patients with severe disabilities, who are socially isolated or geographically remote from specialized respiratory and home ventilation services, may find it difficult to attend regular outpatient clinics. Remote monitoring of NIV for these individuals may overcome current barriers to follow-up. Although many of these signals are yet to be validated [35, 36], monitoring and review of this information can improve the clinician's ability to recognize potential problems early and intervene to optimize ventilation. There is some evidence that remote ventilator monitoring may even provide early recognition of disease exacerbations [37].

Patient Perspective

The patient was keen to use NIV even when aerophagia was limiting how effective therapy was. As she was experiencing daytime breathlessness, "knowing the machine was there to help my breathing really helped my anxiety. It was good to put the mask on as I could relax." The patient reported she still woke up at night "but this was for coughing or going to the toilet. I'm sleeping better and longer now, especially since the machine was set up to give me bigger breaths. When they told me I needed to use a breathing machine for sleep, it upset me a bit. I knew I was getting worse, but that made it real. But I wanted to do anything I could to start to feel better and not have to go to hospital. At first it was a bit hard, but even when I was having problems early on I just told myself I had to do it and when I realized it helped me when I lost my breath, I was happy to use the machine. I was really surprised myself that the higher pressure worked so well. It's really good to have my husband there to help me with the machine, especially all the cleaning stuff. I just leave that to him. I don't want to be without the machine now."

Take-Home Messages

There is increasing evidence of improved clinical outcomes using home NIV in selected patients with stable hypercapnic COPD. However, these benefits are primarily seen in patients exhibiting a stable $PaCO_2$ level ≥ 52 mmHg at least 2–4 weeks following an episode of exacerbation. Titration of settings should be initially undertaken during daytime sessions conducted as an outpatient or in the patient's home, reserving PSG-guided titration to those experiencing issues with therapy including poor adherence or deventilation dyspnea. The goal of titration should be to maximize the reduction in CO_2 clearance, using the highest level of pressure support the patient can comfortably tolerate. Advances in ventilator technology are providing the opportunity to monitor an array of physiological and ventilator parameters remotely to identify early any issues with therapy and adjust settings accordingly.

References

1. Crimi C, Noto A, Princi P, Cuvelier A, Masa JF, Simonds A, et al. Domiciliary noninvasive ventilation in COPD: an International Survey of Indications and Practices. COPD. 2016;13(4):483–90.
2. Lloyd-Owen SJ, Donaldson GC, Ambrosino N, Escarabill J, Farre R, Fauroux B, et al. Patterns of home mechanical ventilation use in Europe: results from the Eurovent survey. Eur Respir J. 2005;25(6):1025–31.
3. Struik FM, Lacasse Y, Goldstein RS, Kerstjens HA, Wijkstra PJ. Nocturnal noninvasive positive pressure ventilation in stable COPD: a systematic review and individual patient data meta-analysis. Respir Med. 2014;108(2):329–37.

4. Osadnik CR, Tee VS, Carson-Chahhoud KV, Picot J, Wedzicha JA, Smith BJ. Non-invasive ventilation for the management of acute hypercapnic respiratory failure due to exacerbation of chronic obstructive pulmonary disease. Cochrane Database Syst Rev. 2017;7(7):CD004104.
5. Casanova C, Celli BR, Tost L, Soriano E, Abreu J, Velasco V, et al. Long-term controlled trial of nocturnal nasal positive pressure ventilation in patients with severe COPD. Chest. 2000;118(6):1582–90.
6. Lin CC. Comparison between nocturnal nasal positive pressure ventilation combined with oxygen therapy and oxygen monotherapy in patients with severe COPD. Am J Respir Crit Care Med. 1996;154(2 Pt 1):353–8.
7. McEvoy RD, Pierce RJ, Hillman D, Esterman A, Ellis EE, Catcheside PG, et al. Nocturnal non-invasive nasal ventilation in stable hypercapnic COPD: a randomised controlled trial. Thorax. 2009;64(7):561–6.
8. Kohnlein T, Windisch W, Kohler D, Drabik A, Geiseler J, Hartl S, et al. Non-invasive positive pressure ventilation for the treatment of severe stable chronic obstructive pulmonary disease: a prospective, multicentre, randomised, controlled clinical trial. Lancet Respir Med. 2014;2(9):698–705.
9. Murphy PB, Rehal S, Arbane G, Bourke S, Calverley PMA, Crook AM, et al. Effect of home noninvasive ventilation with oxygen therapy vs oxygen therapy alone on hospital readmission or death after an acute COPD exacerbation: a randomized clinical trial. JAMA. 2017;317(21):2177–86.
10. Struik FM, Sprooten RT, Kerstjens HA, Bladder G, Zijnen M, Asin J, et al. Nocturnal non-invasive ventilation in COPD patients with prolonged hypercapnia after ventilatory support for acute respiratory failure: a randomised, controlled, parallel-group study. Thorax. 2014;69(9):826–34.
11. Windisch W, Haenel M, Storre JH, Dreher M. High-intensity non-invasive positive pressure ventilation for stable hypercapnic COPD. Int J Med Sci. 2009;6(2):72–6.
12. Ergan B, Oczkowski S, Rochwerg B, Carlucci A, Chatwin M, Clini E, et al. European Respiratory Society guidelines on long-term home non-invasive ventilation for management of COPD. Eur Respir J. 2019;54(3):1901003.
13. Macrea M, Oczkowski S, Rochwerg B, Branson RD, Celli B, Coleman JM, et al. Long-term noninvasive ventilation in chronic stable hypercapnic chronic obstructive pulmonary disease. An official American Thoracic Society clinical practice guideline. Am J Respir Crit Care Med. 2020;202(4):e74–87.
14. Raveling T, Vonk J, Struik FM, Goldstein R, Kerstjens HA, Wijkstra PJ, et al. Chronic non-invasive ventilation for chronic obstructive pulmonary disease. Cochrane Database Syst Rev. 2021;8(8):CD002878.
15. Dreher M, Ekkernkamp E, Walterspacher S, Walker D, Schmoor C, Storre JH, et al. Noninvasive ventilation in COPD: impact of inspiratory pressure levels on sleep quality. Chest. 2011;140(4):939–45.
16. Duiverman ML, Maagh P, Magnet FS, Schmoor C, Arellano-Maric MP, Meissner A, et al. Impact of high-intensity-NIV on the heart in stable COPD: a randomised cross-over pilot study. Respir Res. 2017;18(1):76.
17. Nilius G, Katamadze N, Domanski U, Schroeder M, Franke KJ. Non-invasive ventilation with intelligent volume-assured pressure support versus pressure-controlled ventilation: effects on the respiratory event rate and sleep quality in COPD with chronic hypercapnia. Int J Chron Obstruct Pulmon Dis. 2017;12:1039–45.
18. Oscroft NS, Ali M, Gulati A, Davies MG, Quinnell TG, Shneerson JM, et al. A randomised crossover trial comparing volume assured and pressure preset noninvasive ventilation in stable hypercapnic COPD. COPD. 2010;7(6):398–403.
19. Storre JH, Matrosovich E, Ekkernkamp E, Walker DJ, Schmoor C, Dreher M, et al. Home mechanical ventilation for COPD: high-intensity versus target volume noninvasive ventilation. Respir Care. 2014;59(9):1389–97.
20. Kelly JL, Jaye J, Pickersgill RE, Chatwin M, Morrell MJ, Simonds AK. Randomized trial of 'intelligent' autotitrating ventilation versus standard pressure support non-invasive ventilation: impact on adherence and physiological outcomes. Respirology. 2014;19(4):596–603.

21. Piper AJ. Advances in non-invasive positive airway pressure technology. Respirology. 2020;25(4):372–82.
22. Elliott MW. The interface: crucial for successful noninvasive ventilation. Eur Respir J. 2004;23(1):7–8.
23. Callegari J, Magnet FS, Taubner S, Berger M, Schwarz SB, Windisch W, et al. Interfaces and ventilator settings for long-term noninvasive ventilation in COPD patients. Int J Chron Obstruct Pulmon Dis. 2017;12:1883–9.
24. Lebret M, Leotard A, Pepin JL, Windisch W, Ekkernkamp E, Pallero M, et al. Nasal versus oronasal masks for home non-invasive ventilation in patients with chronic hypercapnia: a systematic review and individual participant data meta-analysis. Thorax. 2021;76(11):1108–16.
25. Ribeiro C, Vieira AL, Pamplona P, Drummond M, Seabra B, Ferreira D, et al. Current practices in home mechanical ventilation for chronic obstructive pulmonary disease: a real-life cross-sectional multicentric study. Int J Chron Obstruct Pulmon Dis. 2021;16:2217–26.
26. Majorski DS, Callegari JC, Schwarz SB, Magnet FS, Majorski R, Storre JH, et al. Oronasal versus nasal masks for non-invasive ventilation in COPD: a randomized crossover trial. Int J Chron Obstruct Pulmon Dis. 2021;16:771–81.
27. Duiverman ML, Vonk JM, Bladder G, van Melle JP, Nieuwenhuis J, Hazenberg A, et al. Home initiation of chronic non-invasive ventilation in COPD patients with chronic hypercapnic respiratory failure: a randomised controlled trial. Thorax. 2020;75(3):244–52.
28. Sheers N, Berlowitz DJ, Rautela L, Batchelder I, Hopkinson K, Howard ME. Improved survival with an ambulatory model of non-invasive ventilation implementation in motor neuron disease. Amyotroph Lateral Scler Frontotemporal Degener. 2014;15(3-4):180–4.
29. Frazier WD, DaVanzo JE, Dobson A, Heath S, Mati K. Early initiation of non-invasive ventilation at home improves survival and reduces healthcare costs in COPD patients with chronic hypercapnic respiratory failure: a retrospective cohort study. Respir Med. 2022;200:106920.
30. Hazenberg A, Kerstjens HA, Prins SC, Vermeulen KM, Wijkstra PJ. Initiation of home mechanical ventilation at home: a randomised controlled trial of efficacy, feasibility and costs. Respir Med. 2014;108(9):1387–95.
31. Lujan M, Moreno A, Veigas C, Monton C, Pomares X, Domingo C. Non-invasive home mechanical ventilation: effectiveness and efficiency of an outpatient initiation protocol compared with the standard in-hospital model. Respir Med. 2007;101(6):1177–82.
32. Hannan LM, Rautela L, Berlowitz DJ, McDonald CF, Cori JM, Sheers N, et al. Randomised controlled trial of polysomnographic titration of noninvasive ventilation. Eur Respir J. 2019;53(5):1802118.
33. Adler D, Perrig S, Takahashi H, Espa F, Rodenstein D, Pepin JL, et al. Polysomnography in stable COPD under non-invasive ventilation to reduce patient-ventilator asynchrony and morning breathlessness. Sleep Breath. 2012;16(4):1081–90.
34. McDowell G, Sumowski M, Toellner H, Karok S, O'Dwyer C, Hornsby J, et al. Assistive technologies for home NIV in patients with COPD: feasibility and positive experience with remote-monitoring and volume-assured auto-EPAP NIV mode. BMJ Open Respir Res. 2021;8(1):e000828.
35. Contal O, Vignaux L, Combescure C, Pepin JL, Jolliet P, Janssens JP. Monitoring of non-invasive ventilation by built-in software of home bilevel ventilators: a bench study. Chest. 2012;141(2):469–76.
36. Stagnara A, Baboi L, Nesme P, Subtil F, Louis B, Guerin C. Reliability of tidal volume in average volume assured pressure support mode. Respir Care. 2018;63(9):1139–46.
37. Borel JC, Pelletier J, Taleux N, Briault A, Arnol N, Pison C, et al. Parameters recorded by software of non-invasive ventilators predict COPD exacerbation: a proof-of-concept study. Thorax. 2015;70(3):284–5.

Chapter 29
Sleep-Disordered Breathing in Concomitant Chronic Obstructive Pulmonary Disease and Obstructive Sleep Apnea: The Overlap Syndrome

Amanda J. Piper (iD)

Introduction

A significant proportion of people with chronic obstructive pulmonary disease (COPD) also have obstructive sleep apnea (OSA) and when this occurs, it is referred to as the overlap syndrome. This co-occurrence of OSA and COPD is associated with a higher burden of health impairments compared to either disorder alone, including poorer quality of life [1], higher risk of hospitalization [2], and reduced survival [3]. However, in many patients with COPD, the presence of OSA goes unrecognized and untreated. While continuous positive airway pressure (CPAP) is the treatment of choice for uncomplicated OSA of moderate or greater severity, the optimal form of positive airway pressure (PAP) therapy in overlap syndrome and its effects on clinical outcomes not been rigorously investigated. The goal of this case study is to highlight current practices and issues to consider when using PAP therapy in patients with overlap syndrome.

Patient Information

A 71-year-old man with previously diagnosed COPD presented to the Emergency Department (ED) with fevers, shortness of breath, lethargy, and decreased appetite. He was hypoxic and the chest X-ray showed right middle and upper zone consolidation. He tested positive for Coronavirus Disease-2019 (COVID-19) and was

A. J. Piper (✉)
Respiratory Support Service, Department of Respiratory and Sleep Medicine, Royal Prince Alfred Hospital, Camperdown, NSW, Australia

C. Frange (ed.), *Clinical Cases in Sleep Physical Therapy*,
https://doi.org/10.1007/978-3-031-38340-3_29

transferred to intensive care unit (ICU) with diagnoses of pneumococcal pneumonia superimposed on COVID-19 and acute infective exacerbation of COPD. During the admission, staff observed loud snoring with periods of apnea and desaturation. As part of his discharge plan, an outpatient diagnostic sleep study was arranged to determine if obstructive sleep apnea was present and if so, its severity.

His past medical history included a 20-pack-year smoking history, having quit 25 years ago, and liver cirrhosis from alcohol and non-alcoholic fatty liver disease. The patient has bilateral total knee replacements, mobilizes with a walking stick, and lives with a carer who assists him in completing some activities of daily living such as cooking, cleaning, and shopping. He experiences significant back pain from time to time, which can impact his sleep. His current regular medications include Frusemide, Spironolactone, Salbutamol, and Umeclidinium/Vilanterol.

Clinical Findings

The physical examination was unremarkable apart from morbid obesity with a body mass index of 40 kg/m^2. His resting SpO_2 was 95% on room air with a heart rate of 82 bpm. He had no signs of lower leg edema, and his jugular venous pressure was not raised. He reported frequent nocturia.

Timeline

August 2022	Presents to ED with fevers and lethargy; diagnosed with pneumococcal pneumonia, COVID-19, and an acute exacerbation of COPD; transferred to ICU and after 10-day hospital admission, discharged home
September 2022	Diagnostic sleep study performed, in laboratory
October 2022	CPAP titration study, in laboratory
February 2023	CPAP review study

Diagnostic Assessment

Subjectively, the patient denied daytime somnolence, recording an Epworth Sleepiness Score of 9 (normal $\leq$10). Lung function testing confirmed moderate airway obstruction with reduced Forced expiratory volume in one second (FEV1) (59% predicted) and Forced vital capacity (FVC) (72% predicted) values, giving an FEV1/FVC ratio of 62%. Expiratory reserve volume was reduced at 0.48 L (47% predicted), reflecting his significant obesity. He declined an arterial blood gas but awake lying stable transcutaneous carbon dioxide monitoring ($TcCO_2$) over a 20-min period showed values within the normal range.

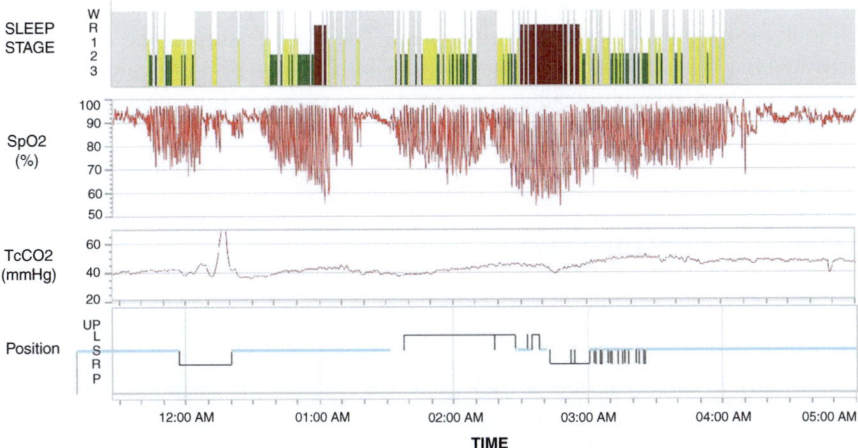

Fig. 29.1 Summary of the overnight diagnostic study. Obstructive events with significant desaturation occurred in all sleep stages and body positions. No N3 (slow wave sleep) was seen on this night. *R* rapid eye movement (REM) sleep, *SpO₂* oxygen saturation measured by pulse oximetry, *TcCO₂* transcutaneous carbon dioxide monitoring, *W* wake. Body positions: *L* left sidelying, *P* prone, *R* right sidelying, *S* supine

A diagnostic polysomnogram was performed in the sleep laboratory. Sleep efficiency was poor (45%) and highly fragmented. No slow wave (N3) sleep was observed. Baseline SpO_2 awake was 95%, with a nadir of 55% during rapid eye movement (REM) sleep and an oxygen desaturation index of 70 events/h. Average SpO_2 in non-REM (NREM) sleep was 86% and 77% in REM sleep, with 63% of total sleep time spent with SpO_2 <90%. Baseline $TcCO_2$ was 44 mmHg and rose no more than 5–6 mmHg across the night (Fig. 29.1).

A diagnosis of overlap syndrome (COPD and severe OSA) was made and, after discussing the results and the potential implications of severe sleep-disordered breathing, he agreed to undergo a trial of positive airway pressure (PAP).

Physiotherapeutic Intervention

Given the severity of the obstructive events and lack of evidence for sleep or daytime hypoventilation ($TcCO_2$ within the normal range), continuous positive airway pressure (CPAP) was set up and titrated overnight. Both nasal and oronasal mask styles were trialed, but he had difficulty breathing comfortably through his nose, and was switched to an oronasal mask. Overnight, the pressure was titrated in increments of 1 cmH₂O to abolish obstructive events, flow limitation, and snoring, with special note taken of gas exchange and airflow morphology when the patient was supine. A pressure of 16 cmH₂O was recommended and he returned home to trial this.

He was asked to use CPAP nightly across the entire sleep period. Initially, he had difficulty using the device due to sinus pain. The ramp feature of the device was activated to aid in acclimation to the pressure with the aim of improving tolerance. In addition, heated humidification was added. Both strategies improved comfort and acceptance of CPAP.

Follow-Up and Outcomes

A review sleep study on CPAP was arranged for 3 months later, although this was not part of usual care. Sleep efficiency remained poor (51%) with long periods awake early in the night due to back pain. He reported his sleep as "worse than usual." REM sleep accounted for 44% of the time he did sleep and N3 sleep was now seen, accounting for 25% of total sleep time. Nadir oxygen saturation was 92% on CPAP, with an average SpO_2 in NREM sleep of 96%, and 97% in REM sleep. CPAP at 16 cmH$_2$O was confirmed as effective pressure in all sleep stages and body positions (Fig. 29.2). His usage over the previous 4 weeks was 7.2 h/night and his Epworth Sleepiness Score had fallen to 5. He was willing to continue CPAP longer term.

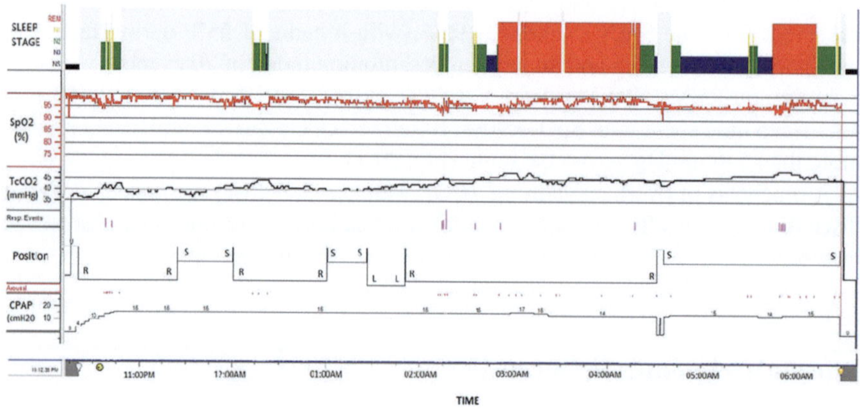

Fig. 29.2 Summary of the follow-up CPAP study. Overnight, CPAP was increased in 1 cmH$_2$O increments to abolish obstructive apneas and hypopneas, snoring, and flow limitation. At 15 cmH$_2$O, CPAP in REM and in the supine position was found to be effective. *R* rapid eye movement (REM) sleep, *SpO$_2$* oxygen saturation measured by pulse oximetry, *TcCO$_2$* transcutaneous carbon dioxide monitoring, *W* wake. Body positions: *L* left sidelying, *P* prone, *R* right sidelying, *S* supine

Discussion

OSA is a highly prevalent disorder in the general population [4] and has been reported to occur in 10–65% of patients with COPD [5, 6]. This wide range in reported prevalence likely reflects differences in how sleep breathing abnormalities were measured and defined, the degree of obesity present, and the population sampled [7]. The presence of overlap represents a severe COPD phenotype, with clinical outcomes of COPD–OSA substantially worse than those seen in either disorder alone, with more impaired quality of life [1, 5], higher risk of acute exacerbations and hospitalizations [3, 5, 8], higher health care costs [9], increased cardiovascular morbidity [10, 11], higher risk of developing cognitive impairment, and reduced survival [3, 10, 12] reported. Gas exchange is also generally more impaired in patients with overlap compared to those with OSA or COPD in isolation [13]. Compared to uncomplicated OSA, patients with overlap are less likely to report symptoms typical of OSA such as snoring, daytime sleepiness, and morning headaches, despite having a similar severity of sleep-disordered breathing [14]. Even when present, these symptoms may be inappropriately attributed to COPD. In others, the symptoms reported may be more atypical such as nocturia [14], resulting in the diagnosis of sleep-disordered breathing not being recognized. In either circumstance, the opportunity to address a modifiable issue contributing to longer-term morbidity and mortality in this population is missed [5].

CPAP is widely recommended in the management of moderate to severe OSA, with several large, randomized trials demonstrating improvements in daytime sleepiness and health-related quality of life with therapy [15]. However, the benefits of CPAP in modifying cardiovascular and metabolic risks associated with OSA are yet to be confirmed [16–18]. Patients with overlap syndrome have generally been excluded from these trials, and despite OSA being highly prevalent in COPD, few high-quality studies have looked at the impact of PAP therapy on long-term outcomes. Recently, this gap in knowledge was formally addressed and ongoing research priorities in this patient population established [7]. Nevertheless, observational studies in patients with overlap syndrome have demonstrated CPAP ameliorates sleep-disordered breathing and improves OSA-related symptoms such as sleepiness, regardless of the severity of the underlying respiratory impairment [19]. However, symptoms more associated with COPD such as breathlessness may not improve with CPAP [19].

Several large longitudinal observational studies have investigated the impact of CPAP and mortality in overlap syndrome. In the first major study, Marin et al. [3] followed 228 overlap patients managed with CPAP, 213 overlap patients not using CPAP therapy, and 210 COPD-only patients over a mean of 9.4 years. In the untreated overlap group, all-cause mortality and mortality from cardiovascular causes were higher than in either the CPAP-treated overlap or the COPD-only groups. In a prospective study of 603 patients with more severe COPD who were already receiving long-term oxygen therapy, Machado et al. [20] identified 95 individuals who had overlap syndrome with moderate to severe OSA. Sixty-one of these patients (64%) agreed to and were adherent to CPAP therapy. In this study, the 5-year survival estimates in the CPAP-adherent overlap patients was 71% compared to 26% in the non-CPAP group ($p < 0.001$), with the cause of death primarily from respiratory failure or cardiovascular disease in both groups. While most studies have not stratified patients according to their level of awake CO_2, Jaoude et al. [12] suggested the reduction in excess mortality in this population may be confined to those individuals who are also hypercapnia, although this is yet to be confirmed by other studies.

Identifying and treating OSA–COPD overlap may also provide a mechanism to reduce avoidable admission and readmissions due to exacerbations of lung disease, and hence improve longer-term health and quality of life outcomes. Several studies have reported a reduction in the risk of hospitalization for an exacerbation of lung disease once CPAP is commenced in these patients [2, 3, 21]. In an analysis of discharge data from more than 1.6 million COPD exacerbations occurring between 2010 and 2016, the presence of OSA increased the odds of a 30-day readmission of patients with COPD, irrespective of whether the patient had obesity or not [2]. However, given the retrospective nature of these studies, there is the potential for confounding factors to bias findings in favor of CPAP.

In the absence of large, well-designed randomized trials [21], clinical management of sleep-disordered breathing in overlap is currently guided by the findings from observational studies and extrapolations from evidence-based recommendations for use of PAP therapy in patients with stable hypercapnic COPD [22] and obesity hypoventilation syndrome [23]. While CPAP is used as initial therapy in most patients [3, 19, 20, 24–26], around 20–25% will likely require bilevel therapy to optimize nocturnal gas exchange [3, 26, 27]. Although not well studied, characteristics of overlap patients most likely to fail CPAP therapy include greater severity of COPD based on spirometric values, more severe obesity, or the presence of hypercapnia during wakefulness [26, 27]. In the only randomized trial to date, Zheng et al. [28] randomized 32 stable hypercapnic patients with overlap syndrome who were morbidly obese to either CPAP or bilevel therapy set in the spontaneous mode for a 3-month period. Both forms of PAP therapy resulted in significant decreases in $PaCO_2$, with bilevel therapy superior to CPAP (9.4 mmHg [95% confidence interval, 4.3–15 mmHg; $p = 0.001$]) in this small study population. However, no between-group differences in other secondary endpoints including adherence to PAP, daytime sleepiness, sleep quality, or neurocognitive function were seen. Larger and longer-term studies comparing different forms of PAP therapy and to no therapy are required in this population [7, 21], and should be stratified for the level of awake hypercapnia, the severity of COPD, and obesity to better appreciate when CPAP or bilevel therapy is most likely to optimize clinical outcomes.

While the "dose" or amount of PAP usage per night to achieve benefit in overlap syndrome is not known, most centers use a definition of adherence of ≥4 h of use per night for ≥70% of nights over a 30-day period [2, 25, 27]. CPAP use has been shown to be an independent predictor of mortality [24, 25], with higher adherence to CPAP associated with longer survival [25]. Lower CPAP usage has also been associated with an increased risk of COPD exacerbations [24]. In a retrospective study of over 6600 overlap patients where PAP usage was monitored remotely and linked to a claims database, a clinically significant reduction in the risk of Emergency Department visits, hospitalizations, compared to health care costs was seen in PAP-adherent compared to non-adherent patients over a 2-year period [2]. Common causes for non-adherence in patients with overlap include claustrophobia, poor mask fit, and excessive leak around the mask [24]. Increasing age and number of comorbid conditions have also been associated with lower usage in this population [25]. Although these latter factors are not modifiable, they may be useful in identifying individuals in whom closer monitoring and support are required to encourage and promote CPAP use.

Take-Home Message

A high level of clinical suspicion regarding the presence of OSA should be used when reviewing patients with COPD given the high prevalence of overlap syndrome and the consequences on morbidity and mortality of not treating OSA in this population. These patients may not present with the traditional symptoms of OSA, and it is important not to simply assume all respiratory symptoms reported are due to their underlying COPD alone. There is significant scope to undertake well-designed studies evaluating the optimal PAP mode in these patients, and how their clinical phenotype may impact on clinical response and adherence to PAP therapy. The management of sleep-disordered breathing is emerging as the new frontier in improving outcomes in patients with COPD.

Patient Perspective

When asked about his perspectives regarding CPAP as long-term therapy, the patient reported it was worthwhile for the benefits he obtained from it. "I am sleeping for much longer now, although I still get up to urinate during the night—I'm on fluid tablets. It can be a bit difficult to put up with when I have the mask on and need to also put my glasses on to read. But I've worked out a way. I have to do both as I don't trust myself not to fall off to sleep without the machine while I'm reading in bed. It took me a bit of time to get used to the pressure, and I used the ramp button a lot when I first started, but now I'm used to the mask and the pressure and haven't used the ramp for a while. I also had some problems with my sinuses early on—I found my mouth and nose became really dry and that caused pain and limited me using the mask. But since adding the humidifier, my sinuses are great. I've got to the point now that if I don't use it for some reason, like when it's really hot at night, I miss it."

References

1. Mermigkis C, Kopanakis A, Foldvary-Schaefer N, Golish J, Polychronopoulos V, Schiza S, et al. Health-related quality of life in patients with obstructive sleep apnoea and chronic obstructive pulmonary disease (overlap syndrome). Int J Clin Pract. 2007;61(2):207–11.
2. Sterling KL, Pepin JL, Linde-Zwirble W, Chen J, Benjafield AV, Cistulli PA, et al. Impact of positive airway pressure therapy adherence on outcomes in patients with obstructive sleep apnea and chronic obstructive pulmonary disease. Am J Respir Crit Care Med. 2022;206(2):197–205.
3. Marin JM, Soriano JB, Carrizo SJ, Boldova A, Celli BR. Outcomes in patients with chronic obstructive pulmonary disease and obstructive sleep apnea: the overlap syndrome. Am J Respir Crit Care Med. 2010;182(3):325–31.
4. Benjafield AV, Ayas NT, Eastwood PR, Heinzer R, Ip MSM, Morrell MJ, et al. Estimation of the global prevalence and burden of obstructive sleep apnoea: a literature-based analysis. Lancet Respir Med. 2019;7(8):687–98.
5. Donovan LM, Feemster LC, Udris EM, Griffith MF, Spece LJ, Palen BN, et al. Poor outcomes among patients with chronic obstructive pulmonary disease with higher risk for undiagnosed obstructive sleep apnea in the LOTT cohort. J Clin Sleep Med. 2019;15(1):71–7.
6. Shawon MS, Perret JL, Senaratna CV, Lodge C, Hamilton GS, Dharmage SC. Current evidence on prevalence and clinical outcomes of co-morbid obstructive sleep apnea and chronic obstructive pulmonary disease: a systematic review. Sleep Med Rev. 2017;32:58–68.
7. Malhotra A, Schwartz AR, Schneider H, Owens RL, DeYoung P, Han MK, et al. Research priorities in pathophysiology for sleep-disordered breathing in patients with chronic obstructive pulmonary disease. An Official American Thoracic Society Research Statement. Am J Respir Crit Care Med. 2018;197(3):289–99.
8. Channick JE, Jackson NJ, Zeidler MR, Buhr RG. Effects of obstructive sleep apnea and obesity on 30-day readmissions in patients with chronic obstructive pulmonary disease: a cross-sectional mediation analysis. Ann Am Thorac Soc. 2022;19(3):462–8.
9. Schwab P, Dhamane AD, Hopson SD, Moretz C, Annavarapu S, Burslem K, et al. Impact of comorbid conditions in COPD patients on health care resource utilization and costs in a predominantly Medicare population. Int J Chron Obstruct Pulmon Dis. 2017;12:735–44.
10. Kendzerska T, Leung RS, Aaron SD, Ayas N, Sandoz JS, Gershon AS. Cardiovascular outcomes and all-cause mortality in patients with obstructive sleep apnea and chronic obstructive pulmonary disease (overlap syndrome). Ann Am Thorac Soc. 2019;16(1):71–81.
11. Luehrs RE, Moreau KL, Pierce GL, Wamboldt F, Aloia M, Weinberger HD, et al. Cognitive performance is lower among individuals with overlap syndrome than in individuals with COPD or obstructive sleep apnea alone: association with carotid artery stiffness. J Appl Physiol. 2021;131(1):131–41.
12. Jaoude P, Kufel T, El-Solh AA. Survival benefit of CPAP favors hypercapnic patients with the overlap syndrome. Lung. 2014;192(2):251–8.
13. Chaouat A, Weitzenblum E, Krieger J, Ifoundza T, Oswald M, Kessler R. Association of chronic obstructive pulmonary disease and sleep apnea syndrome. Am J Respir Crit Care Med. 1995;151(1):82–6.
14. Adler D, Bailly S, Benmerad M, Joyeux-Faure M, Jullian-Desayes I, Soccal PM, et al. Clinical presentation and comorbidities of obstructive sleep apnea-COPD overlap syndrome. PLoS One. 2020;15(7):e0235331.
15. Patil SP, Ayappa IA, Caples SM, Kimoff RJ, Patel SR, Harrod CG. Treatment of adult obstructive sleep apnea with positive airway pressure: an American Academy of Sleep Medicine systematic review, meta-analysis, and GRADE assessment. J Clin Sleep Med. 2019;15(2):301–34.
16. Gottlieb DJ, Punjabi NM. Diagnosis and management of obstructive sleep apnea: a review. J Am Med Assoc. 2020;323(14):1389–400.
17. McEvoy RD, Antic NA, Heeley E, Luo Y, Ou Q, Zhang X, et al. CPAP for prevention of cardiovascular events in obstructive sleep apnea. N Engl J Med. 2016;375(10):919–31.

18. Sanchez-de-la-Torre M, Sanchez-de-la-Torre A, Bertran S, Abad J, Duran-Cantolla J, Cabriada V, et al. Effect of obstructive sleep apnoea and its treatment with continuous positive airway pressure on the prevalence of cardiovascular events in patients with acute coronary syndrome (ISAACC study): a randomised controlled trial. Lancet Respir Med. 2020;8(4):359–67.
19. Adler D, Bailly S, Soccal PM, Janssens JP, Sapene M, Grillet Y, et al. Symptomatic response to CPAP in obstructive sleep apnea versus COPD-obstructive sleep apnea overlap syndrome: insights from a large national registry. PLoS One. 2021;16(8):e0256230.
20. Machado MC, Vollmer WM, Togeiro SM, Bilderback AL, Oliveira MV, Leitao FS, et al. CPAP and survival in moderate-to-severe obstructive sleep apnoea syndrome and hypoxaemic COPD. Eur Respir J. 2010;35(1):132–7.
21. National Guideline Centre (UK). Positive airway pressure therapy variants for OSAHS, OHS and COPD–OSAHS overlap syndrome: obstructive sleep apnoea/hypopnoea syndrome and obesity hypoventilation syndrome in over 16s: evidence review F. London: National Institute for Health and Care Excellence (NICE); 2021. Available from https://www.ncbi.nlm.nih.gov/books/NBK574326/. Accessed Jan 2023.
22. Macrea M, Oczkowski S, Rochwerg B, Branson RD, Celli B, Coleman JM, et al. Long-term noninvasive ventilation in chronic stable hypercapnic chronic obstructive pulmonary disease. An Official American Thoracic Society Clinical Practice Guideline. Am J Respir Crit Care Med. 2020;202(4):e74–87.
23. Mokhlesi B, Masa JF, Brozek JL, Gurubhagavatula I, Murphy PB, Piper AJ, et al. Evaluation and management of obesity hypoventilation syndrome. An Official American Thoracic Society clinical practice guideline. Am J Respir Crit Care Med. 2019;200(3):e6–e24.
24. Jaoude P, El-Solh AA. Predictive factors for COPD exacerbations and mortality in patients with overlap syndrome. Clin Respir J. 2019;13(10):643–51.
25. Stanchina ML, Welicky LM, Donat W, Lee D, Corrao W, Malhotra A. Impact of CPAP use and age on mortality in patients with combined COPD and obstructive sleep apnea: the overlap syndrome. J Clin Sleep Med. 2013;9(8):767–72.
26. Kuklisova Z, Tkacova R, Joppa P, Wouters E, Sastry M. Severity of nocturnal hypoxia and daytime hypercapnia predicts CPAP failure in patients with COPD and obstructive sleep apnea overlap syndrome. Sleep Med. 2017;30:139–45.
27. Schreiber A, Cemmi F, Ambrosino N, Ceriana P, Lastoria C, Carlucci A. Prevalence and predictors of obstructive sleep apnea in patients with chronic obstructive pulmonary disease undergoing inpatient pulmonary rehabilitation. Chronic Obstr Pulm Dis. 2018;15(3):265–70.
28. Zheng Y, Yee BJ, Wong K, Grunstein R, Piper A. A pilot randomized trial comparing CPAP vs bilevel PAP spontaneous mode in the treatment of hypoventilation disorder in patients with obesity and obstructive airway disease. J Clin Sleep Med. 2022;18(1):99–107.

Chapter 30
Long-Term Telemonitoring
in Sleep-Related Breathing Disorders

Carlos Maria Franceschini ⓘ and Mariana Gussoni

Introduction

We are introducing a clinical case whereby we may assess the importance and value of telemonitoring [1], as a tool that provides for properly treating sleep-related breathing disorders (SBD), which require specialized diagnostic and treatment centers—there are few and they are far from patients' homes. Such information entails long waiting times until patients may get an appointment and expense increases [2].

Patient Information

M.B.F., a 38-year-old man, lives 750 km away from the specialized diagnostic center. He has six children (four of them with congenital central alveolar hypoventilation syndrome, two of them use Bilevel machines with oronasal masks, one of them uses a volumetric ventilator with a mask, and the other one uses a volumetric ventilator through a tracheostomy). M.B.F. lives in his house with his children, his wife, his mother, and the nurse responsible for monitoring the medical home care of his son, who is on a ventilator with a tracheostomy. He has a supportive family environment, but he is facing a hard economic and labor situation. At times, he undergoes times of discouragement requiring psychological support.

C. M. Franceschini (✉)
Sleep and Mechanical Ventilation Unit, Cosme Argerich Hospital, Buenos Aires, Argentina

M. Gussoni
Argentine Association of Respiratory Medicine (AAMR) and Argentine Society of Cardiorespiratory Kinesiology (SAKICARE), Buenos Aires, Argentina

C. Frange (ed.), *Clinical Cases in Sleep Physical Therapy*,
https://doi.org/10.1007/978-3-031-38340-3_30

Clinical Findings

The patient had a body mass index (BMI) of 37 kg/m^2, high blood pressure (HBP), non-insulin-dependent diabetes, neck circumference of 47 cm, excessive daytime drowsiness, non-positional snorer, morning headache, memory, and concentration disorders. The blood gases showed hypercapnia and hypoxemia. He was diagnosed with congenital central alveolar hypoventilation syndrome in 2018 due to a PHOX2b gene mutation at the disease reference center. A polysomnography (PSG) test with overnight oximetry was conducted, which showed severe central sleep apnea with continuous desaturation and tachycardia–bradycardia.

Positive airway pressure (PAP) titration was initiated with non-invasive ventilation (NIV), inspiratory support pressure of 15–20 cmH$_2$O, and expiratory positive airway pressure (EPAP) from 10 to 14 cmH$_2$O, with a safe respiratory rate (RR) of 16 breaths/min. An extra-large oronasal mask was used and it was decided to perform PAP titration via telemonitoring along with oximetry during 45 running days, considering the difficulty to tolerate the increasing inspiratory pressure required to reach the saturation rate. The patient adhered to NIV with an improvement in neurocognitive symptoms. In addition, there has been a BMI decrease, and control of HBP and diabetes.

Timeline

July 2018: The hospital staff caring for his children at the sleep-related breathing disorders reference pediatric hospital observed the patient's apneas

August 2018: A polysomnography (PSG) with PAP titration was performed at a sleep center in his province; he was prescribed Bilevel pressure parameters he could not tolerate, and ventilation was never initiated

October 2018: New PSG at the sleep center and reference ventilation with PAP titration; start of NIV with high difficulty and low tolerance

November 2018: Start of PAP titration through telemonitoring and virtual oximetry monitoring

December 2018: Ventilation and lung function testing; started using NIV, stabilizing overnight oximetry levels and improving the neurocognitive symptoms. Final NIV parameters: inspiratory positive airway pressure (IPAP) max: 22 cmH$_2$O; IPAP min: 18 cmH$_2$O; EPAP: 12 cmH$_2$O; RR: 16 breaths/min; inspiratory time: 0.8 s, with an extra-large XL oronasal mask

March 2019: New PSG with Bilevel S/T average volume-assured pressure support (AVAPS)

July 2019: Weight loss, BMI lowering from 36 to 31 kg/m^2, and HBP stabilization with an antihypertensive therapy

September 2019: Patient with acute respiratory insufficiency due to pneumonia admitted to the intensive care unit (ICU), ventilated with NIV, and started with oxygen therapy and antibiotic treatment; he was then changed from an ICU ventilator to his own ventilator, and pressures were titrated again via telemonitoring while in hospital, before transferring the patient to his home

October 2020: He reported excessive daytime drowsiness, and new hypercapnia, bronchial disorder, fever, and mucopurulent secretions were registered; he was treated with antibiotics and 7-day rest

May 2021: Isolated at home because of Coronavirus Disease-2019 (COVID-19) pandemic; NIV with AB filter

July 2021: New PSG under NIV with results within normal parameters

November 2021: New ventilation and lung laboratory within normal parameters; stable with ventilation

May 2022: Stable patient; normal pulse oximetry during sleep and with no neurocognitive symptoms

November 2022: Stable patient adhered to NIV

Diagnostic Test

Several diagnostic tests have been carried out (Tables 30.1, 30.2, 30.3, 30.4, 30.5, and 30.6) and briefly commented below.

Spirometry

Spirometry was within normal limits, without fall in maneuvers on dorsal decubitus position. Bulbar immunity was in terms of peak flow. The maximum static pressures are within normal limits (Table 30.1).

Lung Volumes

Table 30.2 depicts the increase in the expiratory reserve volume, after the significant decrease in BMI and adherence to the use of NIV. Volumes are within normal limits, without air entrapment, but there was a reduced expiratory reserve volume.

Table 30.1 Spirometry

Spirometry	18 September 2018 (%)	15 September 2021 (%)
Seated FVC	95.3	93.3
FVC at rest	96.1	95.4
FEV1	99.5	98.1
FEV1/FVC	86.5	87.1
FEP	119	108

FEP flow expiratory peak, *FEV1* forced expiratory volume in the first second, *FVC* forced vital capacity

Table 30.2 Lung volumes

Slow vital capacity (SVC)	18 September 2018 (%)	15 September 2021 (%)
SVC	89	88
CI	127	122
ERV	15	68
FEV1/SVC	110	103
Volumes		
TLC (N2)	93	89
FRC (N2)	58	61
RV (N2)	96	94
RV/TLC (N2)	102	105

CI capacity inspiratory, *ERV* expiratory reserve volume, *FEV1* forced expiratory volume in the first second, *FRC* functional residual capacity, *N2* nitrogen, *RV* residual volume, *SVC* slow vital capacity, *TLC* total lung capacity

Table 30.3 Carbon monoxide diffusing capacity (DLCO)

CO diffusion	18 September 2018 (%)	15 September 2021 (%)
DLCO unc	140	92
Hgb (g/dL)	15.6	13.1
DLCO cor	125	88
VA	84	77
DL/VA	149	93

CO carbon monoxide, *DL* DLCO, *DLCO unc* carbon monoxide diffusing capacity uncorrected, *DLCO cor* DLCO corrected, *Hgb* hemoglobin, *VA* alveolar volume

Carbon Monoxide Diffusing Capacity

Carbon monoxide diffusing capacity (DLCO) was adjusted for hemoglobin measured at the time of performing this investigation; increased DLCO; alveolar volume measured by the single-breath method within normal limits; the diffusing capacity adjusted to increased alveolar volume; and the reduced expiratory reserve volume are related to obesity (Table 30.3).

Ventilation Control

Arterial blood gases showed a slight increase in hypercapnia, bicarbonate, and base excess, consistent with daytime hypersomnia; the ventilation study showed a flat P01/PetCO$_2$ curve, compatible with an alteration of respiratory centers; new ventilation control in 2021 showed arterial blood gases within normal parameters, with a tendency toward respiratory alkalosis; the ventilation control study along with a response to hypercapnia showed a depressed P0.1/PetCO$_2$ curve, compatible with an alteration of respiratory centers (Table 30.4).

Table 30.4 Ventilation control

Static pressures	18 September 2018 (%)	15 September 2021 (%)
Pi max	146	134
Pe max	192	177
Voluntary apnea		
Check 1		
Apnea time (s)	41	40
$SatO_2$ apnea (%)	97	96
Check 2		
Apnea time (s)	38	36
$SatO_2$ apnea (%)	95	95
Ventilation control		
P01 basal	1.2	1.1
P01 end max	5.3	5.5
PCO_2 basal	45	41
PCO_2 max	67	61
PCO_{2Gap}	22	20
$P01/PCO_{2Slope}$	0.07 (VN: 0.22 ± 0.09)	0.05 (VN: 0.22 ± 0.09)
Borg 1	5	5
Borg 2	5	5
Average Borg test	5	5

Borg Borg Dyspnea scale, *P01* inspiratory occlusion pressure in the first 100 ms, *PCO₂* carbon dioxide blood pressure, *Pe max* maximum expiratory pressure, *Pi max* maximum inspiratory pressure, *SatO₂* oxygen saturation

Cardiorespiratory Oxygen Consumption

There were no electrocardiogram (ECG) changes in ischemia or arrhythmia (Table 30.5); blood pressure was normal; the oxygen consumption (VO_2) was limited by symptoms such as dyspnea and due to a VO_2 plateau; aerobic performance was reduced; there was no cardiovascular or ventilatory limitation; progressive hypercapnia was without limitation as to the ventilatory mechanics, compatible with ventilation control disorders.

Polysomnography Under NIV Titration and Arterial Blood Gases

In the PSG examination, after adherence to the NIV, an increase in slow sleep stage (non-rapid eye movement [NREM] N3) and in $SatO_2$ was observed, and a decrease in apnea–hypopnea index (AHI) and PCO_2 (Table 30.6); sleep fragmentation and increase of arousals were noticed, with increase in light sleep (NREM N1 sleep stage), absence of slow wave sleep (NREM N3 sleep stage), predominant central sleep apneas, and fewer obstructive AHI, 45 ev/h; pulse oximetry was with

Table 30.5 Cardiorespiratory oxygen consumption study

Oxygen consumption study	18 September 2018 (%)	15 September 2021 (%)
Aerobic capacity	AT/VO$_2$ max	VO$_2$ max/theoretical
VO$_2$ (mL/min)	52	61
VO$_2$ (mL/kg/min)	52	61
METs	52	61
Cardiovascular	AT/VO$_2$ max	VO$_2$ max/theoretical
HR (BPM)	80	81
HRR (BPM)	186	165
VO$_2$/HR (mL/beat)	65	75
Ventilatory		
VE BTPS (L/min)	43	33
BR (L/min)	119	119
Tv BTPS (L)	53	68
RR (br/min)	81	84
Ti/tot	98	98
Gas exchange		
VE/VO$_2$	82	78
VE/VCO$_2$	108	74
PETO$_2$	90	91
PETCO$_2$	93	94

AT anaerobic treshold, *BPM* beats per minute, *BR* breathing rate, *BTPS* body temperature, pressure, saturated, *HR* heart rate, *HRR* heart rate reserve, *METs* metabolic equivalent, *PETCO$_2$* transcutaneous carbon dioxide pressure, *PETO$_2$* transcutaneous oxygen pressure, *RR* respiratory rate, *Ti/tot* inspiratory time over total time, *Tv* tidal volume, *VE/VCO$_2$* slope between minute ventilation and carbon dioxide production, *VE/VO$_2$* slope between minute ventilation and oxygen production, *VO$_2$* oxygen consumption

hypoventilation pattern, and saturation index per hour of sleep was 55 desat/h; PAP titration was with continuous positive airway pressure (CPAP), spontaneous mode Bilevel, and S/T for time performed; and finally the best response was obtained under the S/T mode with average volume-assured pressure support (AVAPS); the oximetry could be stabilized with saturations of 90–92%, with max IPAP 20 cmH$_2$O, min IPAP 16 cmH$_2$O, EPAP 11 cmH$_2$O, RR 16 breath/min, tidal volume (Tv) 600 mL, and inspiratory time 0.9 second, with extra-large size oronasal mask.

6-Minute Walking Test

Distance walked: 435 m for a predicted walking distance of 602 m (72.1%); satisfactory effort; reduced walked distance; mild basal oxygen desaturation with the walk.

Table 30.6 Polysomnography under NIV titration and arterial blood gases examinations

Polysomnography under NIV titration	18 October 2018	15 March 2019	15 July 2021
Hypnogram			
NREM N1 sleep stage (% of total sleep time)	2	4	1
NREM N2 sleep stage (% of total sleep time)	76	63	64
NREM N3 sleep stage (% of total sleep time)	0	14	16
REM sleep stage (% of total sleep time)	18	16	17
Arousal (ev/h)	4	3	2
Sleep efficiency (%)	93	95	97
Respiratory indexes (ev/h)			
Apnea–hypopnea index	45	12	2
Obstructive events	16	10	0
Central events	27	2	2
Mixed events	2	0	0
Pulse oximetry			
IDO_3 3% oxygen desaturation index	39	4	1
Average $SatO_2$ (%)	78	91	99
Minimum $SatO_2$ (%)	61	82	86
Average heart rate	92	97	81
Maximum heart rate	127	112	109
Minimum heart rate	42	56	59
Arterial blood gases			
pH	7.33	7.41	7.42
PO_2	69.5	74.9	83.4
PCO_2	53.1	45.5	41.2
BIC	29.9	28.8	26.7
BE	3.3	4.0	2.0
$SatO_{2\,oxygen\,saturation}$ (%)	92.3	94.8	96.4

AHI apnea–hypopnea index, *BIC* bicarbonate, *BE* base excess, *Ev/h* events per hour, *NREM* non-REM, *REM* rapid eye movement, *PO₂* arterial oxygen pressure, *PCO₂* carbon dioxide blood pressure

Doppler Echocardiography

The Doppler echocardiography registered: pulmonary systolic blood pressure of 25 mmHg and enlarged left ventricle with normal biventricular function.

Laboratory Tests

Laboratory tests are shown in Table 30.7.

Table 30.7 Laboratory

	2018	2019	2021
Glucose (mg/dL)	236	94	92
Lactate (mmol/L)	2	1.2	1.7
Hematocrit (%)	44.8	41.1	39.2
Hemoglobin (g/dL)	15.6	13.9	13.1

Congenital Central Alveolar Hypoventilation Syndrome Diagnostic Criteria

A and B criteria must be complied with:

(a) Presence of hypoventilation related to sleep
(b) PHOX2b gene mutation

Hypoventilation during sleep may be related to daytime hypoventilation or normal $PaCO_2$; the PSG shows severe hypercapnia and oxygen desaturation. Some central apneas were observed, but the prevailing pattern was a tidal volume/flow reduction. Although the condition is deemed congenital, some patients with a PHOX2B genotype may present phenotypically later in life (and even in adulthood), especially in the presence of a stressor such as general anesthesia or a severe respiratory infection, pursuant to the *International Classification of Sleep Disorders* [3].

Physiotherapeutic Intervention

M.B.F. managed to lose and control weight, HBP, and diabetes with his local specialized professionals.

Titration and adaptation to NIV were performed under a PSG at the reference hospital, which is 750 km away from his home. For NIV, he received a Bilevel with S/T-AVAPS mode during the PSG, but he did not initially adapt to the titrated pressures, and he had to make some visits to the sleep unit, where attempts were made to adapt and to initiate NIV. However, the NIV was eventually attained via telemonitoring with oximetry added. Telemonitoring enables us to monitor leaks, residual AHI, hours of daily use, tidal volume, respiratory rate, exhaled minute volume, and pulse oximetry, according to the telemonitoring flowchart [2] (Fig. 30.1).

The telemonitoring follow-up consisted in analyzing the ventilation data with oximetry, communicating with the patient by message about the symptoms, and knowing about patient's general condition. With that in mind, we changed the NIV parameters after his authorization (Fig. 30.1).

Despite the attempts to reach tolerance to titrated pressures, he did not adapt, and he remained symptomatic. It was decided to carry out titration and adaptation to NIV via telemonitoring with oximetry of the software added to the ventilator (Figs. 30.2, 30.3, and 30.4).

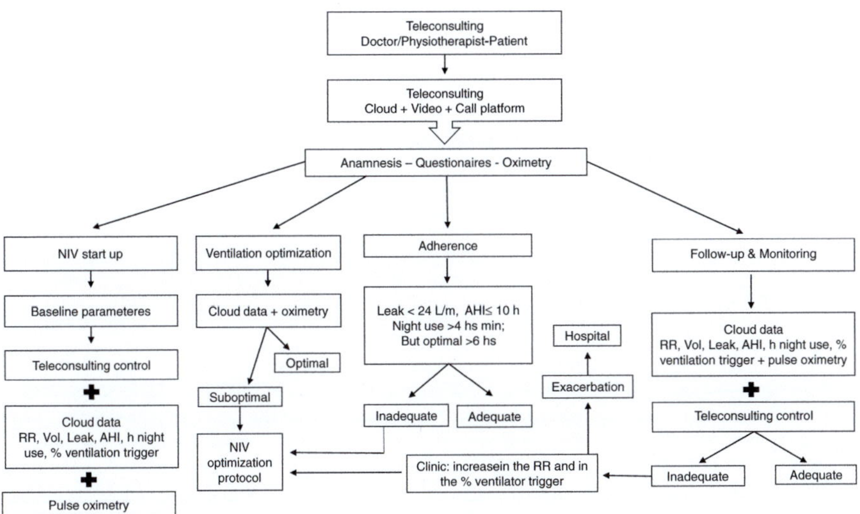

Fig. 30.1 Telemedicine flowchart for non-invasive ventilation support. *AHI* apnea–hypopnea index, *NIV* non-invasive ventilation, *h* hours, *RR* respiratory rate, *Vol* volume

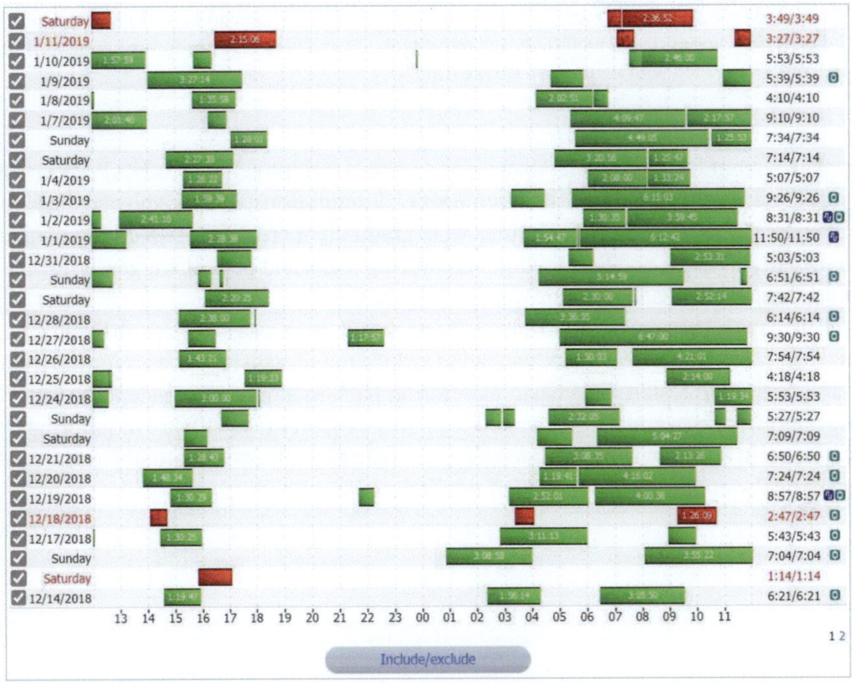

Fig. 30.2 Telemonitoring of non-invasive ventilation use during naptime and at nighttime sleep. Each line represents a 24-hour day. At the bottom a 24-hour time is represented. The green bars represent sleep ≥4 h, and the red bars <4 h. On the right margin, the letter "O" appeared indicating that pulse oximetry was performed during sleep. (Reprinted with permission from I.A.F.)

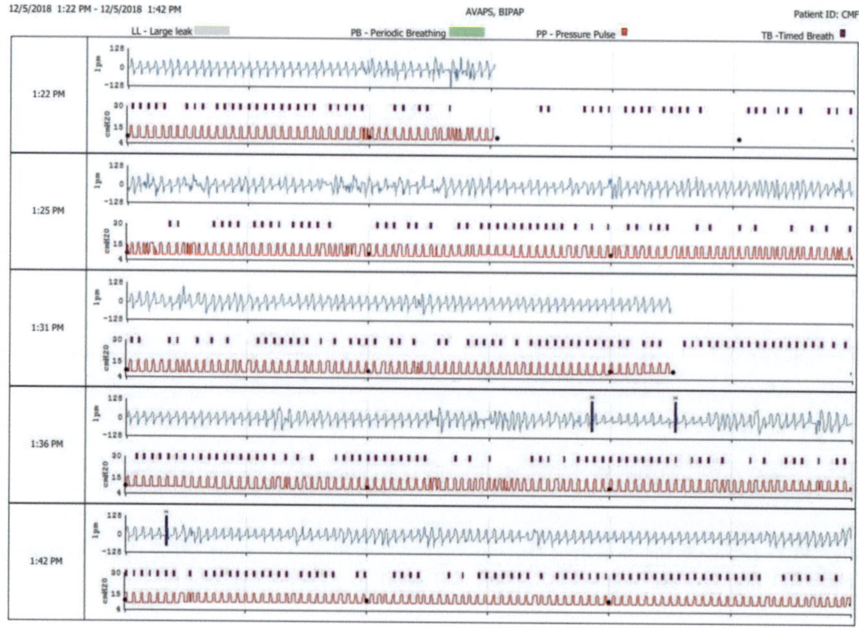

Fig. 30.3 Monitoring of pressure and respiratory flow curves. Examination of leaks and patient-triggered respirations. In the record, the curves of pressure and flow *vs.* time during ventilation are observed. (Reprinted with permission from I.A.F.)

The patient had abdominal distension, nausea, and intolerance to IPAP above 20 cmH$_2$O. Therefore, he was undergoing O$_2$ desaturation, and he showed lack of adherence to NIV. The NIV pressures were gradually increased for 45 days pursuant to patient tolerance and SatO$_2$ while monitoring leaks and patient-triggered respirations through flow and pressure curves (Fig. 30.3).

The days where any intercurrent event occurred, such as a cold, cough, headache, dizziness, or sleep deprivation, we had to reduce the pressures and wait for the right stability time to restart. The basic monitoring pack to attain adherence to NIV during naptime and overnight sleep included pulse oximetry (Fig. 30.4a), monitoring of evolution of symptoms by text message, and control with arterial blood gases. IPAP and EPAP were gradually increased until tolerated.

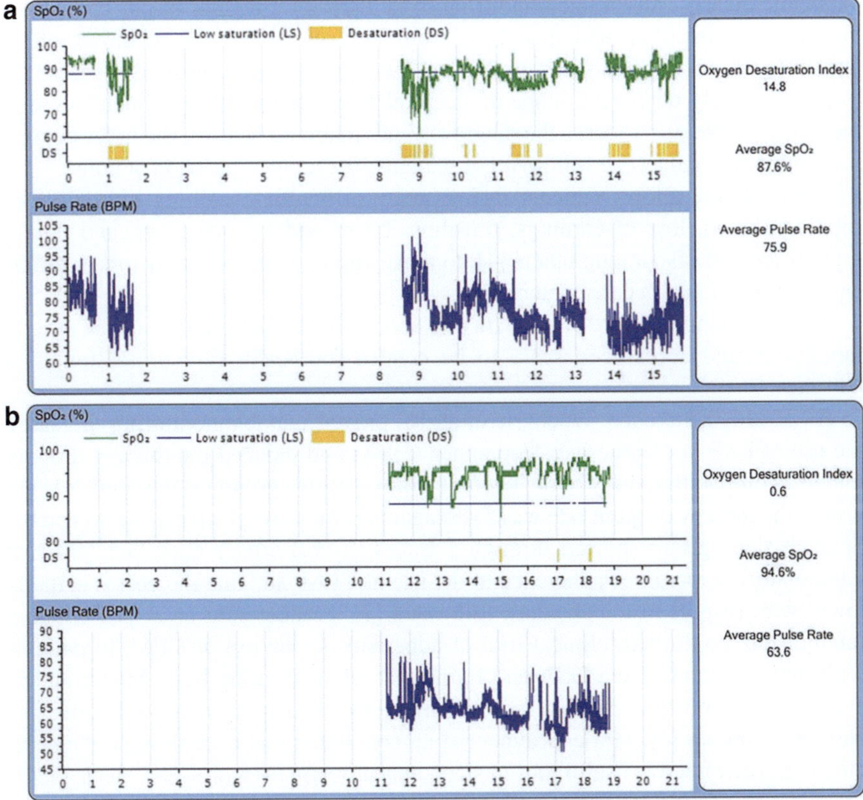

Fig. 30.4 Pulse oximetry result sheet prior (**a**) and post adherence (**b**) to NIV. (Reprinted with permission from I.A.F.)

Follow-Up and Outcomes

The oxygen consumption study (VO_2) was limited by symptoms such as dyspnea and due to a VO_2 plateau. Therefore, aerobic performance was reduced before adherence to NIV. The ventilation control study along with a response to hypercapnia showed a depressed PO.1/PetCO$_2$ curve, compatible with an alteration of respiratory centers before and after adherence to NIV.

Discussion

The use of telemedicine technologies is a way to ensure the timely provision of medical services based on proper quality conditions. Telemonitoring was already used before the COVID-19 pandemic; however, the mobility crisis triggered by the pandemic clearly caused telemonitoring to be used on a regular basis. The access mechanisms, the type and quality of communication, and the reconversion to person-to-person appointments, under specific circumstances, must be ensured.

It is precisely within the scope of sleep medicine that the developments in telemedicine enable us to access the diagnosis and treatment control, the latter being a key option to conduct the follow-up of patients subject to ventilation at home.

Telemedicine allows patients facing many difficulties, such as long-distance trips, workload, loss of earnings, traveling, board and lodging costs, and family organization issues, among others [4], to make appointments with doctors at different specialized health care centers [5].

The confidential nature of the data and access to electronic files must be strictly monitored, and access codes are to be created for health care professionals at all times.

As regards adherence, Woehgrle et al. [6] proved that telemonitoring increased the use of PAP in obstructive sleep apnea (OSA) and reduced the therapy dropout rate in a comparative study of the telemedicine proactive group vs. the standard care group: the therapy dropout rate was 5.4% against 11.0%, respectively. Isseta and the Spanish sleep group showed through a Bayesian cost-effectiveness analysis that telemonitoring increases adherence to the use of CPAP and that the cost is actually lower with respect to the standard follow-up [7]. Franceschini et al. performed a randomized, controlled, clinical trial of adherence to the use of CPAP in patients with moderate and severe OSA and found that telemonitoring has a higher adherence than person-to-person control appointments, and it is equally effective for patient follow-up [8]. Marie Bruyneel et al. concluded that even though telemedicine is a cost-effective useful tool in sleep apnea treatment with CPAP devices, the organization of medical care is undergoing many changes. Telemedicine is going to change the physician–patient relationship, and it may simplify some aspects of diagnosis and care. However, it entails an inherent risk of overdependence on technology and dehumanization of care [9].

The optimization of non-invasive mechanical ventilation, we can of in a study carried out by Mansell SK et al., where the data of tidal volume (Tv), leak, respiratory rate (RR), minute ventilation (MV), patient-triggered respirations, pressures reached, and patient's adherence to therapy were downloaded via telemedicine and card. Telemonitoring proved higher adherence and hours of ventilator use. The use of ventilator data downloading facilitated an early and objective assessment of the leaks and changes in ventilator parameters [10].

Telemedicine may provide to the patients with care and solutions in situations where no person-to-person visits may be made [11]; however, telemedicine also entails some losses in the quality of health care related to the physician and health care providers–patient relationship, which are irreplaceable, such as the time of the appointment with no interruptions, the value of being heard and observed by the health care professional, and on many occasions, a pause in the conversation, shake hands with patients upon receiving them and upon saying goodbye. Sometimes, it is necessary to extend the time of the appointment, and such factors are all advantages of patient-to-patient care, which offers quality support for patients.

There are two works showing conclusions, which are different in part, and they therefore draw the difficulties of arriving at final conclusions in this field. On the one hand, Schoch et al. [12] show how the implementation of telemonitoring over the first month has no positive results on compliance. On the other hand, by working on a sleep virtual unit in a fully telematic way in which patients are always cared for remotely (including the initial diagnosis, treatment, and follow-up), Lugo et al. [13] showed the usefulness and cost-effectiveness of telemonitoring as a new technological tool.

Despite the limitations due to the few studies published, it may be broadly stated that the data extracted from the ventilators are taken for mere guiding purposes, but they have proved to be useful under different clinical conditions for follow-up. Some documents have been published by scientific societies about the positioning of telemedicine as regards SBD and mechanical ventilation [14, 15]. Therefore, it is necessary to perform further studies addressing such short-term and long-term telemonitoring to reach consensus based on evidence levels.

Patient's Perspective

My experience was really good. It helped me get controlled day after day and adjust ventilation without modifying my routine. It really changed my life and made me feel better and much safer. I had never thought about using a ventilator. Even more so, I did not want to use a ventilator, but the truth is that it was the solution to my disease. I could find the way to gradually adapt to ventilation, to be in contact with the doctor, who told me the adjustments he made in the Bilevel and why he did such adjustment, and that made me feel safe.

References

1. Isetta V, Negrín MA, Monasterio C, Masa JF, Feu N, Álvarez A, et al. A Bayesian cost-effectiveness analysis of a telemedicine-based strategy for the management of sleep apnoea: a multicentre randomised controlled trial. Thorax. 2015;70(11):1054–61.
2. Franceschini CM, y Smurra, M. Telemedicine in sleep-related breathing disorders and treatment with positive airway pressure devices. Learnings from SARS-CoV-2 pandemic times. Sleep Sci. 2022;15(1):118–27.
3. American Academy of Sleep Medicine. International classification of sleep disorders. Darien: American Academy of Sleep Medicine; 2014.
4. Franceschini C, Rodriguez J, Ferrufino R, Nievas S, Torres Boden M. Cost analysis in telemonitoring of adherence to the use of CPAP in apnea moderate and severe obstructive sleep. RESPIRAR. 2020;12:13.
5. Singh J, Chair M, Badr S, Epstein L, Fields B, Hwang D, et al. Sleep telemedicine implementation guide. Darien: American Academy of Sleep Medicine (AASM); 2017.
6. Woehrle H, et al. Telemedicine-based proactive patient management during positive airway pressure therapy. Impact on therapy termination rate. Somnologie. 2017;21:121–7.
7. Isetta V, et al. A Bayesian cost-effectiveness analysis of a telemedicine-based strategy for the management of sleep apnoea: a multicentre randomised controlled trial. Thorax. 2015;70:1054–61.

8. Franceschini CM, et al. Tele-monitoring of adherence to the use of CPAP in patients with moderate and severe obstructive sleep apnea. RAMR. 2019;2019:130–1.
9. Bruyneel M, et al. Telemedicine in the diagnosis and treatment of sleep apnoea. Eur Respir Rev. 2019;28:180093.
10. Mansell SK, et al. Using domiciliary non-invasive ventilator data downloads to inform clinical decision-making to optimize ventilation delivery and patient compliance. BMJ Open Respir Res. 2018;5(1):e000238.
11. World Health Organization. Maintaining essential health services: operational guidance for the COVID-19 context: interim guidance. Geneva: WHO; 2020.
12. Schoch OD, Baty F, Boesch M, Benz G, Niedermann J, Brutsche MH. Telemedicine for continuous positive airway pressure in sleep apnea. A randomized controlled study. Ann Am Thorac Soc. 2019;16:1550–7.
13. Lugo VM, Garmendia O, Suarez-Girón M, Torres M, Vázquez-Polo FJ, Negrín MA, et al. Comprehensive management of obstructive sleep apnea by telemedicine: clinical improvement and cost-effectiveness of a virtual sleep unit. A randomized controlled trial. PLoS One. 2019;14:e0224069.
14. Montserrat Canal JM, Suárez-Giróna M, Egea C, Embida C, Matute-Villacís M, de Manuel L, Martínez ÁO, González-Cappa J, Mediano MTCO, et al. Positioning of the Spanish Society of Pneumology and Surgery Thoracic in the use of telemedicine in respiratory disorders sleep and mechanical ventilation. Arch Bronconeumol. 2021;57(4):281–90.
15. Vidigal TA, Brasil EL, Ferreira MN, Mello-Fujita LL, Moreira GA, Drager LF, Soster LA, Genta PR, Poyares D, Haddad FLM. Proposed management model for the use of tele-monitoring of adherence to positive airway pressure equipment - position paper of the Brazilian Association of Sleep Medicine - ABMS. Sleep Sci. 2021;14(1):31–40. https://doi.org/10.5935/1984-0063.20200086. PMID: 34917271; PMCID: PMC8663734.

Index

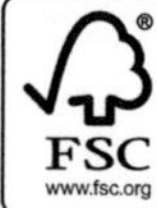